The IMA Volumes in Mathematics and its Applications

Volume 125

Series Editor
Willard Miller, Jr.

Springer
New York
Berlin
Heidelberg
Barcelona
Hong Kong
London
Milan
Paris
Singapore
Tokyo

Institute for Mathematics and its Applications IMA

The **Institute for Mathematics and its Applications** was established by a grant from the National Science Foundation to the University of Minnesota in 1982. The IMA seeks to encourage the development and study of fresh mathematical concepts and questions of concern to the other sciences by bringing together mathematicians and scientists from diverse fields in an atmosphere that will stimulate discussion and collaboration.

The IMA Volumes are intended to involve the broader scientific community in this process.

Willard Miller, Jr., Professor and Director

* * * * * * * * * * *

IMA ANNUAL PROGRAMS

1982–1983	Statistical and Continuum Approaches to Phase Transition
1983–1984	Mathematical Models for the Economics of Decentralized Resource Allocation
1984–1985	Continuum Physics and Partial Differential Equations
1985–1986	Stochastic Differential Equations and Their Applications
1986–1987	Scientific Computation
1987–1988	Applied Combinatorics
1988–1989	Nonlinear Waves
1989–1990	Dynamical Systems and Their Applications
1990–1991	Phase Transitions and Free Boundaries
1991–1992	Applied Linear Algebra
1992–1993	Control Theory and its Applications
1993–1994	Emerging Applications of Probability
1994–1995	Waves and Scattering
1995–1996	Mathematical Methods in Material Science
1996–1997	Mathematics of High Performance Computing
1997–1998	Emerging Applications of Dynamical Systems
1998–1999	Mathematics in Biology
1999–2000	Reactive Flows and Transport Phenomena
2000–2001	Mathematics in Multimedia
2001–2002	Mathematics in the Geosciences
2002–2003	Optimization
2003–2004	Probability and Statistics in Complex Systems: Genomics, Networks, and Financial Engineering

Continued at the back

Carlos Castillo-Chavez
with
Sally Blower, Pauline van den Driessche,
Denise Kirschner, and Abdul-Aziz Yakubu
Editors

Mathematical Approaches for Emerging and Reemerging Infectious Diseases: An Introduction

With 82 Illustrations

Springer

Carlos Castillo-Chavez, Director
Mathematical and Theoretical Biology Institute
and member, Departments of Biometrics, Statistics and Theoretical and Applied Mechanics
Cornell University
Ithaca, NY 14853-7801
USA
cc32@cornell.edu
http://www.biom.cornell.edu/Homepages/Carlos_Castillo-Chavez/

Sally Blower
Department of Biomathematics
UCLA School of Medicine
Los Angeles, CA 90095-1766
USA
SBlower@biomath.medsch.ucla.edu

Abdul-Aziz Yakubu
Department of Mathematics
Howard University
Washington, DC 20059
USA
ayakubu@fac.howard.edu
or Biometrics Department
Cornell University
Email: ay32@cornell.edu

Pauline van den Driessche
Department of Math and Stats
University of Victoria
Victoria, British Columbia
V8W 3P4
Canada
pvdd@math.uvic.ca

Series Editor:
Willard Miller, Jr.
Institute for Mathematics and its Applications
University of Minnesota
Minneapolis, MN 55455
USA

Denise Kirschner
Dept. of Microbiology and Immunology
University of Michigan Medical School
Ann Arbor, MI 48109-0620
USA
kirschne@umich.edu

Mathematics Subject Classification (2000): 92-01, 92-02, 92-06, 92B05, 92D25, 92D30, 92D40, 37N25, 34C60, 34D23, 37C75, 34K60, 39A11, 39-06, 45-06, 60J80

Library of Congress Cataloging-in-Publication Data
Mathematical approaches for emerging and reemerging infectious diseases. An introduction / editors, Carlos Castillo-Chavez . . . [et al.].
p. cm. — (The IMA volumes in mathematics and its applications ; 125)
Includes bibliographical references and index.
ISBN 0-387-95354-X (alk. paper)
1. Communicable diseases—Epidemiology—Mathematical models. I. Castillo-Chávez, Carlos. II. IMA volumes in mathematics and its applications ; v. 125.
RA643 .M35 2001
614.5′01′51—dc21 2001053054

Printed on acid-free paper.

Production managed by A. Orrantia; manufacturing supervised by Jeffrey Taub.
Camera-ready copy prepared by the IMA.
Printed and bound by Sheridan Books, Inc., Ann Arbor, MI.
Printed in the United States of America.

9 8 7 6 5 4 3 2 1

ISBN 0-387-95354-X SPIN 10850708

Springer-Verlag New York Berlin Heidelberg
A member of BertelsmannSpringer Science+Business Media GmbH

FOREWORD

This IMA Volume in Mathematics and its Applications

MATHEMATICAL APPROACHES FOR EMERGING AND REEMERGING INFECTIOUS DISEASES: AN INTRODUCTION

is based on the proceedings of a successful tutorial on "Introduction to Epidemiology and Immunology." The two-day tutorial provided an overview to the IMA workshop on "Mathematical Approaches for Emerging and Reemerging Infectious Diseases: Models, Methods and Theory" to be published as IMA Volume 126. The tutorial and the workshop are integral parts of the September 1998 to June 1999 IMA program on "MATHEMATICS IN BIOLOGY."

I would like to thank Carlos Castillo-Chavez (Director of the Mathematical and Theoretical Biology Institute and a member of the Departments of Biometrics, Statistics and Theoretical and Applied Mechanics, Cornell University), Sally M. Blower (Biomathematics, UCLA School of Medicine), Pauline van den Driessche (Mathematics and Statistics, University of Victoria), and Denise Kirschner (Microbiology and Immunology, University of Michigan Medical School) for their superb roles as organizers of the meetings and editors of the proceedings. Carlos Castillo-Chavez, especially, made a major contribution by spearheading the editing process. I am also grateful to Kenneth L. Cooke (Mathematics, Pomona College), for being one of the workshop organizers and to Abdul-Aziz Yakubu (Mathematics, Howard University) for serving as co-editor of the proceedings. I thank Simon A. Levin (Ecology and Evolutionary Biology, Princeton University) for providing an introduction.

Finally, I take this opportunity to thank the National Science Foundation (NSF), whose financial support of the IMA made the Mathematics in Biology program possible, and the National Institute of General Medical Sciences of the National Institutes of health (NIH), for providing partial support for the workshop.

Willard Miller, Jr., Professor and Director
Institute for Mathematics and its Applications
University of Minnesota
400 Lind Hall, 207 Church St. SE
Minneapolis, MN 55455-0436
612-624-6066, FAX 612-626-7370
miller@ima.umn.edu
World Wide Web: http://www.ima.umn.edu

PREFACE

MATHEMATICAL APPROACHES FOR EMERGING AND REEMERGING INFECTIOUS DISEASES: AN INTRODUCTION

The research collected in the volumes, *Mathematical Approaches for Emerging and Reemerging Infectious Diseases: An Introduction* and *Mathematical Approaches for Emerging and Reemerging Infectious Diseases: Models, Methods, and Theory*, grew out of the discussions and presentations instigated by the Workshop on Emerging and Reemerging Diseases sponsored by the Institute for Mathematics and its Applications (IMA) at the University of Minnesota in May 17-21, 1999. This workshop included a two day tutorial session directed to ecologists, epidemiologists, immunologists, mathematicians and scientists interested in being exposed to some of the modeling and mathematical approaches used in the study of disease dynamics. Tutorial papers presented at this workshop or requested, in response to the nature of the contributions of workshop participants, have been included (mostly) in this first volume. The contributions to this volume, IMA Volume 125, are geared towards beginning graduate students in applied mathematics, scientists in the biological sciences or mathematicians who want to enter the field of mathematical or theoretical epidemiology. Specific applications to the study of Cancer, HIV, Pertussis and Tuberculosis are addressed in some of the articles in this volume.

Tutorial and research contributions focus on the use of dynamical systems (discrete, delay, PDEs and ODEs) and stochastic models in the study of disease dynamics. Although the modeling approaches presented in both volumes are highlighted in the context of specific diseases, their growth and development, as pointed by Simon Levin's introduction, are the result of the marriage between mathematics and population biology. Hence, the methods and approaches presented here should be also of interest to researchers interested in population biology.

These volumes are dedicated to Fred Brauer and Kenneth Cooke on their retirement from their academic positions at the University of Wisconsin-Madison and Pomona College, respectively. The leading articles in each volume take a personal look at their contributions to mathematics, mathematical biology and epidemiology over the past five decades. It is but a small gesture of our appreciation as we continue to learn from our personal and professional association to these leading researchers and extraordinary teachers and mentors.

The last two contributions in this volume are co-authored by Angel Capurro who died suddenly in a car accident on December 10, 2000. Angel was a leading researcher at the Departamento de Investigaciones of the Universidad de Belgrano in Buenos Aires Argentina for the past six years. Angel, in a very short time, established one of the most active research groups on the study of tuberculosis. He was not only a leading researcher in the field of tuberculosis but also active in ecology with an appointment at the Universidad Nacional in Lujan, Argentina. Angel was a wonderful individual with friends all over the world. He was a close friend of many of us, and we will miss him.

We want to thank Simon A. Levin for writing the introduction and for encouraging and supporting the completion of these two volumes. We spent various amounts of time at the IMA in 1998 and 1999 and earlier during the preparation of many of the activities associated with the organization of the 1998-99 IMA Special Year in Mathematical Biology. We also want to express our gratitude to those individuals who were responsible not only for the support of the activities associated with the preparation of these volumes but also to those members of IMA's staff who made our visit to this institute a wonderfully productive experience. The leadership and support of Willard Miller and Fred Dulles are highly appreciated. We also want to acknowledge the help and friendliness of Kathy Boyer, Inés Foss, Michelle Glubke, Dzung Nguyen and all the IMA staff who are responsible for the IMA's first rate operation. Special thanks to Patricia V. Brick for her professionalism in the production of these two volumes.

The Workshop on Emerging and Reemerging Diseases and the preparation of these volumes were partially supported by NSF and NIH grants to IMA. We want to thank these agencies for their support although we must re-state that the views and research presented in these volumes are the direct responsibility of the authors and the editorial group, that is, they do not represent the views of the funding agencies or the IMA.

Carlos Castillo-Chavez (Cornell University)

Sally Blower (University of California at Los Angeles)

Pauline van den Driessche (University of Victoria)

Denise Kirschner (University of Michigan)

Abdul-Aziz Yakubu (Howard University)

CONTENTS

NEW DIRECTIONS IN THE MATHEMATICS OF INFECTIOUS DISEASE

SIMON A. LEVIN*

The study of infectious diseases represents one of the oldest and richest areas in mathematical biology. Infectious diseases have fascinated mathematicians for a century, and with good reason. Most seductive, of course, is the possibility of using mathematics to make a positive contribution to the world. In the study of infectious diseases, the essential elements are quickly grasped, and well-captured within mathematical representations. As new epidemics, from AIDS to bovine spongiform encephalopathy (mad-cow) to foot-and-mouth, make their appearances on the world stage, mathematical models are essential to inform decision-making. Governments and health agencies turn to the leading modelers for advice, and news services seek them out for the clarity they can bring. It is a rare opportunity for relevance for those who spend so much of their time in otherwise abstract and esoteric exercises.

Among the problems of biology, those involving the transmission dynamics of infectious diseases are among the most accessible to those not trained as biologists. There is a standard and well-established mathematical framework, expanded and given credibility by the work of many over the past century (see Anderson and May, 1991). For specific situations, this general framework always requires tailoring or more substantial modification, but that is part of the attraction for the researcher. The usual equations also have easily-identified control parameters, or intervention points, such as vaccination strategies or contact rates, which determine the dynamics and provide handles for decision-making. Furthermore, crisp, powerful and robust results, such as the existence of critical thresholds, emerge naturally from the analyses, and can be translated very directly into lessons for control.

Add to these attractive features the dynamical richness of epidemiological problems, and the appeal to mathematicians is irresistible. The basic epidemiological equations are sufficiently nonlinear to make things interesting, but still simple enough to provide sharp results. They provide wonderful vehicles for the techniques of dynamical systems theory, especially bifurcation analysis. Furthermore, straightforward elaborations of them, to account say for age structure or latent periods, take one immediately into the world of integral or partial differential equations, and into the study of delay equations. Management issues are naturals for control theory; and game theory is essential both for understanding the evolution

*Department of Ecology and Evolutionary Biology, Princeton University, Princeton, NJ 08544-1003.

of infectious agents, as well as for a full treatment of management issues. Finally, disease transmission is a fundamentally stochastic process, meaning that the techniques of probability and statistics undergird the entire subject.

These two remarkable volumes explore the subject very broadly, from the classical roots to the frontiers of the subject. The impressive collection of contributors includes many who have been in the forefront of the development of the subject, and the warmth with which the volumes and individual articles have been dedicated to Fred Brauer and Ken Cooke is obvious. That is also not hard to understand. Not only have both of these outstanding mathematicians been seminal contributors to the literature, but both are wonderful human beings who evoke good feelings in all who interact with them. It is therefore my pleasure to join in the chorus, and to wish both Fred and Ken continued good health and productivity

In the following sections, I will touch upon some of the problems at the frontier of the subject, as seen through my own idiosyncratic filter. Many of these are explored within the individual contributions in this volume; others undoubtedly will find their way into the sequels to these works.

Frontiers in the study of infectious diseases. Any selection of frontiers in any subject is necessarily somewhat speculative, a bit like trying to predict the next variant of a virus. Still, a number of classes of problems seem to me to be ripe for exploration, and fundamentally important in their implications. My own bias is often to look for problems at the ecotones between disciplines, because it is there that cross-fertilization has the potential to lead to rich harvests in short amounts of time. Many of these involve the integration of phenomena across scales, problems whose analysis has been facilitated by recent advances in methodology and technology (Levin et al., 1997).

One of the most important of the interfaces, of course, is that between epidemiology and immunology. This has received much attention recently by problems associated with the AIDS epidemic (Nowak et al., 1991; Perelson et al., 1996), and the interplay between viral evolution and the immune dynamics of hosts. It is, however, a fundamental aspect of understanding the dynamics of any disease. In the case of AIDS, the immune system must play a fundamental role in the progression of the disease, and mathematical models have elucidated the role of cytotoxic T cells (Nowak et al., 1995a; Nowak et al., 1995b). Evolutionary issues also intrude here, such as in the evolution of resistance in HIV to antiretroviral drugs, and the implications for treatment strategies (McLean and Nowak, 1992; Ho et al., 1995; Wei et al., 1995). Immunology has long been a rich but speculative area of theoretical biology, with milestones such as in the work of the late George Bell, a pioneer in scaling real and intellectual mountain peaks. In recent years, especially since the landmark contributions to AIDS research, the subject has achieved prominence, especially in terms of its interfaces with epidemiology. Surely this activity will expand, and include the interplay of the immune system with hormonal systems, and how factors such as stress, nutrition and general health affect responses to infectious agents.

The evolutionary issues mentioned in the previous paragraph just scratch the surface. The importance of heterogeneous transmission in the dynamics of disease directs attention to genetic variation in infectivity and transmissibility, and ultimately to the evolution of these properties (Dushoff and Levin, 1995; Dushoff, 1999). Aspects of the evolution of infectious agents are central to understanding the dynamics of diseases such as malaria (Gupta et al., 1994) and influenza (Andreasen et al., 1997), with attention to the evolution of patterns of cross-reactivity and the self-organization of strain structure. Fitch et al. (1991; 1997) have done remarkable work on the evolution of influenza, with implications for the development of vaccines. The integration of all of these processes cross scales from the cellular to the ecological to the evolutionary, and require the efforts of a broad spectrum of scientists. Bacterial evolution poses particularly important problems: The evolution of antibiotic resistance is one of the greatest threats facing society today (Daily and Ehrlich, 1996). Finally, host-parasite systems provide ideal vehicles for the study of coevolution (Levin and Pimentel, 1981; Anderson and May, 1982; Levin, 1983a). The central issues certainly involve the interplay between host resistance and the pathogen infectivity (Anderson and May, 1982; Futuyma and Slatkin, 1983; Levin, 1983b; Levin et al., 1999), but also extend to issues such as plasmid evolution, the competitive dynamics of strains, and the interplay between interacting diseases.

Another interface likely to see more attention in the coming decade will be that between epidemiology and economics, with ethics also lurking not so far in the background. Like it or not, many of the management challenges have economic overtones, and furthermore introduce problems of the global commons. How should the cost of treatment be factored into decisions to vaccinate, or even to treat? What are the tradeoffs between using particular antibiotics to treat individuals, and the risks of the development of antibiotic resistance? What are the incentives for drug companies to develop genuinely novel antibiotics? Can we determine optimal global and regional management strategies for antibiotic use, accounting for the costs and benefits of multiple antibiotics, and balancing adequately the rights of individuals and the needs of societies? These non-traditional areas for mathematical investigation are likely to receive much more attention in the near future.

Climatology provides another venue for investigation of disease interactions. With global warming, there will undoubtedly be implications for the spread of disease. Changing climate will affect the diseases themselves, the health and habits of potential hosts, and most importantly the population biology of vectors. Malaria, dengue and cholera are all diseases attracting considerable attention as regards the potential effects of global warming and habitat alteration.

The issue of habitat alteration is one aspect of a suite of spatial problems demanding attention. Understanding the spread of infectious diseases is a problem that long has been of interest to theoreticians, but more recently much has been learned about the coupling of the dynamics of disease among different cities (Bolker and Grenfell, 1993). The degree of synchronization among local oscillations can affect the persistence of diseases (Lloyd and May, 1996; Earn et al., 2000), and have profound implications for management. Furthermore, globalization and the changing connectivity of local populations can affect these dynamics, and also lead to reinterpretation of the critical thresholds for persistence. Indeed, many of the emergent and re-emergent diseases threatening our societies today were likely well-contained as endemics locally when communities were more isolated (see Levin, 1999).

All of these issues and more will receive increased attention in the coming years, and many have already been broached in these volumes. Castillo-Chavez and Yakubu examine the importance of patchy environments, and Allen and Ernest look at problems of spread. Ferguson and Andreasen look at links to the immune system, and patterns of cross-reactivity within evolving families of strains. Hsu Schmitz introduces genetic heterogeneity, and explores its consequences. It is clear that these are just a start, and that the study of infectious diseases will continue to be one of the most rewarding areas for mathematical investigation for years to come. These volumes provide an important step along that path.

REFERENCES

ANDERSON, R.M. AND MAY, R.M. 1982. Coevolution of hosts and parasites. *Parasitology,* **85**:411–426.

ANDERSON, R.M. AND MAY, R.M. 1991. *Infectious Diseases of Humans: Dynamics and Control.* Oxford, UK: Oxford University Press.

ANDREASEN, V., LIN, J., AND LEVIN, S.A. 1997. The dynamics of cocirculating influenza strains conferring partial cross-immunity. *Journal Mathematical Biology,* **35**:825–842.

BOLKER, B.M. AND GRENFELL, B.T. 1993. Chaos and biological complexity in measles dynamics. *Proc. R. Soc. Lond. B*, **251**:75–81.

DAILY, G.C. AND EHRLICH, P.R. 1996. Global change and human susceptibility to disease. *Ann. Rev. Energy Environ.,* **21**:125–144.

DUSHOFF, J. 1999. Host heterogenity and disease endemicity: A moment-based approach. *Theoretical Population Biology,* **56**.

DUSHOFF, J. AND LEVIN, S.A. 1995. The effects of population heterogeneity on disease spread. *Mathematical Biosciences,* **128**:25–40.

EARN, D.J.D., LEVIN, S.A., AND ROHANI, P. 2000. Coherence and conservation. *Science,* **290**:1360–64.

FITCH, W.M., BUSH, R.M., BENDER, C.A., AND COX, N.J. 1997. Long term trends in the evolution of H(3) HA1 human influenza type A. *Proceedings of the National Academy of Sciences, USA,* **94**:7712–7718.

FITCH, W.M., LEITER, J.M.E., LI, X., AND PALESE, P. 1991. Positive Darwinian evolution in human influenza A viruses. *Proceedings of the National Academy of Sciences, USA,* **88**:4270–4274.

FUTUYMA, D. AND SLATKIN, M., eds. 1983. *Coevolution.* Sunderland, MA: Sinauer.

GUPTA, S., SWINTON, J., AND ANDERSON, R.M. 1994. Theoretical studies of the effects of heterogeneity in the parasite population on the transmission dynamics of malaria. *Proc. R. Soc. Lond., B,* **256**:231–238.

HO, D.D., NEUMANN, A.U., PERELSON, A.S., CHEN, W., LEONARD, J.M., AND MARKOWITZ, M. 1995. Rapid turnover of plasma virons and CD4 lymphocytes in HIV-1 infections. *Nature,* **373**.

LEVIN, B.R., LIPSITCH, M., AND BONHOEFFER, S. 1999. Population biology, evolution, and infectious disease: Convergence and synthesis. *Science,* **283**:806–809.

LEVIN, S.A. 1983a. Coevolution. In *Population Biology,* Lecture Notes in Biomathematics (H. Freedman and C. Strobeck, eds.), pp. 328–334, Berlin: Springer-Verlag.

LEVIN, S.A. 1983b. Some approaches to the modelling of coevolutionary interactions. In *Coevolution* (M. Nitecki, ed.), pp. 21–65 Chicago, Illinois: University of Chicago Press.

LEVIN, S.A. 1999. *Fragile Dominion: Complexity and the Commons.* Reading, MA: Perseus Books.

LEVIN, S.A., GRENFELL, B., HASTINGS, A., AND PERELSON, A.S. 1997. Mathematical and computational challenges in population biology and ecosystem science. *Science,* **275**:334–343.

LEVIN, S.A. AND PIMENTEL, D. 1981. Selection of intermediate rates of increase in parasite-host systems. *American Naturalist,* **117**:308–315.

LLOYD AND MAY, R.M. 1996. Spatial heterogeneity in epidemic models. *J. Theoretical Biology,* **179**:1–11.

MCLEAN, A.R. AND NOWAK, M.A. 1992. Competition between zidovudine sensitive and resistant strains of HIV. *AIDS,* **6**:71–79.

NOWAK, M.A., ANDERSON, R.M., MCLEAN, A.R., WOLFS, T., GOUDSMIT, J., AND MAY, R.M. 1991. Antigenic diversity thresholds and the development of AIDS. *Science,* **254**:963–966.

NOWAK, M.A., MAY, R.M., PHILLIPS, R.E., ROWLAND-JONES, S., LALLOO, D.G., MCADAM, S., KLENERMAN, P., KÖPPE, B., SIGMUND, K., BANGHAM, C.R.M., AND MCMICHAEL, A.J. 1995a. Antigenic oscillations and shifting immunodominance in HIV-1 infections. *Nature,* **375**:606–611.

NOWAK, M.A., MAY, R.M., AND SIGMUND, K. 1995b. Immune responses against multiple epitopes. *J. Theoretical Biology,* **175**:325–353.

PERELSON, A.S., NEUMANN, A.U., MARKOWITZ, M., LEONARD, J.M., AND HO, D.D. 1996. HIV-1 dynamics in vivo: Virion clearance rate, infected cell life-span, and viral generation time. *Science,* **271**:1582–1586.

WEI, X., GHOSH, S.K., TAYLOR, M.E., JOHNSON, V.A., EMINI, E.A., DEUTSCH, P., LIFSON, J.D., BONHOEFFER, S., NOWAK, M.A., HAHN, B.H., SAAG, M.S., AND SHAW, G.M. 1995. Viral dynamics in HIV-1 infection. *Nature,* **373**:117–122.

FRED BRAUER: THE MAN AND HIS MATHEMATICS

CHRISTOPHER M. KRIBS-ZALETA*

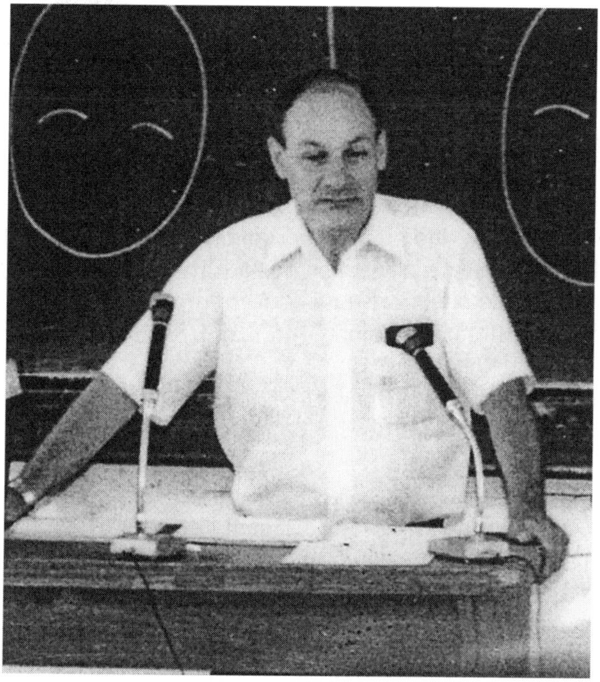

Fred Brauer†

Introduction. When I first met Fred Brauer, he was warning a class of first-semester calculus students about the dangers of applying techniques without thinking. As an example, he wrote on the chalkboard the expression $\frac{\sin x}{n}$. He then proceeded to cancel the n's from numerator and denominator:

$$\frac{\text{si}\not{n}x}{\not{n}},$$

leaving *six*.

At the time, I, a first-semester graduate student, knew nothing of the vast body of work he had produced in rather more advanced mathematics,

*Department of Mathematics, University of Texas at Arlington, Arlington, TX 76019-0408.

†Department of Mathematics University of British Columbia, Vancouver, B.C V6T 1Z2, Canada.

but his thoughtful approaches to solving problems, coupled with his sense of humor, appealed to me. He later encouraged those same calculus students, "Lions in the Serengeti Desert solve optimization problems — and they don't even know calculus."‡

That semester we (I was one of the TAs assigned to his lecture) were using a new calculus text§ which began somewhat unconventionally, using discrete-time population models. Perhaps that should have given me a clue as to what to expect a year later, when I went to him in search of a Ph.D. advisor. In the past fifty years, Fred's research has spanned the gamut of population biology, from theoretical work in differential and integral equations to applied studies of the relationship between demographic processes and the spread of diseases. He has collaborated with dozens of mathematicians, written over 100 books and papers, performed research in such places as Brazil, Israel, and the Netherlands, and lectured in Italy, China, Mexico, and many places in between. In addition to his own doctoral students, he has fostered the work and careers of many young scientists. He is (to steal indiscriminately from Gilbert and Sullivan) the very model of a mathematics modeller.

Fred Brauer, who grew up with mathematics in his family, received his Ph.D. from MIT in 1956 under Norman Levinson. After teaching at the University of Chicago and the University of British Columbia, he came in 1960 to the University of Wisconsin. During his tenure in Madison he became a cornerstone of the department, serving as chair among other positions, and instituting the departmental seminar in "spherical trigonometry" to show that mathematicians can also play basketball. (He continues to do so.) In two terms as associate chair he made important developments to the undergraduate curriculum, including sequences of precalculus courses and mathematics courses for biologists as well as the infusion of differential equations into multivariable calculus, linear algebra and the upper-level curriculum. It was in Madison that he formed a long-term collaboration with John Nohel, also a student of Levinson; in the early 1960's the two wrote what has become a classic textbook on qualitative theory of ODEs. A year or two later, Hans Schneider (also in the department) joined them to write a second text unifying linear algebra and linear systems of ODE's. John and Fred wrote several more books together in the years that followed, and worked together on some of the aforementioned curriculum development.

Fred's recent return to his native Canada with wife Esther brought them close not only to his old stomping grounds at UBC but to one of their three children — and, consequently, to grandchildren as well. It doesn't hurt that Vancouver is a nice place to live — and to visit.

---

‡Fred attributes this observation to Colin Clark.

§Frank Wattenberg's *Calculus in a Real and Complex World*

Differential equations. With Norman Levinson as his advisor, it is not surprising that Fred's early work concentrated on properties of differential equations. From the completion of his dissertation in 1956 until the early 1970's, his papers addressed topics including spectral theory for linear systems, uniqueness and convergence of successive approximations, and asymptotic behavior of perturbed nonlinear systems. Three papers on the first topic in the late 1950's investigated the expansion in eigenfunctions of operators (with associated boundary conditions) for systems of linear differential equations. Three other papers in the same time period [1, 2, 3, 4] explored a duality between local uniqueness and global existence of solutions, by viewing global existence as a kind of uniqueness at infinity. These papers also compared local uniqueness with the convergence of successive approximations, of the type

$$x_j(t) = \int_0^t f[x_{j-1}(s), s]\, ds,$$

presenting various conditions for them and noting (via counterexamples) that although the two notions are independent — neither implies the other — most criteria which guarantee one also guarantee the other.

Four papers in the *Journal of Mathematical Analysis and Applications* from 1966 to 1972 [5, 6, 7, 8] described an alternative method for considering perturbations to nonlinear systems of DEs. Rather than using a Lyapunov function for the unperturbed equation, the articles adapted Alekseev's nonlinear variation of constants formula to determine the effects of perturbation on solutions, as a function of the stability properties of the solutions to the original system. The result was an extended hierarchical look at different kinds of stability. As Fred noted, some kind of stability information must be known about the solutions of the unperturbed system in order to know the effects of perturbations. A number of different types of (or criteria for) stability, several of which are identical for linear systems (and some of which were new), provided different results, and a ranking by implication:

exponential stability → asymptotic stability in variation
→ asymptotic stability
→ uniform stability in variation
→ integral stability
→ uniform stability
→ stability

In addition, uniform asymptotic stability also implies asymptotic stability, but is independent of asymptotic stability in variation (neither implies the other).

Population biology. It was in the early 1970's that Fred turned his eye to population biology, and for the next twenty years he studied problems related to predator-prey systems and harvesting. A series of papers, many co-authored by A. C. Soudack, considered managed nonlinear predator-prey systems of the form

$$x' = x\,f(x,y) - F,$$
$$y' = y\,g(x,y) - G,$$

where F and G represent constant harvesting (if positive) or stocking (if negative) terms, x the prey and y the predators, and with the biologically-motivated constraints $f_x < 0$ (limited resources for prey), $g_x > 0$ (predator reliance on prey), $g_y \leq 0$ (limited resources for predators), and $f_x g_y - f_y g_x > 0$ for $x, y > 0$. Results [9, 10] showed that excessive harvesting of predators would cause the predator population to crash (reach zero in finite time), and excessive harvesting of prey would cause both populations to crash. On the other hand, stocking had the possibility of destabilizing the system, and excessive "enrichment" of the prey environment (by raising the prey's carrying capacity) could give rise to limit cycles. One case where the system was asymptotically stable only in a limited basin of attraction underscored the need for careful management of such populations.

Another research area involved the forms used to describe biological processes. Models in population biology have traditionally assumed exponential distributions in most of the processes involved — births, deaths, and even infections and recoveries in epidemic models — in order that the models be systems of differential equations. However, the quantitative biological justification for this assumption is weak, and Fred recognized that there were times when other forms would more accurately model the biological processes involved. In particular, processes with fixed duration can be represented by step functions, which lead to systems of difference equations, or delay differential equations. More generally, the models can be written as systems of Volterra integral equations, with the function describing the rate at which the process in question occurs serving as a kind of convolution kernel. Consequently, a number of Fred's models considered the effects of delays and more general rate distributions. The analysis of such models is, of course, more complex, but the results are worth the fuss: If, on the one hand, results match those for the ODE model, a robust principle has been derived, which holds regardless of the form of the distribution. If, on the other hand, as conventional wisdom has it, delays are more conducive to instability of equilibria, then one must make some effort to determine how the process in question can best be described.

His first such papers extended earlier results, such as the application of Alekseev's nonlinear variation of constants formula and the effects of constant-effort harvesting, to systems described by Volterra integral equations. In 1987 a paper in *Natural Resource Modeling* [11] described how delays and a generalized lifespan (mortality) distribution interact to affect the stability of an equilibrium: for the simple system

$$x(t) = p_0 \int_0^\infty g\big(x(t-s-\tau)\big)P(s)\,ds,$$

where $g(x)$ is the birth rate as a function of population x, τ is age to adulthood ($x(t)$ counts only adults), and p_0 is the probability of survival to adulthood (age τ). $P(s)$ is a nonnegative, nonincreasing, integrable function (with $P(0) = 1$) representing the probability of surviving to age $\tau + s$, given survival to age τ. The delay τ and mortality distribution P interact in the following way:

(i) If $-1 < p_0 g'(x_\infty) \int_0^\infty P(s)ds < 1$, then the equilibrium x_∞ is stable regardless of τ;

(ii) if $p_0 g'(x_\infty) \int_0^\infty P(s)ds > 1$, then the equilibrium x_∞ is unstable regardless of τ;

(iii) if $p_0 g'(x_\infty) \int_0^\infty P(s)ds < -1$, then there is a finite value of τ past which the equilibrium x_∞ is unstable.

Here we see that the delay in recruitment and the expected lifetime do affect the stability of the population. Also in this paper an application to a previously studied epidemic model for an SIR (recovery with immunity) disease with fixed incubation and infective periods gave a hint of the direction in which Fred's research would next turn.

Epidemic models. Like the interaction between recruitment delay and mortality distribution in general population models, disease transmission and (other) demographics can affect each other in important ways. These effects have been one of the most prominent aspects of Fred's research in the realm of infectious diseases. In particular, models he studied with Carlos Castillo-Chávez, Jorge Velasco-Hernández, Steve Blythe and others focused on the influence of disease state on the size of the at-risk population, and the effects in turn of this recruitment on the disease itself. In the study of sexually transmitted diseases, the notion of a core group has been established [12] as central to understanding disease dynamics. It has also been observed that the perceived prevalence of the disease may affect individuals' decision whether or not to enter the at-risk population (by increasing their activity level). The aforementioned models considered both one-sex (homosexual) and two-sex (heterosexual) transmission of diseases — some universally fatal, such as HIV/AIDS, and others of more limited duration, such as gonorrhea — in which the rate at which new individuals entered the core was a (nonincreasing) function of the disease prevalence.

Initial results using exponentially distributed recovery times (as usual, leading to ODE models) and core recruitment influenced by the total number of infected individuals mirrored the prototypical R_0 threshold behavior, but more detailed models [13, 14, 15], in which recruitment was a function of the *proportion* of either infected individuals, or treated infected individuals, or in which the noncore population was also active (but at a lower rate than the core), or in which the recovery rate was not exponentially distributed, allowed for the possibility of Hopf bifurcations with $R_0 > 1$, which led to sustained oscillations. As these oscillations could have very long periods, their empirical observation might be difficult. In general, as the level of infection increased, the recruitment into the core would damp down, until the infection began to die out. Once the infection level was low, however, recruitment would return to a higher rate, with the infection level rising behind it. This sort of behavior and subsequent rise in infection prevalence has been observed in some cases. These results suggest that in order to develop robust principles regarding disease transmission and control, we must consider a variety of distributions for the biological processes we model (or, at least, consider which distributions are most appropriate, rather than most convenient), as well as different ways to model the influence of perceived disease prevalence.

Conclusion. In the past forty years Fred has been active not only in producing and fostering research but in developing college-level mathematics education, to a large extent on a local level, but also in developing courses and authoring textbooks which present relevant mathematics to biologists, such as probability and dynamical systems. Tailoring of mathematical content to biologists and those interested in investigating phenomena such as infectious diseases is a rising trend which helps to prepare — and perhaps attract — the mathematical biologists of tomorrow, and it is an important part of leadership for the mathematical biologists of today to take part in this development.

For all his contributions: research in systems of differential and integral equations, in population biology and in mathematical epidemiology; fostering in the large and on the individual level education and productivity in these areas; and for his keen humor and being an exemplary colleague, we make this dedication to Fred Brauer.

Note: The references below are intended as a sample rather than an extensive list. They were chosen as representative of the results discussed in this article. Further references can be identified by search engines such as MathSciNet, or by checking citations in these articles.

REFERENCES

[1] Fred Brauer and Shlomo Sternberg (1958). Local uniqueness, existence in the large, and the convergence of successive approximations, *Amer. J. Math.* 80: 421–430.

[2] Fred Brauer and Shlomo Sternberg (1959). Errata to our paper "Local uniqueness, etc.", *Amer. J. Math.* 81: 797.

[3] Fred Brauer (1959). A note on uniqueness and convergence of successive approximations, *Canad. Math. Bull.* 2: 5–8.

[4] Fred Brauer (1959). Some results on uniqueness and successive approximations, *Canad. J. Math.* 11: 527–533.
[5] Fred Brauer (1966). Perturbations of nonlinear systems of differential equations, *J. Math. Anal. Appl.* 14: 198–206.
[6] Fred Brauer (1967). Perturbations of nonlinear systems of differential equations. II, *J. Math. Anal. Appl.* 17: 418–434.
[7] Fred Brauer and Aaron Strauss (1970). Perturbations of nonlinear systems of differential equations. III, *J. Math. Anal. Appl.* 31: 37–48.
[8] Fred Brauer (1972). Perturbations of nonlinear systems of differential equations. IV, *J. Math. Anal. Appl.* 37: 214–222.
[9] Fred Brauer and A. C. Soudack (1978). Response of predator-prey systems to nutrient enrichment and proportional harvesting, *Internat. J. Control* 27(1): 65–86.
[10] Fred Brauer and A. C. Soudack (1982). On constant effort harvesting and stocking in a class of predator-prey systems, *J. Theor. Biol.* 95(2): 247–252.
[11] Fred Brauer (1987). A class of Volterra integral equations arising in delayed-recruitment population models, *Natur. Resource Modeling* 2(2): 259–278.
[12] Herbert W. Hethcote and James A. Yorke (1984). *Gonorrhea transmission dynamics and control.* Lecture Notes in Biomathematics 56. New York: Springer-Verlag.
[13] S. P. Blythe, Fred Brauer, Carlos Castillo-Chávez and Jorge X. Velasco-Hernández (1995). Models for sexually transmitted diseases with recruitment, in *Mathematical Population Dynamics: Analyses of Heterogeneity* (O. Arino, D. Axelrod, M. Kimmel, M. Langlais, eds.). Winnipeg: Wuerz Publishing Co. Vol. 1, pp. 197–207.
[14] Fred Brauer, Carlos Castillo-Chávez and Jorge X. Velasco-Hernández (1996). Recruitment effects in heterosexually transmitted disease models, *Int. J. App. Science & Computation* 3: 78–90.
[15] Fred Brauer, Carlos Castillo-Chávez and Jorge X. Velasco-Hernández (1997). Recruitment with a core group and its effect on the spread of a sexually transmitted disease, in *Advances in Mathematical Population Dynamics — Molecules, Cells, and Man* (O. Arino, D. Axelrod, M. Kimmel, eds.). Singapore: World Scientific Press. pp. 477–486.

Papers by Fred Brauer

1. Fred Brauer (1958). Singular self-adjoint boundary value problems for the differential equation $Lx = \lambda Mx$, *Trans. Amer. Math. Soc.* 88: 331–345.
2. Fred Brauer (1958). Spectral theory for the differential equation $Lu = \lambda Mu$, *Can. J. Math.* 10: 431–446.
3. Fred Brauer and Shlomo Sternberg (1958). Local uniqueness, existence in the large, and the convergence of successive approximations, *Amer. J. Math.* 80: 421–430; errata, same journal, 81: 797 (1959).
4. Fred Brauer (1959). A note on uniqueness and convergence of successive approximations, *Can. Math. Bulletin* 2: 5–8.
5. Fred Brauer (1959). Some results on uniqueness and successive approximations, *Can. J. Math.* 11: 527–533.
6. Fred Brauer (1960). Spectral theory for linear systems of differential equations, *Pacific J. Math.* 10: 17–34.
7. Fred Brauer (1961). Global behavior of solutions of ordinary differential equations, *J. Math. Anal. Appl.* 2: 145–158.

8. Fred Brauer (1962). Asymptotic equivalence and asymptotic behavior of linear systems, *Mich. Math. J.* 9: 33–43.
9. Fred Brauer (1963). Lyapunov functions and comparison theorems, in *International Symposium on Nonlinear Differential Equations and Nonlinear Mechanics* (J. P. LaSalle & S. Lefschetz, eds.). New York: Academic Press. pp. 435–441.
10. Fred Brauer (1963). Bounds for solutions of ordinary differential equations, *Proc. Amer. Math. Soc.* 14: 36–43.
11. Fred Brauer (1963). On the asymptotic behavior of Bessel functions, *Amer. Math. Monthly* 70: 954–957.
12. Fred Brauer (1964). Nonlinear differential equations with forcing terms, *Proc. Amer. Math. Soc.* 15: 758–765.
13. Fred Brauer (1964). On the completeness of biorthogonal systems, *Mich. Math. J.* 11: 379–383; errata, same journal, 12: 127–128 (1965).
14. Fred Brauer (1965). Some refinements of Lyapunov's second method, *Can. J. Math.* 17: 811–819.
15. Fred Brauer (1966). Perturbations of nonlinear systems of differential equations, *J. Math. Anal. Appl.* 14: 198–206.
16. Fred Brauer (1966). The use of comparison theorems for ordinary differential equations, in *Stability Problems of Solutions of Diff. Equations* (Proc. NATO Advanced Study Inst., Padua, 1965). Gubbio: Edizione "Oderisi". pp. 29–50.
17. Fred Brauer (1966). The asymptotic behavior of perturbed nonlinear systems, in *Stability Problems of Solution of Diff. Equations* (Proc. NATO Advanced Study Inst., Padua, 1965). Gubbio: Edizione "Oderisi". pp. 51–56.
18. Fred Brauer (1966). The solution of non-homogeneous systems of differential equations by undetermined coefficients, *Can. Math. Bull.* 9: 81–87.
19. Fred Brauer (1967). Green's functions for singular ordinary differential operators, *Can. J. Math.* 19: 571–582.
20. Fred Brauer (1967). Perturbations of nonlinear systems of differential equations, II., *J. Math. Anal. Appl.* 17: 418–434.
21. Fred Brauer (1968). A class of nonlinear eigenvalue problems, in *U.S.-Japan Seminar on Differential & Functional Equations.* New York: W. A. Benjamin, Inc. pp. 429–433.
22. Fred Brauer (1968). Nonlinear perturbations of Sturm-Liouville boundary-value problems, *J. Math. Anal. Appl.* 22: 591–598.
23. Fred Brauer and James S. W. Wong (1969). On asymptotic behavior of perturbed linear systems, *J. Diff. Equations* 6: 142–153.
24. Fred Brauer and James S. W. Wong (1969). On the asymptotic relationships between solutions of two systems of ordinary differential equations, *J. Diff. Equations* 6: 527–543.
25. Fred Brauer and Aaron Strauss (1970). Perturbations of nonlinear

systems of differential equations, III, *J. Math. Anal. Appl.* 31: 37–48.

26. Fred Brauer (1972). Perturbations of nonlinear systems of differential equations, IV, *J. Math. Anal. Appl.* 37(1): 214–222.
27. Fred Brauer (1972). A nonlinear variation of constants formula for Volterra equations, *Math. Systems Theory* 6: 226–235.
28. Fred Brauer (1972). A nonlinear predator-prey problem, *Ordinary differential equations*, Proc. 1971 NRL-MRC Conference (L. Weiss, ed.). New York: Academic Press. pp. 371–377.
29. Fred Brauer (1972). The nonlinear simple pendulum, *Ann. Math. Monthly* 79: 348–355.
30. Fred Brauer (1974). On the populations of competing species, *Math. Biosci.* 19: 299–306.
31. Fred Brauer (1975). On a nonlinear integral equation for population growth problems, *SIAM J. Math. Anal.* 6: 312–317.
32. Fred Brauer and David A. Sánchez (1975). Constant rate population harvesting: equilibrium and stability, *Theor. Pop. Biol.* 8: 12–30.
33. Fred Brauer and David A. Sánchez (1975). Some models for population growth with harvesting, in *Proc. International Conference on Differential Equations*, Univ. of Southern Calif., Los Angeles, 1974 (H. A. Antosiewicz, ed.). New York: Academic Press. pp. 53–64.
34. Fred Brauer and David A. Sánchez (1976). Cosecha de poblaciones en competencia [Harvesting of competing populations], in *Mathematical Notes and Symposia, Vol. 2: Ecuaciones Differenciales* (Proc. Third Mexico-U.S. Symposium) (C. Imaz, ed.). Mexico City: Fondo de Cultura Económica. pp. 171–176.
35. Fred Brauer (1976). Constant rate harvesting of populations governed by Volterra integral equations, *J. Math. Anal. Appl.* 56: 18–27.
36. Fred Brauer (1976). Some applications of the theory of ordinary differential equations to population growth problems, *Ann. Acad. Brasil de Ciencias* 48: 369–385.
37. Fred Brauer (1976, October). Perturbations of the nonlinear renewal equation, *Advances in Math.* 22(1): 32–51.
38. Fred Brauer (1976). Destabilization of predator-prey systems under enrichment, *Int. J. Control* 23: 541–552.
39. Fred Brauer, A. C. Soudack and H. S. Jarosch (1976). Stabilization and destabilization of predator-prey systems under harvesting and nutrient enrichment, *Int. J. Control* 23: 553–573.
40. Fred Brauer (1977). Stability of some population models with delay, *Math. Biosciences* 33: 345–358.
41. Fred Brauer (1977). Periodic solutions of some ecological models, *J. Theor. Biol.* 69: 143–152.

42. Fred Brauer and A. C. Soudack (1978). Response of predator-prey systems to nutrient enrichment and proportional harvesting, *Int. J. Control* 27: 65–86.
43. Fred Brauer (1978). Asymptotic stability of a class of integro-differential equations, *J. Differential Equations* 28: 180–188.
44. Fred Brauer (1979). Harvesting strategies for population systems, *Rocky Mountain J. Math.* 19: 19–26.
45. Fred Brauer (1979). Decay rates for solutions of a class of differential-difference equations, *SIAM J. Math. Anal.* 10: 783–788.
46. Fred Brauer and A. C. Soudack (1979). Stability regions and transitions phenomena for harvested predator prey systems, *J. Math. Biol.* 7: 319–337.
47. Fred Brauer (1979). Boundedness of solutions of predator-prey systems, *Theor. Pop. Biol.* 15: 268–273.
48. Fred Brauer (1979). Characteristic return times for harvested population models with time-lag, *Math. Biosci.* 45: 295–311.
49. Fred Brauer and A. C. Soudack (1979). Stability regions in predator-prey systems with constant-rate prey harvesting, *J. Math. Biol.* 8: 55–71.
50. Fred Brauer and A. C. Soudack (1981). Constant-rate stocking of predator-prey systems, *J. Math. Biol.* 11(1): 1–14.
51. Fred Brauer and A. C. Soudack (1981). Coexistence properties of some predator-prey systems under constant rate harvesting and stocking, *J. Math. Biol.* 12: 101–114.
52. Fred Brauer and A. C. Soudack (1981). Constant-rate effort harvesting and stocking in a class of predator-prey systems, in *Differential Equations and Applications in Ecology, Epidemics and Population Problems* (Stavros N. Busenberg and Kenneth L. Cooke, eds.). New York: Academic Press. pp. 131–144.
53. Fred Brauer and A. C. Soudack (1982). On constant effort harvesting and stocking in a class of predator-prey systems, *J. Theor. Biol.* 95: 247–252.
54. Fred Brauer (1983). Constant-rate harvesting of age-structured populations, *SIAM J. Math Anal.* 14 (1983), 947–961.
55. Fred Brauer (1983). Nonlinear age-dependent population growth under harvesting, *Int. J. Computers and Math. with Appl.* 9: 345–352.
56. Fred Brauer (1984). The effect of harvesting on population systems, in *Trends in Theory & Practice of Nonlinear Differential Equations* (Proc., Arlington, TX, 1982, V. Lakshmikantham, ed.). New York: Marcel Dekker. pp. 81–89.
57. Fred Brauer (1984). Constant-yield harvesting of population systems, in *Mathematical Ecology*, Proc. Trieste 1982 (S. A. Levin and T. G. Hallam, eds.), Lec. Notes in Biomathematics 54. Berlin: Springer-Verlag. pp. 238–246.

58. Fred Brauer and A. C. Soudack (1985). Optimal harvesting in predator-prey systems, *Int. J. Control* 41(1): 111–128.
59. Fred Brauer and A. C. Soudack (1985). Mutualism models with nonlinear growth rates, *Int. J. Control* 41(6): 1601–1612.
60. Fred Brauer and Ma Zhien (1987). Stability of stage-structured population models, *J. Math. Anal. Appl.* 126: 301–315.
61. Fred Brauer (1987). A class of Volterra integral equations arising in delayed-recruitment population models, *Nat. Res. Modeling* 2(2): 259–278.
62. Fred Brauer (1987). Absolute stability in delay equations, *J. Differential Equations* 69: 185–191.
63. Fred Brauer (1987). A simplification of Taylor's theorem, *Amer. Math. Monthly* 94: 453–455.
64. Fred Brauer (1987). Harvesting in delayed-recruitment population models, in *Proc. Canadian Mathematical Society 1986 Seminar on Oscillation, Bifurcation and Chaos.* Providence, RI: Amer. Math. Soc. pp. 317–327.
65. Fred Brauer, Stephen Ellner and M. D. Krom (1988). Modeling and management for seawater fishponds, in *Proc. 1986 Trieste Research Conference on Mathematical Ecology* (T. G. Hallam, S. A. Levin, and L. J. Gross, eds.). Teaneck, NJ: World Scientific Press. pp. 215–235.
66. Fred Brauer (1988). Coexistence and survival of invading species, in *Proc. 1986 Trieste Research Conference on Mathematical Ecology* (T. G. Hallam, S. A. Levin, and L. J. Gross, eds.). Teaneck, NJ: World Scientific Press. pp. 599–610.
67. Fred Brauer, David Rollins and A. C. Soudack (1988). Harvesting in population models with delayed recruitment and age-dependent mortality, *Nat. Res. Modeling* 3(1): 45–62.
68. Fred Brauer (1988). Some topics in population biology involving delay equations, 38 pp.; translated into Chinese by Ma Zhien. Xian, China: Department of Mathematics, Xian Jiaotong University. 58 pp.
69. Fred Brauer (1989). Epidemic models in populations of varying size, in *Mathematical Approaches to Problems in Resource Management and Epidemiology* (C. Castillo-Chávez, S. Levin, and C. Shoemaker, eds.), Lecture Notes in Biomathematics 81. Berlin: Springer-Verlag. pp. 109–123.
70. Fred Brauer (1989). Multi-species interactions and coexistence, in *Proc. Int. Conf. on Theory and Applications of Differential Equations* (A.R. Aftabizadeh, ed.). Athens, OH: Ohio Univ. Press. pp. 91–96.
71. Fred Brauer (1990). Models for the spread of universally fatal diseases, *J. Math. Biology* 28: 451–462.
72. Fred Brauer (1990). Some infectious disease models with popula-

tion dynamics and general contact rates, *J. Diff. Integral Equations* 5: 827–836.

73. Fred Brauer (1991). Stability of equilibria in some infectious disease models, in *Differential Equations: Stability and Control* (S. Elaydi, ed.). New York: Marcel Dekker. pp. 53–62.
74. Fred Brauer and Hao Dun-Yuan (1991). Analysis of a characteristic equation, *J. Integral Equations and Appl.* 3: 239–254.
75. Fred Brauer (1991). Models for the spread of universally fatal diseases II, in *Differential Equations Models in Biology, Epidemiology, and Ecology*, Proc. Claremont 1990 (Stavros Busenberg and Mario Martelli, eds.), Lec. Notes in Biomathematics 92. Berlin: Springer-Verlag. pp. 57–69.
76. S. P. Blythe, Fred Brauer and Carlos Castillo-Chávez (1995). Demographic recruitment in sexually transmitted disease models, in *Computational Medicine, Public Health and Biotechnology: Building a Man in the Machine* (M. Witten, ed.). Singapore: World Scientific Press. pp. 1438–1457.
77. Fred Brauer (1995). Models for diseases with exposed period, *Rocky Mountain J. Math.* 25: 57–66.
78. S. P. Blythe, Fred Brauer, Carlos Castillo-Chávez, and Jorge X. Velasco-Hernández (1995). Models for sexually transmitted diseases with recruitment, in *Mathematicl Population Dynamics: Analyses of Heterogeneity* (O. Arino, D. Axelrod, M. Kimmel, and M. Langlais, eds.). Vol 1. Winnipeg: Wuerz Publishing Co. pp. 197–207.
79. Fred Brauer (1995). Models for diseases with vertical transmission and nonlinear population dynamics, *Math. Biosci.* 128: 13–24.
80. Fred Brauer (1996). Variable infectivity in communicable disease models, in *Proc. First World Congress of Nonlinear Analysts*, Tampa, Florida, 1992 (V. Lakshmikantham, ed.). Berlin: de Gruyter. Vol 4, pp. 3201–3210.
81. Fred Brauer, Carlos Castillo-Chávez and Jorge X. Velasco-Hernández (1996). Recruitment effects in heterosexually transmitted diseases, *Int. J. App. Science & Computation* 3: 78–90.
82. Fred Brauer and Carlos Castillo-Chávez (1995). Basic models in epidemiology, in *Ecological Time Series* (T.M. Powell and J.H. Steele, eds.). Chapman & Hall. pp. 410–447.
83. Fred Brauer, Jorge X. Velasco-Hernández and Carlos Castillo-Chávez (1996). Effects of treatment and prevalence-dependent recruitment on the dynamics of a fatal disease, *IMA J. Math. Applied to Medicine and Biology* 13: 175–192.
84. Fred Brauer (1996). A characteristic equation arising in models for diseases with vertical transmission and without immunity, in *Differential Equations and Applications to Biology and to Industry* (M. Martelli, K. Cooke, E. Cumberbatch, B. Tang, and H. Thieme,

eds.). Singapore: World Scientific Press. pp. 41–48.

85. Fred Brauer (1996). A model for populations with variable maturation period, *Dynamics of Continuous, Discrete, and Impulsive Systems* 2: 41–50.
86. Fred Brauer, Carlos Castillo-Chávez and Jorge X. Velasco-Hernández (1997). Recruitment with a core group and its effect on the spread of a sexually transmitted disease, in *Advances in Mathematical Population Dynamics: Molecules, Cells, and Man* (O. Arino, D. Axelrod, and M. Kimmel, eds.). Singapore: World Scientific Press. pp. 477–486.
87. Fred Brauer (1997). Continuous and discrete delayed, recruitment population models, *Dynamics of Continuous, Discrete and Impulsive Systems* 3: 245–252.
88. Fred Brauer (1999). General recruitment models for sexually transmitted diseases, in *Differential Equations with Applications to Biology* (S. Ruan, G. S. K. Wolkowicz, and J. Wu, eds.), Fields Institute Communications No. 21. Providence, RI: Amer. Math. Soc. pp. 45–50.
89. Fred Brauer (1999). Continuous and discrete population models with age-dependent mortality, *Dynamics of Continuous, Discrete, and Impulsive Systems* 5: 107–113.
90. Fred Brauer (in press). Time lags in disease models with recruitment, *Mathematical and Computer Modelling*, to appear.
91. Fred Brauer (in press). Infectious disease models with chronological age structure, this volume.
92. Fred Brauer (in press). Basic ideas of mathematical epidemiology, this volume.
93. Fred Brauer (in press). Extensions of the basic models, this volume.
94. Fred Brauer and Pauline van den Driessche (in press). Models for the transmission of disease with immigration of infectives, to appear.
95. Fred Brauer (in press). What goes up must come down, eventually, *American Mathematical Monthly*, to appear.
96. Fred Brauer (in press). A model for an SI disease in an age-structured population, to appear.

Books by Fred Brauer

1. Fred Brauer and John A. Nohel (1967). *Ordinary Differential Equations: A first course.* New York: W. A. Benjamin, Inc. 1st ed. xvi + 457 pp. 2nd ed., 1973, ix + 470 pp.
2. Fred Brauer and John A. Nohel (1968). *Elementary Differential Equations: Principles, problems, solutions.* New York: W. A. Benjamin, Inc. xi + 222 pp.
3. Fred Brauer and John A. Nohel (1968). *Problems and Solutions in Ordinary Differential Equations.* New York: W. A. Benjamin,

Inc. x + 267 pp.
4. Fred Brauer and John A. Nohel (1969). *Qualitative Theory of Ordinary Differential Equations.* New York: W. A. Benjamin, Inc. xi + 314 pp. Reprinted, Dover, 1989.
5. Fred Brauer, John A. Nohel and Hans Schneider (1970). *Linear Mathematics.* New York: W. A. Benjamin, Inc. xii + 347 pp.
6. Fred Brauer (1976). *Some Stability and Perturbation Problems for Differential and Integral Equations*, Monografias de Matemática no. 25. Rio de Janeiro: Instituo de Matemática Pura e Aplicada. iii + 163 pp.
7. Fred Brauer and John A. Nohel (1985). *An Introduction to Differential Equations with Applications.* New York: Harper & Row. xii + 620 pages.
8. Fred Brauer and Carlos Castillo-Chávez (2001). *Mathematical Models in Population Biology and Epidemiology.* (Texts in Applied Mathematics 40), Springer-Verlag, New York, (c) 2001, 416 pages, ISBN 0-387-98902-1.

KENNETH L. COOKE: RESEARCHER, EDUCATOR PAR EXCELLENCE

P. VAN DEN DRIESSCHE*

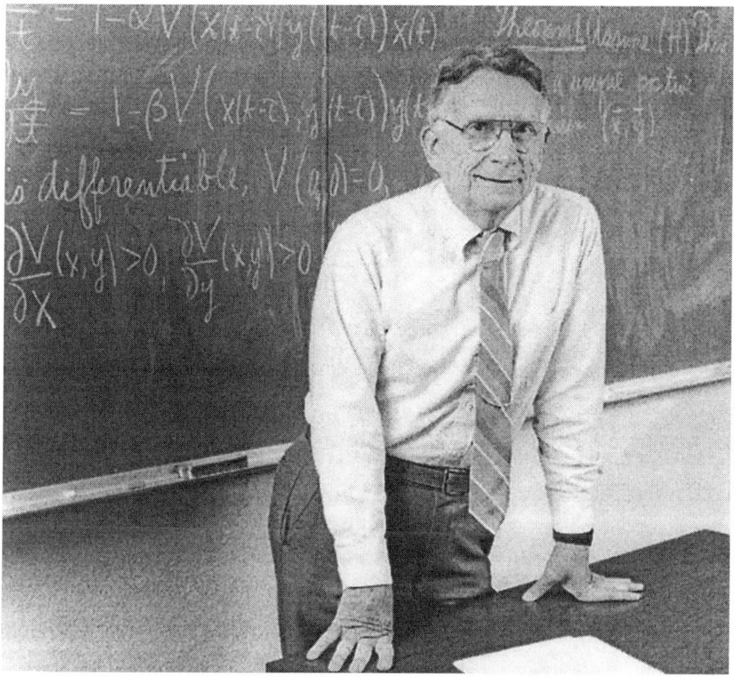

Kenneth L. Cooke†

It was fifty years ago that Kenneth Cooke (Ken) started as an instructor at the State College of Washington while studying for his PhD degree at Stanford University. From there he went to Pomona College, Claremont, where he advanced through the ranks, and where he is now Professor Emeritus. During this time he has been Chairman of the Department, and he has held research positions and visited many institutions, including Brown University, IMA Minnesota, Cornell University, England, Italy, Brazil and Mexico.

Ken's professional work during these years has had a profound effect on the areas of functional differential equations (especially delay-differential

*Department of Math and Stats, University of Victoria, Victoria, British Columbia, V8W 3P4 Canada.

†Mathematics Department, Pomona College, Claremont, CA 91711. Photograph is a courtesy of J.L. Harlan.

equations) and population biology (especially epidemic models). He has published five books and co-edited four volumes on these topics. His 1963 book *Differential-difference Equations*, co-authored with R. Bellman (his PhD advisor), has become a classic. His 1993 book *Vertically Transmitted Diseases*, co-authored with S. Busenberg, provides a marvellous single source for work in this recently developed area.

Sometime in the late 1960s, Ken's interests in differential equations expanded to include classes of equations that can be interpreted as models of biological processes. His 1967 paper *Functional differential equations: some models and perturbation problems* emphasized the "threshold" type equations and state dependent delays, with biological models as examples. His seminal 1973 paper with J. Yorke (which has been influential among modelers) studies the delay-differential equation

$$x' = g[x(t)] - g[x(t-L)]$$

and its generalization that allows for a distribution of life spans

$$x'(t) = g[x(t)] + \int_0^L g[x(t-s)]P'(s)ds.$$

Here $x(t)$ is the number of individuals in a population at time t, $g[x(t)]$ is the number of births per unit time, $P(a)$ is the proportion surviving to age a, and L is the maximum life span. Under realistic assumptions on g and P, they proved that any bounded solution approaches a limit as $t \to \infty$. More recently he has worked on various models of HIV/AIDS with several collaborators, including D.A. Allers, S. Busenberg, C. Castillo-Chavez, Y.-H. Hsieh, W. Huang (a former PhD student), S.A. Levin and H. Thieme.

Bellman and Cooke 1963 was one of my "bibles" when I met Ken at the University of Utah in 1978 at a summer school on Nonlinear Oscillations in Biology. One morning in the cafeteria, I plucked up courage to talk to this Professor whose book I so much admired, and was surprised to find him both approachable and enthusiastic about ideas. This conversation led to collaboration, and our first joint paper in 1986 on delay-differential equations. Lest it be misunderstood, it is not Ken who works slowly, but there were delays in our work! Since that time, I have come to value Ken as a collaborator and friend. He embodies superb qualities as a mathematician, which he applies to biological systems. On a more personal level, he shows patience, understanding and obviously enjoys many collaborations. He and his wife Margaret are very generous in hosting guests who visit Claremont to give talks or to attend meetings.

In January 1990, nearly two hundred research workers participated in an international meeting in Claremont for the celebration of Ken's 65th birthday. From this conference, two volumes of papers were published. One, devoted to models in mathematical biology, epidemiology and ecology, is published as volume 92 in the series Lecture Notes in Biomathematics.

The second, devoted to delay-differential equations, is published in the companion series Lecture Notes in Mathematics. The breadth, depth and interdisciplinary scope of Ken's work is well mirrored in these two volumes, and in the list of Ken's refereed articles given below.

In 1994, Ken was a member of the organizing committee of the Claremont International Conference "Differential Equations and Applications to Biology and to Industry". This was dedicated to the memory of his collaborator and great friend, Stavros Busenberg, who had tragically died the previous year. Ken gave generously in both time and effort to ensure the tremendous success of this conference and its proceedings.

This past year, Ken has been Chair of the Southern California Section of the Mathematical Association of America. This position fits his role as educator and leader. He has presented uncountably many excellent lectures, which are full of insight, enthusiasm and inspiration. He has advised six PhD students at Claremont Graduate University and been a mentor to countless other students and colleagues. Ken's humility and deep respect for all individuals and cultures is unparalleled. Hence, Ken's accomplishments cannot be completely understood without providing an explicit and typical example of the type of mentoring that he has carried out over the last fifty years. Carlos Castillo-Chavez vividly remembers his first interactions with Ken while both shared an office at Cornell in 1987. Carlos was a postdoc working with S.A. Levin when Ken came to spend his sabbatical leave. Ken almost immediately, actually on the second day, instigated a collaboaration (that still continues) on the transmission dynamics of HIV. The long and variable period of incubation of HIV naturally brought the use of functional differential equations into play. *The expert* taught Carlos functional differential equations during their working sessions, and now, many years later, Carlos realizes that Ken taught him a lot more than functional differential equations.

For his role as researcher, educator, and for his generous, warm personality we make this dedication to Kenneth L. Cooke.

Refereed Articles of Kenneth L. Cooke

(1953): The asymptotic behavior of the solutions of linear and non-linear differential-difference equations. Trans. Amer. Math. Soc., **75**, 80-105.

(1954): The rate of increase of real continuous solutions of algebraic differ ential-difference equations of the first order. Pacific J. Math., **4**, 483-501.

(1955): A non-local existence theorem for systems of ordinary differential equations. Rend. Circ. Mat. Palermo, Ser. II, Tomo **4**, 301-308.

(1955): Forced periodic solutions of a stable non-linear differential-difference equation. Annals of Math. **61**, 387-391.

(1957): Hadamard matrices. With J.L. Brenner, Rev. Ci. Lima **59**, 5-13.

(1958): A symbolic method for finding integrals of linear difference and

differential-difference equations. Math. Magazine, 121-126.
(1959): Stability theory and adjoint operators for linear differential-difference equations. With R. Bellman, Trans. Amer. Math. Soc. **92**, 470-500.
(1959): On the limit of solutions of differential-difference equations as the retardation approaches zero. With R. Bellman, Proc. Nat. Acad. Sci. **45**, 1026-1028.
(1959): The rate of increase of real continuous solutions of certain algebraic functional equations. Trans. Amer. Math. Soc. **92**, 106-124.
(1960): Stability and asymptotic theory for linear differential-difference equations. Proc. Symposium on Ordinary Differential Equations at Mexico City, September 1959, Boletin de la Sociedad Mat. Mexicana, 277-283.
(1962): On transcendental equations related to differential-difference equations. J. Math. Anal. Appl. **4**, 65-71.
(1963): Differential-difference equations, in *Nonlinear Differential Equations and Nonlinear Mechanics*, J.P. LaSalle and S. Lefschetz, eds., Academic Press, 155-171.
(1965): Existence and uniqueness theorems in invariant imbedding - I: conservation principles. With R. Bellman, R. Kalaba, G.M. Wing, J. Math. Anal. Appl. **10**, 243-244.
(1965): Existence and uniqueness theorems in invariant imbedding - II: convergence of a new difference algorithm. With R. Bellman, J. Math. Anal. Appl. **12**, 247-253.
(1965): The condition of regular degeneration for singularly perturbed linear differential-difference equations. J. Differential Equations **1**, 39-94.
(1965): Convergence of successive approximations in the shortest route problem. With D.L. Bentley, J. Math. Anal. Appl. **10**, 269-274.
(1965): On the computational solution of a class of functional differential equations. With R. Bellman, J. Math. Anal. Appl. **12**, 495-500.
(1966): The condition of regular degeneration for singularly perturbed systems of linear differential-difference equations. With K.R. Meyer, J. Math. Anal. Appl. **14**, 83-106.
(1966): The shortest route through a network with time- dependent internodal transit times. With E. Halsey, J. Math. Anal. Appl. **14**, 493-498.
(1966): Graphical solution of difficult crossing puzzles. With P. Detrick, R. Fraley, Math. Mag. **39**, 151-157.
(1966): Functional differential equations close to differential equations. Bull. Amer. Math. Soc. **72**, 285-288.
(1967): Functional differential equations with asymptotically vanishing lag. Rend. Circ. Mat. di Palermo, series II, XVI, 39-56.
(1967): Functional differential equations: some models and perturbation problems, in *Differential Equations and Dynamical Systems*, J.K. Hale and J.P. LaSalle, eds., Academic Press, 167-183.
(1967): Asymptotic theory for the delay-differential equation $u'(t) = -au(t - r(u(t)))$. J. Math. Anal. Appl. **19**, 160-173.
(1967): Some recent work on functional-differential equations, in *Proc.*

U.S. Japan Seminar on Differential and Functional Equations, W.A. Harris, Jr., Y. Sibuya, eds., W.A. Benjamin, 27-47.
(1968): Difference-differential equations and nonlinear initial-boundary value problems for linear hyperbolic partial differential equations. With D. Krumme, J. Math. Anal. Appl. **24**, 372-387.
(1969): The Königsberg bridges problem generalized. With R. Bellman, J. Math. Anal. Appl. **25**, 1-7.
(1970): Linear functional differential equations of asymptotically autonomous type. J. Diff. Eq. **7**, 154-174.
(1971): A linear mixed problem with derivative boundary conditions. *Seminar on Differential Equations and Dynamical Systems, III*, D. Sweet and J.A. Yorke, eds., University of Maryland, College Park, 11-17.
(1972): Equations modelling population growth, economic growth, and gonorrhea epidemiology. With J. Yorke, 1971 NRL-MRC Conference, *Ordinary Differential Equations*, L. Weiss, ed., Academic Press, New York.
(1973): Some equations modelling growth processes and gonorrhea epidemics. With J. Yorke, Math. Biosciences **16**, 75-101.
(1973): On a class of hereditary processes in biomechanics. With N. Distefano, B. Kashef, Math. Biosciences **16**, 359-373.
(1974): A linear hyperbolic problem all of whose solutions are constant after finite time. SIAM J. Math. Anal. **5, No. 3**, 482-488.
(1975): Asymptotic equivalence of an ordinary and a functional differential equation. J. Math. Anal. Appl. **51**, 187-207, Abstract in *International Conference on Differential Equations*, H.A. Antonsiewicz, ed., Academic Press, New York, 808-809.
(1975): A discrete-time epidemic model with classes of infectives and susceptibles. Theor. Population Biol. **7**, 175-196.
(1975): A discrete-time epidemic model with classes of infectives and susceptibles (Summary). *Epidemiology*, Proceedings of SIMS Conference, D. Ludwig, K. Cooke, eds., SIAM, Philadelphia, 132-138.
(1976): An epidemic equation with immigration. Math. Biosciences **29**, 135-158.
(1976): A periodicity threshold theorem for epidemics and population growth. With J.L. Kaplan, Math. Biosciences **31**, 87-104.
(1977): Stability or chaos in discrete epidemic models. With D.F. Calef, E.V. Level, *Nonlinear Systems and Applications*, V. Lakshmikantham, ed., Academic Press, New York, 73-93.
(1978): Periodic solutions of a periodic nonlinear delay differential equation. With S. Busenberg, SIAM J. Applied Math. **35**, 704-721.
(1979): Periodic solutions of delay differential equations arising in some models of epidemics. With S. Busenberg, *Applied Nonlinear Analysis*, V. Lakshmikantham, ed., Academic Press, New York, 67-78.
(1979): Mathematical approaches to culture change, in *Transformations: Mathematical Approaches to Culture Change*, C. Renfrew, K. Cooke, eds., Academic Press, New York, 45-81.

(1979): Stability analysis for a vector disease model. Rocky Mountain J. of Math. **9**, 31-42.
(1979): An experiment on the simulation of culture changes. With C. Renfrew, in *Transformations: Mathematical Approaches to Culture Change*, C. Renfrew, K. Cooke, eds., Academic Press, New York, 327-348.
(1980): The effect of integral conditions in certain equations modelling epidemics and population growth. With S. Busenberg, J. Math. Biology **10**, 13-32.
(1981): On the construction and evaluation of mathematical models, in *Simulations in Archaeology*, J.A. Sabloff, ed., Univ. New Mexico Press, Albuquerque.
(1981): Stability of a functional differential equation for the motion of a radiating charged particle. With J.L. Kaplan, M. Sorg, Nonlinear Analysis: TMA **5**, 1133-1139.
(1981): Delay differential equations, in *Mathematics of Biology*, M. Iannelli, ed., Liguori editore, Napoli, 5-80.
(1982): Vertically transmitted diseases. With S. Busenberg, in *Nonlinear Phenomena in the Mathematical Sciences*, V. Lakshmikantham, ed., Academic Press, New York, 189-197.
(1982): Models of vertically transmitted diseases with sequential continuous dynamics. With S. Busenberg, in *Nonlinear Phenomena in the Mathematical Sciences*, V. Lakshmikantham, ed., Academic Press, New York, 179-187.
(1982): Discrete delay, distributed delay and stability switches. With Z. Grossman, J. Math. Anal. Appl. **86**, 592-627.
(1982): Models for endemic infections with asymptomatic cases I. One group. Mathematical Modelling **3**, 1-15.
(1983): Analysis of a model of a vertically transmitted disease. With S. Busenberg, M.A. Pozio, J. Math. Biol. **17**, 305-329.
(1983): Stability conditions for linear retarded functional differential equations. With J.M. Ferreira, J. Math. Anal. Appl. **96**, 480-504.
(1984): Distributional and analytic solutions of functional differential equations. With J. Wiener, J. Math. Anal. Appl. **98**, 111-129.
(1984): Retarded differential equations with piecewise constant delays. With J. Wiener, J. Math. Anal. Appl. **99**, 265-297.
(1984): Stability conditions for linear non-autonomous delay differential equations. With S. Busenberg, Quart. Appl. Math., **42**, 295-306.
(1984): Mathematical models of vertical transmission of infection, in *Mathematical Ecology*, S.A. Levin, T.G. Hallam, eds., Lecture Notes in Biomathematics **54**, Springer- Verlag, 344-355.
(1984): Stability of non-autonomous delay differential equations by Liapunov functionals, in *Infinite-Dimensional Systems*, F. Kappel, W. Schappacher, eds., Lecture Notes in Mathematics **1076**, Springer-Verlag.
(1985): Infection models with asymptomatics, in *Mathematics and Computers in Biomedical Applications*, J. Eisenfeld, C. De Lisi, eds., Elsevier

Science Publ., 277-282.
(1985): Stability of delay differential eqations with applications in biology and medicine, in *Mathematics in Biology and Medicine*, V. Capasso, E. Grosso, S.L. Paveri-Fontana, eds., Lecture Notes in Biomathematics **57**, Springer-Verlag, 439-446.
(1986): Stability regions for linear equations with piecewise continuous delay. With J. Wiener, Comp. & Math. with Appl. **12A**, 695-701.
(1986): One-dimensional linear and logistic harvesting models. With M. Witten, Math. Modelling **7**, 301-340.
(1986): On zeroes of some transcendental equations. With P. van den Driessche, Funkcialaj Ekvacioj **29**, 77-90.
(1987): An equation alternately of retarded and advanced type. With J. Wiener, Proc. Amer. Math. Soc. **99**, 726-732.
(1987): Neutral differential equations with piecewise constant arguments. With J. Wiener, Bollettino UMI **7**, 321-346.
(1987): Analysis of the complicated dynamics of some harvesting models. With H.E. Nusse, J. Math Biol. **25**, 521-542.
(1988): Harvesting procedures with management policy in iterative density-dependent population models. With R. Elderkin, M. Witten, Natural Resource Modeling **2**, No.3, 383-420.
(1988): A nonlinear equation with piecewise continuous argument. With L.A.V. Carvalho, Diff. and Integral Eqns. **1**, 359-367.
(1988): The population dynamics of two vertically transmitted infections. With S. Busenberg, Theoretical Population Biology **33**, 181-198.
(1988): Endemic thresholds and stability in a class of age-structured populations. With S. Busenberg, M. Iannelli, SIAM J. Applied. Math. **48**, 1379-1395.
(1988): Oscillation in systems of differential equations with piecewise constant argument. With J. Wiener, J. Math. Anal. Appl. **137**, 221-239.
(1989): On the role of long incubation periods in the dynamics of acquired immunodeficiency syndrome (AIDS) Part 1: Single population models. With C. Castillo-Chavez, W. Huang, S.A. Levin, J. Math. Biol. **27**, 373-398.
(1989): Stability and thresholds in some age-structured epidemics. With S. Busenberg and M. Iannelli, in *Mathematical Approaches to Problems in Resource Management and Epidemiology*, C. Castillo-Chavez, S.A. Levin, C.A. Shoemaker, eds., Lecture Notes in Biomathematics **81**, Spring-Verlag, 124-141.
(1989): Results on the dynamics for models of the sexual transmission of the human immunodeficiency virus. With C. Castillo-Chavez, W. Huang, S.A. Levin, Appl. Math. Lett. **2**, No. 4, 327-331.
(1989): On the modelling of epidemics. With C. Castillo- Chavez and S.A. Levin, in *High Performance Computing*, J.L. Delhaye, E. Glenebe, eds., North-Holland, Amsterdam-New York-Oxford-Tokyo, 389-402.
(1989): The role of long periods of infectiousness in the dynamics of ac-

quired immunodeficiency syndrome (AIDS). With C. Castillo-Chavez, W. Huang, S.A. Levin, in *Mathematical Approaches to Problems in Resource Management and Epidemiology*, C. Castillo-Chavez, S.A. Levin, C.A. Shoemaker, eds., Lecture Notes in Biomathematics **81**, Springer-Verlag, 177-189.
(1989): On the role of long incubation periods in the dynamics of acquired immunodeficiency syndrome (AIDS) Part 2: Multiple group models. With C. Castillo-Chavez, W. Huang, S.A. Levin, in *Mathematical and Statistical Approaches to AIDS Epidemiology*, Lecture Notes in Biomathematics **83**, C. Castillo-Chavez, ed., 200-217.
(1990): Coexistence of analytic and distributional solutions for linear differential equations, I. With J. Wiener, J. Math. Anal. Appl. **148**, 390-421.
(1991): On dichotomic maps for a class of differential-difference equations. With L.A.V. Carvalho, Proc. Roy. Soc. Edinburgh **117A**, 317-328.
(1991): Mixing patterns in models of AIDS. With D.A. Allers and C. Castillo-Chavez, in *Mathematical Population Dynamics*, O. Arino, D.E. Axelrod, M. Kimmel, eds., Lecture Notes in Pure and Applied Mathematics **131**, Marcel Dekker, New York-Basel-Hong Kong, 297-309.
(1991): Demographic change and persistence of HIV/AIDS in a heterogeneous population. With S. Busenberg and H. Thieme, SIAM J. Applied Math **51**, 1030-1052.
(1991): Coexistence of analytic and distributional solutions for linear differential equations, II. With J. Wiener and S.M. Shah, J. Math. Anal. Appl. **159**, 271-289.
(1991): A survey of differential equations with piecewise continuous arguments. With J. Wiener, in *Delay Differential Equations and Dynamical Systems*, Lecture Notes in Mathematics **1475**, S. Busenberg and M. Martelli, eds., 1-15.
(1992): Stability and bifurcation for a multiple-group model for the dynamics of HIV/AIDS transmission. With W. Huang, C. Castillo-Chavez, SIAM J. Appl. Math. **52**, 835-854.
(1992): A theorem of George Seifert and an equation with state-dependent delay. With Wenzhang Huang, in *Delay and Differential Equations* (Proceedings in Honor of George Seifert on his Retirement), ed. A.M. Fink, Richard K. Miller, and Wolfgang Kliemann. World Scientific, Singapore-New Jersey-London-Hong Kong, 65-77.
(1992): Liapunov functionals and stability of certain differential-difference equations. With L.A.V. Carvalho, in *Functional Differential Equations*, T. Yoshizawa and J. Kato, eds., World Scientific, Singapore-New Jersey-London-Hong Kong, 32-42.
(1993): Spectral conditions and an explicit expression for the stabilization of hybrid systems in the presence of feedback delays. With J. Turi and G. Turner, Quarterly Appl. Math. **51**, 147-159.
(1993): Distributional and small solutions for linear time-dependent delay equations. With S.M. Verduyn Lunel, Differential and Integral Equations,

1101-1117.
(1994): Numerical approximation of the solutions of delay differential equations on an infinite interval using piecewise constant arguments. With I. Györi, Computers Math. Applic. **28**, 81-92.
(1994): Stability, instability in delay equations modeling human respiration. With J. Turi, J. Math. Biol. **32**, 535-543.
(1995): A Model for HIV in Asia. With S. Busenberg and Y.-H. Hsieh, Math. Biosci. **128**, 185-210.
(1995): Remembering Stavros Busenberg. With C. Castillo-Chavez and H. Thieme, Math. Biosci. **128**, 3-11.
(1995): Two problems on differential-delay equations, in *Ordinary Differential Equations and their Applications*, Proceedings of International Meeting in Firenze, Italy, Sept. 20-24. 1993, published in Bologna.
(1995): A boundary value problem for a functional-differential equation with a linearly transformed argument. With L.E. Rossovskii and A.L. Skubachevskii. Differential Equations **31**, 1294-1299. (Translated from Differentsial'nye Uravneniya **31** (August, 1995), 1348-1352.)
(1996): On the sharpness of a theorem by Cooke and Verduyn Lunel. With G. Derfel, J. Math. Anal. Appl. **197**, 379-391.
(1996): Applying Carvalho's method to find periodic solutions of difference equations. With L.A.C. Ladeira, J. Difference Equations & Applications, **2**, 105-115.
(1996): Modeling antiviral immune response: a negative feedback control approach. With B. Tang and D. Babai, Int. J. of Appl. Sc. & Computations, **3** no. 1, 48-56.
(1996): On the problem of linearization for state-dependent delay differential equations. With W. Huang. Proc. Amer. Math. Soc. **124**, 1417-1426.
(1996): Analysis of an SEIRS epidemic model with two delays. With P. van den Driessche. J. Math. Biol. **35**, 240-260.
(1997): Three lectures on mathematical modeling of diseases, in Three Lectures, Colóquio de Equações Diferenciais, L. A. V. Carvalho and L.A.V. Ladeira, eds. Sào Carlos, Brazil.
(1998): Collapsible backward continuation and numerical approximations in a functional differential equation. With L. A.V. Carvalho. J. Differential Equations **143**, 96-109.
(1998): Analyses of an antiviral immune response model with time delays. With Y. Kuang and B. Li. Canadian Appl. Math. Quarterly **6** no. 4, 321-354.
(1999): Interaction of maturation delay and nonlinear birth in population and epidemic models. With P. van den Driessche and X. Zou. J. Math. Biology **39**, 332-352.
(1999): On periodic solutions for a class of linear scaled differential equations I. With L.A.V. Carvalho and L.A.C. Ladeira. Communications in Applied Analysis **3**, no. 3, 399-413.
(1999): On periodic solutions for a class of linear scaled differential equa-

tions II. With L.A.V. Carvalho and L.A.C. Ladeira. Communications in Applied Analysis **3**, no. 3, 415-431.
(2000): On the discretization of a delay differential equation. With A. F. Ivanov. Journal of Difference Equations and Applications, **6**, 105-119.
(2000): Behaviour change and treatment of core groups: its effect on the spread of HIV/AIDS. With Ying-Hen Hsieh. IMA Journal Math. Appl. Med. Biol., Vol. 17: 213-241.

BASIC IDEAS OF MATHEMATICAL EPIDEMIOLOGY

FRED BRAUER*

1. Introduction. Communicable diseases are an important part of modern life. The AIDS epidemic and outbursts of diseases such as the Ebola virus are events of concern and interest to many people. The prevalence and effects of many diseases in less developed countries are probably less well-known but may be of even more importance. Every year millions of people die of measles, respiratory infections, diarrhoeas and other diseases which are easily treated and not considered dangerous in the Western world. Diseases such as malaria, typhus, cholera, schistosomiasis, and sleeping sickness are endemic (always present) in many parts of the world. The effects of high disease mortality on the mean life span and of disease debilitation and mortality on the economy in countries afflicted by them are considerable.

Epidemics, which may be described as sudden outbreaks of diseases which infect a substantial fraction of the population in a region before disappearing while leaving many members untouched have probably been occurring since human beings began to form communities. Often, these attacks have recurred with intervals of several years between outbreaks, possibly diminishing in severity as populations developed some immunity.

The Book of Exodus describes the plagues that Moses brought down upon Egypt, and there are several other Biblical descriptions of epidemics. Descriptions of epidemics in ancient and mediaeval times frequently used the term plague because of a general belief that epidemics were divine retribution for sinful living. More recently, some have described AIDS as punishment for sinful activities, and such views have delayed attempts to control this modern epidemic.

The historian W.H. McNeill argues, especially in his book [18], that the spread of communicable diseases has frequently been an important influence in history. For example, there was a sharp population increase throughout the world in the eighteenth century; the population of China increased from 150,000,000 in 1760 to 313,000,000 in 1794 and the population of Europe increased from 118,000,000 in 1700 to 187,000,000 in 1800. There were many factors involved in this increase, including changes in marriage age and technological improvements leading to increased food supplies, but these are not sufficient to explain the increase. Demographic studies indicate that a satisfactory explanation requires recognition of a decrease in the mortality caused by periodic epidemic infections. This decrease came about partly through improvements in medicine, but a more

*Department of Mathematics, University of British Columbia, Vancouver, B.C., V6T 1Z2, CANADA.

important influence was probably that more people developed immunities against infection as increased travel intensified the circulation of diseases.

There are many Biblical references to diseases as historical influences, such as the decision of Sennacherib, the king of Assyria to abandon his attempt to capture Jerusalem about 700 B.C. because of the illness of his soldiers (Isaiah 37, 36–38). The fall of empires has been attributed directly or indirectly to epidemic diseases. In the second century A.D. the so-called Antonine plagues (possibly measles and smallpox) invaded the Roman Empire, causing drastic population reductions and economic hardships, leading to disintegration of the empire because of disorganization which facilitated invasions of barbarians. The Han empire in China collapsed in the third century A.D. after a very similar sequence of events. The defeat of a population of millions of Aztecs by Cortez and his 600 followers can be explained by a smallpox epidemic which devastated the Aztecs but had almost no effect on the invading Spaniards because of the immunities they had developed in Europe. The Aztecs were not only weakened by disease but also confounded by what they interpreted as a divine favouring of the invaders. Smallpox then spread southward to the Incas in Peru and was an important factor in the success of Pizarro's invasion a few years later. Smallpox was followed by other diseases such as measles and diptheria imported from Europe to North America. In some regions, the indigenous populations were (literally) decimated by these diseases. Between 1519 and 1530 the Indian population of Mexico was reduced from 30,000,000 to 3,000,000.

The Black Death (bubonic plague) spread from Asia throughout Europe several times during the fourteenth century, beginning in 1346 and is estimated to have caused the death of as much as one third of the population of Europe between 1346 and 1350. The disease recurred regularly in various parts of Europe for more than 300 years, notably in the Great Plague of London of 1665–1666 and then gradually withdrew from Europe. As the plague struck some regions harshly while avoiding others, it had a profound effect on political and economic developments in mediaeval times. In the last epidemic in France (1720–1722), half the population of Marseilles, 60 per cent of the population in nearby Toulon, 44 per cent of the population of Arles and 30 per cent of the population of Aix and Avignon died, but the epidemic did not spread beyond Provence.

There are many questions which are of interest to public health physicians confronted with a possible epidemic. For example, how severe will the epidemic be? This question may be interpreted in a variety of ways. For example, how many people will be affected altogether and thus require treatment? What is the maximum number of people needing care at any particular time? How long will the epidemic last? How much good would quarantine of victims do in reducing the severity of the epidemic?

For diseases which are endemic in some region, public health physicians need to be able to estimate the number of infectives at a given time as well as the rate at which new infections arise. Just as for epidemics, the effects of quarantine or vaccine in reducing the number of victims are of importance. In addition, the possibility of defeating the endemic nature of the disease and thus controlling the disease are worthy of study. How can such questions be answered?

Scientific experiments usually are designed to obtain information and to test hypotheses. Experiments in epidemiology with controls are often difficult or impossible to design and even if it is possible to arrange an experiment there are serious ethical questions involved in withholding treatment from a control group. Sometimes data may be obtained after the fact from reports of epidemics or of endemic disease levels, but the data may be incomplete or inaccurate. In addition, data may contain enough irregularities to raise serious questions of interpretation, such as whether there is evidence of chaotic behaviour [9]. This makes parameter estimation and model fitting very difficult, and raises the question of whether mathematical modelling in epidemiology is of value.

We believe that mathematical modelling is of considerable importance in epidemiology because it may provide understanding of the underlying mechanisms which influence the spread of disease and may suggest control strategies. Even if it is not possible to verify hypotheses accurately, agreement with hypotheses of a qualitative nature may be valuable. Models may indicate behaviour which is obscured by the experimental data. This apparently foolish statement may be justified if the indication can be justified by closer examination of the qualitative behaviour of the actual data. For example, one of the fundamental results in mathematical epidemiology is that there is generally a "threshold" behaviour. If a dimensionless quantity known as the basic reproductive number and representing the average number of secondary infections caused by an average infective is less than 1, a disease will die out and if the basic reproductive number exceeds 1 there will be an epidemic or the disease will become endemic. This broad principle is consistent with observations. Estimates of the basic reproductive number may lead to predictions about the course of the disease. If there is a vaccine which will provide immunity against the disease, it may be possible to estimate how widespread vaccination must be to prevent the spread of disease.

In the mathematical modelling of disease transmission, as in most other areas of mathematical modelling, there is always a trade-off between simple models which omit many aspects of a situation and are designed only to explain the general qualitative behaviour and more complex models which attempt to incorporate more detail about a specific situation. Such complex models are designed to make short term quantitative predictions but are generally difficult or impossible to solve analytically and limited in their usefulness. Our approach here will be to begin with simple possible models in order to try to establish broad principles and to introduce more detailed structure primarily to see whether this can lead to differences in qualitative behaviour.

We may think of a disease as an invasion of a host population, consisting of separate patches (individuals) by a pathogen. An epidemic is a successful invasion, meaning that the number of patches increases over time after the initial.introduction of the pathogen into the host population.

The idea of invisible living creatures as agents of disease goes back at least to the writings of Aristotle (384 B.C.–322 B.C.) and developed as a theory in the sixteenth century. The existence of micro-organisms was demonstrated by Leeuwenhoek (1632–1723) with the aid of the first microscopes. The first expression of the germ theory of disease by Jacob Henle (1809–1885) came in 1840 and was developed by Robert Koch (1843–1910), Joseph Lister (1827–1912), and Louis Pasteur (1827–1875) in the latter part of the nineteenth century and the early part of the twentieth century.

The mechanism of transmission of infections is now known for most diseases. Generally, diseases transmitted by viral agents, such as influenza, measles, rubella (German measles), and chicken-pox confer immunity against re-infection, while diseases transmitted by bacteria, such as meningitis and gonorrhea confer no immunity against re-infection. Other diseases, such as malaria, are transmitted not directly from human to human but by vectors, agents (usually insects) who are infected by humans and who then transmit the disease to humans.

Many of the early developments in the mathematical modelling of communicable diseases are due to public health physicians. The first known result in mathematical epidemiology is a defense of the practice of inoculation against smallpox in 1760 by Daniel Bernouilli, a member of a famous family of mathematicians (eight spread over three generations) who had been trained as a physician. The first contributions to modern mathematical epidemiology are due to P.D. En'ko between 1873 and 1894, and the foundations of the entire approach to epidemiology based on compartmental models were laid by public health physicians such as Sir R.A. Ross, W.H. Hamer, A.G. McKendrick, and W.O. Kermack between 1900 and 1935, along with important contributions from a statistical perspective by J. Brownlee. A particularly instructive example is the work of Ross on malaria. Dr. Ross was awarded the second Nobel Prize in medicine for his demonstration of the dynamics of the transmission of malaria between mosquitoes and humans. Although his work received immediate acceptance in the medical community, his conclusion that malaria could be controlled by controlling mosquitoes was dismissed on the grounds that it would be impossible to rid a region of mosquitoes completely and that in any case mosquitoes would soon re-invade the region. After Ross formulated a mathematical model which predicted that malaria outbreaks could be avoided if the mosquito population could be reduced below a critical threshold level, field trials supported his conclusions and led to brilliant successes in malaria control.

We will formulate our descriptions as *compartmental models*, with the population under study being divided into compartments and with assumptions about the nature and time rate of transfer from one compartment to another. Diseases which confer immunity will have a different compartmental structure from diseases without immunity and for diseases transmitted by vectors it will be necessary to divide both populations into compartments. The rates of transfer between compartments are expressed mathematically as derivatives with respect to time of the sizes of the compartments, and as a result our models will be formulated initially as *differential equations*, relations between the derivatives of unknown functions and the functions. The crucial mathematical idea here is that the derivative of a function represents the rate of change of that function. Later, when we study models in which the rates of transfer depend on the sizes of compartments over the past as well as at the instant of transfer, we will be led to more general types of functional equations such as differential-difference equations or integral equations.

Simple differential equations may sometimes be "solved in closed form" (expressed in terms of specific functions), but this is seldom possible for more general functional equations. We will de-emphasize solutions in closed form and focus on qualitative analysis which gives less specific information but which may be applied much more broadly. In qualitative analysis we try to determine whether solutions approach a limit as the independent variable (usually time in our context) becomes large or whether solutions are periodic. We will give a description of the procedures of this qualitative analysis with statements of the principal mathematical results to be used but will refer the reader to more mathematically advanced source for their proofs. Fortunately, application of these results is usually a much easier task than analytic solution.

It is not possible to avoid technical mathematics completely in the qualitative study of differential equations. We will need to make use of some of the basic properties of the exponential function. The derivative of an exponential function e^{at} is proportional to the function,

$$\frac{d}{dt}(e^{at}) = a\,e^{at} \ .$$

Another way of expressing this property is to say that the function $y = e^{at}$ is a solution of the differential equation $y' = ay$. In fact, every solution of this differential equation is of the form $y = c\,e^{at}$ for some constant c. The particular constant c is specified by some additional requirement, usually an *initial condition*, a specification of the value of the solution for some value of t (often $t = 0$). We will make frequent use of this result, whose proof may be found in any differential equations text. It will also be important to note that as $t \to \infty$, the function e^{at} approaches zero if $a < 0$ and grows unbounded if $a > 0$.

2. A simple epidemic model. In the nineteenth century recurrent invasions of cholera killed millions in India. The influenza epidemic of 1918–1919 killed 20 million people overall, more than half a million in the United States. One of the questions which first attracted the attention of scientists interested in the study of the spread of communicable diseases was an explanation why diseases would suddenly develop in a community and then disappear just as suddenly without attacking the entire community. One of the early triumphs of mathematical epidemiology [16] was the formulation of a very simple model which predicted behavior very similar to the behavior observed in countless epidemics. We will begin our mathematical presentation with a description of this model and its analysis.

Perhaps the first epidemic to be examined from a modelling point of view was the Great Plague in London (1665–1666). The Plague was one of a sequence of attacks beginning in the year 1346 of what came to be known as the Black Death. It is now identified as bubonic plague, which had actually invaded Europe as early as the sixth century during the reign of the Emperor Justinian of the Roman Empire and continued for four centuries after the Black Death. The Great Plague killed about one sixth of the population of London. One of the few good features of the Plague is that it caused Cambridge University to be closed for two years and while Isaac Newton was at home because of this he discovered his law of gravitation.

The characteristic features of the Great Plague were that it appeared quite suddenly, grew in intensity, and then disappeared, leaving part of the population untouched. The same features have been observed in many other epidemics, both of fatal disease and of diseases whose victims recovered with immunity against re-infection.

In order to model such an epidemic, we divide the population being studied into three classes labelled S, I, and R. We use primes ($'$) to denote derivative of functions of t with respect to t; more generally we will use primes to denote differentiation whenever it is clear from the context what is the independent variable. We let $S(t)$ denote the number of individuals who are susceptible to the disease, that is, who are not (yet) infected at time t. $I(t)$ denotes the number of infected individuals, assumed infectious and able to spread the disease by contact with susceptibles. $R(t)$ denotes the number of individuals who have been infected and then removed from the possibility of being infected again or of spreading infection, through isolation from the rest of the population or through immunization against infection or through recovery from the disease with full immunity against re-infection or through death caused by the disease. These characterizations of removed members are very different from an epidemiological perspective but are equivalent from a modelling point of view which takes into account only the state of an individual with respect to the disease.

In formulating models in terms of the derivatives of the sizes of each compartment, we are assuming that the number of members in a compartment is a differentiable function of time. This may be a reasonable approximation if there are many members in a compartment but is certainly suspect otherwise. In formulating models as differential equations, we are assuming that they are *deterministic*, that is, the behaviour of a model is determined completely by its history and by the rules which govern the development of the model. For small compartment sizes, the behaviour of the compartment size may be strongly influenced by random perturbations and other types of models (stochastic) are more appropriate.

The model proposed by Kermack and McKendrick in 1927 to describe this situation is

$$\begin{aligned} S' &= -\beta SI \\ I' &= \beta SI - \alpha I \\ R' &= \alpha I \ . \end{aligned}$$

It is based on the following assumptions:

(i) An average infective makes contact sufficient to transmit infection with βN others in unit time, where N represents total population size.

(ii) A fraction α of infectives leave the infective class in unit time.

(iii) There is no entry into or departure from the population, except possibly through death from the disease.

According to (i), since the probability that a contact by an infective will be with a susceptible and thus can transmit infection is S/N, the number of new infections in unit time is $(\beta N)(S/N)I = \beta SI$. We need not give an algebraic expression for N since it cancels out of the final model, but we should note that for a disease which is fatal to all who are infected $N = S + I$, while for a disease from which all infected members recover with immunity $N = S + I + R$. The hypothesis (iii) really says that the time scale of the disease is much faster than the time scale of births and deaths so that demographic effects on the population may be ignored. In a later section we shall consider a model which is the same as the one considered here except for the incorporation of demographic effects (births and deaths) along with the epidemiological assumptions.

The assumption (ii) requires a fuller mathematical explanation as the assumption of a recovery rate proportional to the number of infectives has no epidemiological meaning. We consider the "cohort" of members who were all infected at one time and let $u(s)$ denote the number of these who are still infective s time units after having been infected. If a fraction α of these leave the infective class in unit time, then

$$u' = -\alpha u$$

and the solution of this elementary differential equation is

$$u(s) = u(0)\, e^{-\alpha s} .$$

Thus the fraction of infectives remaining infective s time units after having become infective is $e^{-\alpha s}$, so that the length of the infective period is distributed exponentially with mean $\int_0^\infty e^{-\alpha s} ds = 1/\alpha$, and this is what (ii) really assumes.

The assumptions of a rate of contacts proportional to population size and of a recovery rate which is exponentially distributed are unrealistically simple. Later, we shall consider more general models, but our goal here is to show what may be deduced from an extremely simple model. It will turn out that more realistic models may exhibit very similar behaviour.

In our model R is determined once S and I are known, and we can drop the R' equation from our model, leaving the system of two equations

$$\begin{aligned} S' &= -\beta S I \\ I' &= \left(\beta S - \alpha\right) I . \end{aligned} \tag{2.1}$$

We are unable to solve this system analytically but we may learn a great deal about the behaviour of its solutions by the following elementary qualitative approach. We observe that $S' < 0$ for all t and $I' > 0$ if and only if $S > \frac{\alpha}{\beta}$. Thus I increases so long as $S > \frac{\alpha}{\beta}$ but since S decreases for all t, I ultimately decreases and approaches zero. If $S(0) < \frac{\alpha}{\beta}$, I decreases to zero (no epidemic), while if $S(0) > \frac{\alpha}{\beta}$, I first increases to a maximum attained when $S = \frac{\alpha}{\beta}$ and then decreases to zero (epidemic). We think of introducing a small number of infectives into a population of susceptibles and ask whether there will be an epidemic. The quantity $\beta S(0)/\alpha$ is a threshold quantity called the basic reproductive number and denoted by R_0 which determines whether there is an epidemic or not. If $R_0 < 1$ the infection dies out, while if $R_0 > 1$ there is an epidemic.

Instead of trying to solve for S and I as functions of t, we could divide the two equations of the model to give

$$\frac{I'}{S'} = \frac{dI}{dS} = \frac{\left(\beta S - \alpha\right) I}{-\beta S I} = -1 + \frac{\alpha}{\beta S}$$

and integrate to find the orbits (curves in the S-I plane, or phase plane),

$$I = -S + \frac{\alpha}{\beta} \log S + c \tag{2.2}$$

with c an arbitrary constant of integration and log denoting the natural logarithm. Another way to describe the orbits is to define the function

$$V(S, I) = S + I - \frac{\alpha}{\beta} \log S$$

and to note that each orbit is a curve given implicitly by the equation $V(S, I) = c$ for some choice of the constant c. The constant c is determined by the initial values S_0, I_0 of S and I respectively because $c = V(S_0, I_0) = S_0 + I_0 - \frac{\alpha}{\beta} \log S_0$. We think of a population of size K into which a small number of infectives is introduced, so that $S_0 \approx K$, $I_0 \approx 0$ and $R_0 = \beta K/\alpha$. We know that $\lim_{t\to\infty} I(t) = 0$, and we let $S_\infty = \lim_{t\to\infty} S(t)$. Then the relation $V(S_0, I_0) = V(S_\infty, 0)$ gives

$$K - \frac{\alpha}{\beta} \log S_0 = S_\infty - \frac{\alpha}{\beta} \log S_\infty$$

from which we obtain an expression for β/α in terms of the measurable quantities S_0 and S_∞, namely

$$\beta/\alpha = \frac{\log \dfrac{S_0}{S_\infty}}{K - S_\infty} \tag{2.3}$$

It is generally difficult to estimate the contact rate β which depends on the particular disease being studied but may also depend on social and behavioural factors. The quantities S_0 and S_∞ may be determined by serologic studies (measurements of immune responses in blood samples) before and after an epidemic, and from this data the basic reproductive number R_0 may be determined.

The maximum number of infectives at any time is the number of infectives when $S = \alpha/\beta$, given by

$$I_{max} = S_0 + I_0 - \frac{\alpha}{\beta} \log S_0 - \frac{\alpha}{\beta} + \frac{\alpha}{\beta} \log \frac{\alpha}{\beta} \tag{2.4}$$

obtained by substituting $S = \frac{\alpha}{\beta}$, $I = I_{max}$ into (2.2).

EXAMPLE 1. A study of Yale University freshmen [10] reported in [14] reported an influenza epidemic with $S_0 = 0.911$, $S_\infty = 0.513$. Here we are measuring the number of susceptibles as a fraction of the total population size, or using the population size K as the unit of size. Substitution into (2.3) gives the estimate $\beta/\alpha = 1.44$ and $R_0 = 1.44$. Since we know that τ is approximately 3 days for influenza, we see that the contact rate β is approximately 0.48 contacts per day per member of the population.

EXAMPLE 2 (The Great Plague in Eyam). The village of Eyam near Sheffield, England suffered an outbreak of bubonic plague in 1665–1666, whose source is generally believed to be the Great Plague of London, survived by only 83 of an initial population of 350 persons. As detailed records were preserved and as the community was persuaded to quarantine itself to try to prevent the spread of disease to other communities, the disease in Eyam has been used as a case study for modelling [21]. Detailed examination of the data indicates that there were actually two outbreaks of which the first was relatively mild. Thus we shall try to fit the model (2.1) over the period from mid-May to mid-October 1666, measuring time in months with an initial population of 7 infectives and 254 susceptibles, and a final population of 83. The relation (2.3) with $S_0 = 254$, $I_0 = 7$, $S_\infty = 83$ gives $\beta/\alpha = 6.54 \times 10^{-3}$, $\alpha/\beta = 153$. The infective period was 11 days, or 0.3667 months, so that $\alpha = 2.73$ Then $\beta = 0.0178$. The relation (2.4) gives an estimate of 30.4 for the maximum number of infectives.

We use the values obtained here for the parameters β and τ in the model (2.1) for simulations of both the phase (S-I) plane and for graphs of S and I as functions of t.

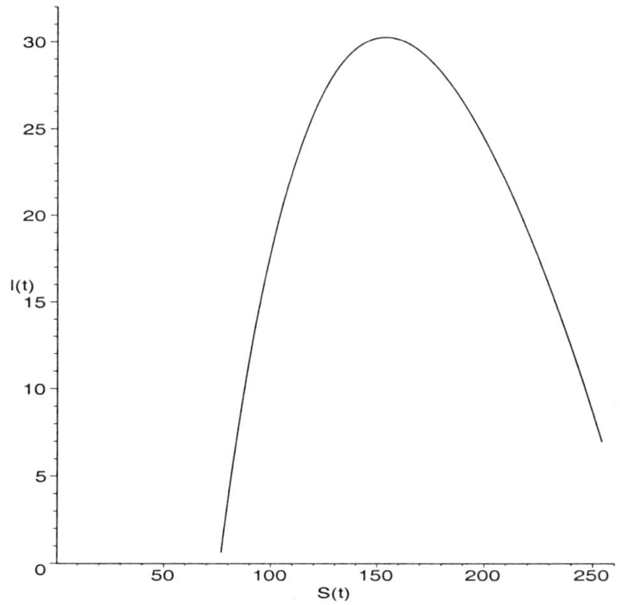

FIG. 1. *The S-I plane.*

The actual data for the Eyam epidemic is remarkably close to the predictions of this very simple model. However, the model is really too good to be true. Our model assumes that infection is transmitted directly between people. While this is possible, bubonic plague is transmitted mainly by rat fleas. When an infected rat is bitten by a flea, the flea becomes extremely hungry and bites the host rat repeatedly, spreading the infection in the rat. When the host rat dies, its fleas move on to other rats, spreading the disease further. As the number of available rats decreases, the fleas move to human hosts, and this is how the plague starts in a human population (although the second phase of the epidemic may have been the pneumonic form of bubonic plague, which can be spread from person to person) . One

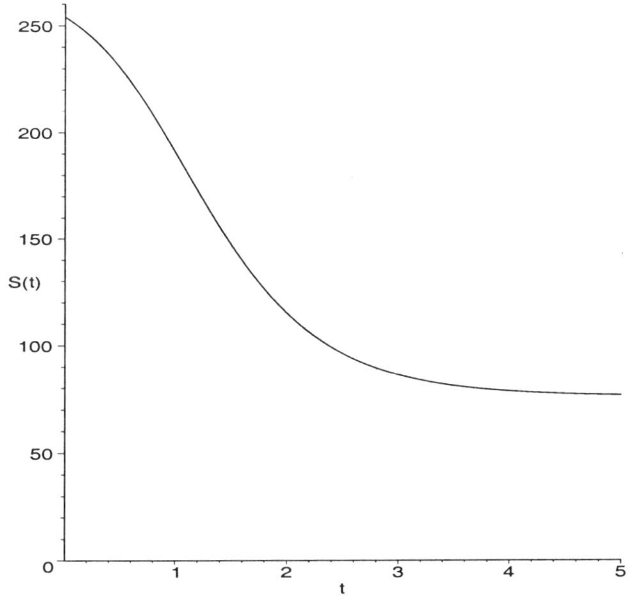

FIG. 2. *S as a function of t.*

of the main reasons for the spread of plague from Asia into Europe was the passage of many trading ships; in mediaeval times ships were invariably infested with rats. An accurate model of plague transmission would have to include flea and rat populations, as well as movement in space. Such a model would be extremely complicated and its predictions might well not be any closer to observations than our simple unrealistic model. In the village of Eyam, the rector persuaded the entire community to quarantine itself to prevent the spread of disease to other communities. One effect of this policy was to increase the infection rate in the village by keeping fleas, rats, and people in close contact with one another, and the mortality rate from bubonic plague was much higher in Eyam than in London. Further, the quarantine could do nothing to prevent the travel of rats and thus did little to prevent the spread of disease to other communities. One message this suggests to mathematical modellers is that control strategies based on false models may be harmful, and it is essential to distinguish between simplifying assumptions which do not alter the predicted effects substantially and wrong assumptions.

In order to prevent the occurrence of an epidemic if infectives are introduced into a population it is necessary to reduce the basic reproductive number R_0 below 1. This may sometimes be achieved by immunization, which has the effect of transferring members of the population from the

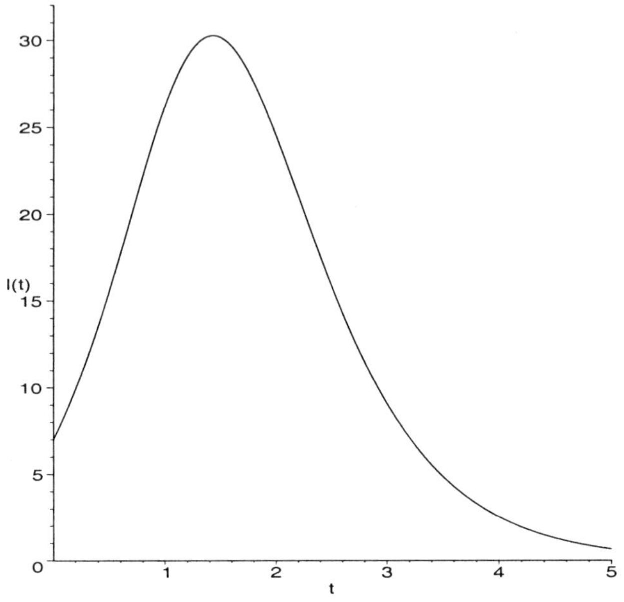

FIG. 3. *I as a function of t.*

susceptible class to the removed class and thus of reducing $S(0)$. If a fraction p of the population is successfully immunized, the effect is to replace $S(0)$ by $S(0)(1-p)$, and thus to reduce the basic reproductive number to $\beta S(0)(1-p)/\alpha$. The requirement $\beta S(0)(1-p)/\alpha < 1$ gives $1-p < \dfrac{\alpha}{\beta S(0)}$, or

$$p > 1 - \frac{\alpha}{\beta S(0)} = 1 - \frac{1}{R_0} \, .$$

A large basic reproductive number means that the fraction which must be immunized to prevent the spread of infection is large. This relation is connected to the idea of herd immunity which we shall introduce in Section 4.

3. A model for diseases with no immunity. The model in the preceding section is an example of a model in which the population is divided into different compartments and the transitions between compartments are modelled. It is described as an S-I-R model because the transitions are from susceptible to infective to removed, with the removal coming through recovery with full immunity (as in measles) or through death from the disease (as in plague, rabies and many other animal diseases). Another type of model is an S-I-S model, in which infectives return to the susceptible class on recovery because the disease confers no immunity against re-infection. Such models are appropriate for most diseases transmitted by bacterial or helminth agents, and most sexually transmitted diseases (including gonorrhea, but not such diseases as AIDS from which there is no recovery).

The simplest S-I-S model, due to Kermack & McKendrick [17], is

$$\begin{aligned} S' &= -\beta SI + \gamma I \\ I' &= \beta SI - \gamma I \,. \end{aligned} \tag{3.1}$$

This differs from the S-I-R model only in that the recovered members return to the class S at a rate γI instead of passing to the class R. The total population $S+I$ is a constant, since $(S+I)' = 0$. We call this constant K; sometimes population size is measured using K as the unit so that the total population size is 1. We may reduce the model to a single differential equation by replacing S by $K - I$, to give the single differential equation

$$I' = \beta I(K-I) - \gamma I = (\beta K - \gamma)I - \beta I^2 = (\beta K - \gamma)I\left(1 - \frac{I}{K - \frac{\gamma}{\beta}}\right). \tag{3.2}$$

In order to study this model, we make a digression about the logistic differential equation which is of considerable importance in population biology.

The logistic differential equation. The differential equation

$$y' = ry\left(1 - \frac{y}{L}\right) \tag{3.3}$$

where r and L are positive constants first arose in population biology in 1838 [24, 20]. It is possible to solve the logistic equation analytically either by separation of variables or by recognizing it as an equation of Bernouilli type and using the change of variable $y = 1/z$ to reduce it to a linear differential equation. By either method, one finds that every solution with a non-negative initial value $y(0)$ except the constant solution $y = 0$ is a member of the family

$$y = \frac{L}{1 + ce^{-rt}} \,. \tag{3.4}$$

The member of this family with a given initial value $y(0)$ is determined by the relation $y(0) = \dfrac{L}{1+c}$, or $c = \dfrac{L - y_0}{y_0}$, provided $y_0 \neq 0$. This is valid whether the constants r and L are positive or negative, but if $r < 0$, $L > 0$ or $r > 0$, $L < 0$ there are solutions with non-negative initial values which are unbounded and fail to exist for all t. The basic qualitative result that we wish to use is the following:

> If $r > 0$, $L > 0$, every solution of the logistic differential equation (3.2) is bounded for all t and every solution except the constant solution $y = 0$ approaches the limit L as

$t \to \infty$. If $r < 0$, $L < 0$, every solution is bounded for all t and every solution except the constant solution $y = L$ $(c = 0)$ approaches the limit 0 as $t \to \infty$.

As an introduction to one of the main approaches to qualitative analysis of differential equations, we now describe another way to obtain this information about limits of solutions of the logistic differential equation which does not make use of the explicit representation (3.4) of the solutions. This method will be of great value in obtaining information about the behaviour of solutions of a differential equation which we are unable to solve in closed form. We will present it in a form which is also suitable for systems of differential equations, although there is a simpler geometric approach which may be used for first order differential equations. The method is restricted to differential equations which do not depend explicitly on the independent variable; such differential equations are said to be *autonomous*.

The first step is to determine the constant solutions, or equilibria, of the differential equation. A constant function $y = a$ is a solution if and only if it makes the right side of the differential equation equal to zero; thus the constant solutions of (3.3) are $y = 0$ and $y = L$. The next step is to approximate the differential equation near an equilibrium by a linear differential equation. This is done by finding the linear approximation to the right side of the differential equation near the equilibrium and replacing the right side of the differential equation by this linear approximation. In general, the linear approximation to a function $f(y)$ near $y = y_0$ is $f(y_0) + f'(y_0)(y - y_0)$. Thus, near $y = 0$, the linear approximation to $ry(1 - \frac{y}{L})$ is ry, and near $y = L$, the linear approximation to $ry(1 - \frac{y}{L})$ is $-r(y - L)$. The linear approximation to the logistic differential equation near $y = 0$ is $y' = ry$ and the linear approximation to the logistic differential equation near $y = L$ is $y' = -r(y - L)$.

The basic theorem which we shall cite without proof (a proof may be found in any text which describes the qualitative study of differential equations; our favourite example is [5, Section 4.4]) is that if all solutions of the linear approximation to an autonomous differential equation near an equilibrium approach the equilibrium, then all solutions of the differential equation with initial value sufficiently close to the equilibrium also approach the equilibrium. As the linear approximation to an autonomous differential equation or system of differential equations is a system with constant coefficients which may be solved in closed form, this criterion may be verified in practice.

It is easy to apply this result to the logistic differential equation. We observe that since the solutions of $y' = ry$ form the family of functions $y = ce^{rt}$ solutions starting near 0 move away from 0 if $r > 0$ and approach 0 if $r < 0$. Since the solutions of $y' = -r(y - L)$ form the family of functions $y = L + ce^{-rt}$ solutions starting near L approach L if $r < 0$ and move away from L if $r > 0$. In fact, it is not difficult to show that the result is global, that is, that it holds for all solutions and not only for solutions starting sufficiently close to the equilibrium.

We now return to the infectious disease model (3.2). As it is a logistic differential equation with $r = \beta K - \gamma$ and $L = K - \frac{\gamma}{\beta}$, our qualitative result tells us that if $\beta K - \gamma < 0$, or $\frac{\beta K}{\gamma} < 1$, then all solutions of the model (3.2) with non-negative initial values except the constant solution $I = K - \frac{\beta}{\gamma}$ approach the limit 0 as $t \to \infty$, while if $\frac{\beta K}{\gamma} > 1$, then all solutions with non-negative initial values except the constant solution $I = 0$ approach the limit $K - \frac{\gamma}{\beta} > 0$ as $t \to \infty$. Thus there is always a single limiting value for I but the value of the quantity $\frac{\beta K}{\gamma}$ determines which limiting value is approached regardless of the initial state of the disease. In epidemiological terms, this says that if the quantity $\frac{\beta K}{\gamma}$ is less than 1 the infection dies out in the sense that the number of infectives approaches zero. For this reason, the equilibrium $I = 0$, which corresponds to $S = K$ is called the disease-free equilibrium. On the other hand, if the quantity $\frac{\beta K}{\gamma}$ exceeds 1, the infection persists. The equilibrium $I = K - \frac{\gamma}{\beta}$, which corresponds to $S = \frac{\gamma}{\beta}$, is called an *endemic* equilibrium.

The dimensionless quantity $\frac{\beta K}{\gamma}$ is called the basic reproductive number or contact number for the disease, and it is usually denoted by R_0. In studying an infectious disease, the determination of the basic reproductive number is invariably a vital first step. The value 1 for the basic reproductive number defines a threshold at which the course of the infection changes between disappearance and persistence. Since βK is the number of contacts made by an average infective in unit time and $1/\gamma$ is the mean infective period, R_0 represents the average number of secondary infections caused by each infective over the course of the infection. Thus it is intuitively clear that if $R_0 < 1$ the infection should die out while if $R_0 > 1$ the infection should establish itself. In more highly structured models than the simple one we have developed here the calculation of the basic reproductive number may be much more complicated but the essential concept of the basic reproductive number as the number of secondary infections caused by an average infective over the course of the disease remains.

We were able to reduce the system of two differential equations (3.1) to the single equation (3.2) because of the assumption that the total population $S + I$ is constant. If there are deaths due to the disease, this assumption is violated, and it would be necessary to use a two-dimensional system as a model. We shall consider this in a more general context in the next section.

4. Models with demographic effects. Measles is a disease for which endemic equilibria have been observed in many places, frequently with sustained oscillations about the equilibrium. As recovery from measles provides immunity against re-infection, the S-I-S model of the preceding section is inappropriate. The epidemic model of Section 2 assumes that the epidemic time scale is so short relative to the demographic time scale that demographic effects may be ignored. For measles, however, the reason for the endemic nature of the disease is that there is a flow of new susceptible members into the population, and in order to try to model this we must include births and deaths in the model. The simplest way to incorporate births and deaths in an infectious disease model is to assume a constant number of births and an equal number of deaths in unit time so that the total population size remains constant. This is, of course, feasible only if there are no deaths due to the disease. In developed countries there are few deaths from measles and such an assumption is plausible. In less-developed countries there is often a very high mortality rate for measles and other assumptions are necessary. The first attempt to formulate an S-I-R model with births and deaths to describe measles was given by H.E. Soper [23], who assumed a constant birth rate μK in the susceptible class and a constant death rate μK in the removed class.

$$\begin{aligned} S' &= -\beta SI + \mu K \\ I' &= \beta SI - \gamma I \\ R' &= \gamma I - \mu K \end{aligned}$$

This model is unsatisfactory biologically because the linkage of births of susceptibles to deaths of removed members is unreasonable. It is also an improper model mathematically because if $R(0)$ and $I(0)$ are sufficiently small, then $R(t)$ will become negative. For any disease model to be plausible, it is essential that the problem be properly posed in the sense that the number of members in each class must remain non-negative. A model which does not satisfy this requirement can not be a proper description of a disease model and therefore must contain some assumption which is biologically unreasonable. A full analysis of a model should include the verification of this property.

A model of Kermack and McKendrick [17] includes births in the susceptible class proportional to total population size and a death rate in each class proportional to the number of members in the class. This model allows the total population size to grow exponentially or die out exponentially if the birth and death rates are unequal. It is applicable to questions of whether a disease may control the size of a population which would otherwise grow exponentially. We shall return to this topic, which is important in the study of many diseases in less-developed countries with high birth rates. For the moment we shall follow the approach suggested by H.W. Hethcote [12], in which the total population size is held constant by making birth and death rates equal. Such a model is

$$\begin{aligned} S' &= -\beta SI + \mu(K - S) \\ I' &= \beta SI - \gamma I - \mu I \\ R' &= \gamma I - \mu R \,. \end{aligned}$$

Because $S + I + R = K$, we can eliminate R and consider the two-dimensional system

$$\begin{aligned} S' &= -\beta SI + \mu(K - S) \\ I' &= \beta SI - \gamma I - \mu I \,. \end{aligned}$$

We shall examine a slightly more general S-I-R model with births and deaths for a disease which may be fatal to some infectives. For such a disease the class R of removed members should contain only recovered members, not members removed by death from the disease. It is not possible to assume that the total population size remains constant if there are deaths due to disease and a plausible model for a disease which may be fatal to some infectives must allow the total population to vary in time. The simplest assumption to allow this is a constant birth rate. Let us analyze the model

$$\begin{aligned} S' &= \mu K - \beta SI - \mu S \\ I' &= \beta SI - \mu I - \alpha I - \gamma I \\ R' &= \gamma I - \mu R \end{aligned} \tag{4.1}$$

with a constant number of births μK in unit time, a proportional death rate μ in each class, and with a fraction α of infectives dying from infection and a fraction γ of infectives recovering with immunity against re-infection. In this model, if $\alpha > 0$ the total population size is not constant and K represents a carrying capacity, or maximum possible population size, rather than the population size. Just as in the case $\alpha = 0$ we may drop the third equation but the reasoning is somewhat different. We view the first two equations as determining S and I, and then consider the third equation as determining R once S and I are known. This is possible because R does not enter into the first two equations.

We shall analyze the model (4.1) qualitatively and then make some inferences, or predictions which follow from the model, about herd immunity, mean age at infection, and inter-epidemic period. These inferences may be of value in testing the model or in estimating parameters. Our approach will be analogous to the method used in the previous section to study the

S-I-S model. This method involved identifying equilibria (constant solutions) and then determining the asymptotic stability of each equilibrium (i.e., learning whether every solution with initial value close to an equilibrium approaches that equilibrium as $t \to \infty$). To find equilibria, we set the right side of each of the two equations equal to zero. The second of the resulting algebraic equations factors, and gives two alternatives. The first alternative is $I = 0$, which will give a disease-free equilibrium, and the second alternative is $\beta S = \mu + \gamma + \alpha$, which will give an endemic equilibrium, provided $\beta S = \mu + \gamma + \alpha < \beta K$. If $I = 0$, the other equation gives $S = K$. For the endemic equilibrium, the first equation gives

$$I = \frac{\mu K}{\mu + \gamma + \alpha} - \frac{\mu}{\beta} . \tag{4.2}$$

To linearize about an equilibrium (S_∞, I_∞), we let $y = S - S_\infty$, $z = I - I_\infty$ and write the system in terms of the new variables y and z. Because (S_∞, I_∞) is an equilibrium, the constant terms will cancel. We discard the quadratic terms and retain only the linear terms, obtaining a system of two linear differential equations

$$\begin{aligned} y' &= -(\beta I_\infty + \mu) y - \beta S_\infty z \\ z' &= \beta I_\infty y + (\beta S_\infty - \mu - \gamma - \alpha) z . \end{aligned}$$

This linear system has coefficient matrix

$$\begin{bmatrix} -\beta I_\infty - \mu & -\beta S_\infty \\ \beta I_\infty & \beta S_\infty - \mu - \gamma - \alpha \end{bmatrix} .$$

We then look for solutions whose components are constant multiples of $e^{\lambda t}$; this means that λ must be an eigenvalue of the coefficient matrix. The condition that all solutions of the linearization at an equilibrium tend to zero as $t \to \infty$ is that all eigenvalues of this coefficient matrix have negative real part. At the disease-free equilibrium the matrix is

$$\begin{bmatrix} -\mu & -\beta K \\ 0 & \beta K - \mu - \gamma - \alpha \end{bmatrix}$$

which has eigenvalues $-\mu$ and $\beta K - \mu - \gamma - \alpha$. Thus the disease-free equilibrium is asymptotically stable if $\beta K < \mu + \gamma + \alpha$ and unstable if $\beta K > \mu + \gamma + \alpha$. Note that this condition for instability of the disease-free equilibrium is the same as the condition for the existence of an endemic equilibrium.

In general, the condition that the eigenvalues of a 2×2 matrix have negative real part is that the determinant must be positive and the trace (the sum of the diagonal elements) must be negative. Since $\beta S_\infty = \mu + \gamma + \alpha$

at an endemic equilibrium, the matrix of the linearization at an endemic equilibrium is

$$\begin{bmatrix} -\beta I_\infty - \mu & -\beta S_\infty \\ \beta I_\infty & 0 \end{bmatrix} \tag{4.3}$$

and this matrix has positive determinant and negative trace. Thus the endemic equilibrium, if there is one, is always asymptotically stable. If the quantity

$$R_0 = \frac{\beta K}{\mu + \gamma + \alpha} = \frac{K}{S_\infty} \tag{4.4}$$

is less than one, the system has only the disease-free equilibrium and this equilibrium is asymptotically stable. In fact, it is not difficult to prove that this asymptotic stability is *global*, that is, that every solution approaches the disease-free equilibrium. If the quantity R_0 is greater than one, then the disease-free equilibrium is unstable but there is an endemic equilibrium which is asymptotically stable. The quantity R_0 is called the basic reproductive number. It depends on the particular disease (determining the parameters γ and α) and on the rate of contacts, which may depend on the population density in the community being studied. The disease model exhibits a *threshold behaviour*: If the basic reproductive number is less than one the disease will die out but if the basic reproductive number is greater than one the disease will be endemic. Our first model, in Section 2, also exhibited a threshold behaviour but of a slightly different kind. For this model, which was an S-I-R model without births or natural deaths, the threshold distinguished between dying out of the disease and an epidemic, or short-term spread of disease.

The S-I-R model with births and deaths and the S-I-S model both support endemic equilibria. This suggests that a requirement for an endemic equilibrium is a flow of new susceptibles, either through births or through recovery without immunity against re-infection.

If we add the three equations of the model we obtain

$$N' = \mu K - \mu N - \alpha I\ .$$

From this we see that at the endemic equilibrium, $N = K - \dfrac{\alpha}{\mu} I$, and the reduction in the population size from the carrying capacity K is

$$\frac{\alpha}{\mu} I = \frac{\alpha K}{\mu + \gamma + \alpha} - \frac{\alpha}{\beta}\ .$$

The parameter α in the S-I-R model may be considered as describing the pathogenicity of the disease. If α is large, it is more difficult to achieve $R_0 >$ 1. If α is small, then the total population size at the endemic equilibrium is close to the carrying capacity K of the population. Thus the maximum population decrease caused by disease will be for diseases of intermediate pathogeneity.

We now make some predictions implied by this model about some qualitative aspects of the spread of a disease.

Herd immunity. In order to prevent a disease from becoming endemic it is necessary to reduce the basic reproductive number R_0 below 1. This may sometimes be achieved by immunization. If a fraction p of the μK newborn members in unit time of the population is successfully immunized, the effect is to replace K by $K(1-p)$, and thus to reduce the basic reproductive number to $R_0(1-p)$. The requirement $R_0(1-p) < 1$ gives $1 - p < \frac{1}{R_0}$, or

$$p > 1 - \frac{1}{R_0} .$$

A population is said to have *herd immunity* if a large enough fraction has been immunized to assure that the disease can not become endemic. The only disease for which this has actually been achieved worldwide is smallpox for which R_0 is approximately 5 so that 80 % immunization will provide herd immunity.

For measles, epidemiological data in the United States indicates that R_0 for rural populations ranges from 5.4 to 6.3, requiring vaccination of 81.5 % to 84.1 % of the population. In urban areas R_0 ranges from 8.3 to 13.0, requiring vaccination of 88.0 % to 92.3 % of the population. In Great Britain, R_0 ranges from 12.5 to 16.3, requiring vaccination of 92 % to 94 % of the population. The measles vaccine is not always effective and vaccination campaigns are never able to reach everyone. As a result, herd immunity against measles has not been achieved (and probably can never be achieved). Since smallpox is viewed as more serious and requires a lower percentage of the population to be immunized, herd immunity is attainable for smallpox. In fact, smallpox has been eliminated; the last known case was in Somalia in 1977, and the virus is maintained now only in laboratories. The eradication of smallpox was actually more difficult than expected because high vaccination rates were achieved in some countries but not everywhere, and the disease persisted in some countries. It was possible to eradicate smallpox only after an intensive campaign for vaccination worldwide [13].

Age at infection. In order to calculate the basic reproductive number R_0 for a disease, we need to know the values of the parameters β, μ, γ, and α. The parameters μ, γ, and α can usually be measured experimentally but the contact rate β is difficult to determine directly. There is an indirect means of estimating R_0 in terms of the life expectancy and the mean age at infection [8].

Consider the "age cohort" of members of a population born at some time t_0 and let a be the age of members of this cohort. If $y(a)$ represents the fraction of members of the cohort who survive to age (at least) a, then the assumption that a fraction μ of the population dies in unit time means that $y'(a) = -\mu y(a)$. Since $y(0) = 1$, we may solve this first order initial value problem to obtain $y(a) = e^{-\mu a}$. The fraction dying at (exactly) age a is $-y'(a) = \mu y(a)$. The mean life span is the average age at death, which is $\int_0^\infty a[-y'(a)]\, da$, and if we integrate by parts we find that this life expectancy is

$$\int_0^\infty a[-y'(a)]\, da = \Big[-ay(a)\Big]_0^\infty + \int_0^\infty y(a)\, da = \int_0^\infty y(a)\, da$$

and since $y(a) = e^{-\mu a}$, this reduces to $\frac{1}{\mu}$. The life expectancy is often denoted by L, so that we may write

$$L = \frac{1}{\mu}\ .$$

The rate at which surviving susceptible members of the population become infected at age a, time $t_0 + a$, is $\beta I(t_0 + a)$. Thus if $z(a)$ is the fraction of the age cohort alive and still susceptible at age a, $z'(a) = -[\mu + \beta \mathrm{I}(t_0)]\ z(a)$. Solution of this first linear order differential equation gives

$$z(a) = e^{-[\mu a + \int_0^a \beta I(t_0+b)db]} = y(a)e^{-\int_0^a \beta I(t_0+b)db}$$

The mean length of time in the susceptible class for members who may become infected, as opposed to dying while still susceptible, is

$$\int_0^\infty e^{-\int_0^a \beta I(t_0+b)db}\, da$$

and this is the mean age at which members become infected. If the system is at an equilibrium I_∞, this integral may be evaluated, and the mean age at infection, denoted by A, is given by

$$A = \int_0^\infty e^{-\beta I_\infty a}\, da = \frac{1}{\beta I_\infty}\ .$$

For our model we have found the endemic equilibrium

$$I_\infty = \frac{\mu K}{\mu + \gamma + \alpha} - \frac{\mu}{\beta}$$

and this implies

$$\frac{L}{A} = \frac{\beta I_\infty}{\mu} = R_0 - 1\ .$$

This relation is very useful in estimating basic reproductive numbers. For example, in some urban communities in England and Wales between 1956 and 1969 the average age of contracting measles was 4.8 years. If life expectancy is assumed to be 70 years, this indicates $R_0 = 15.6$.

The relation between age at infection and basic reproductive number indicates that measures such as inoculations which reduce R_0 will increase the average age at infection. For diseases such as rubella (German measles) whose effects may be much more serious in adults than in children, this indicates a danger which must be taken into account. While inoculation of children will decrease the number of cases of illness, it will tend to increase the danger to those who are not inoculated or for whom the inoculation is not successful. Nevertheless, the number of older cases of infection will be reduced although the fraction of cases which are in older people will increase.

The inter-epidemic period. Many common childhood diseases, such as measles, whooping cough, chicken-pox, diptheria, and rubella exhibit variations from year to year in the number of cases. These fluctuations are frequently regular oscillations, suggesting that the solutions of a model might be periodic. This does not agree with the predictions of the model we have been using in this section, but would not be inconsistent with solutions of the characteristic equation which are complex conjugate with small negative real part, corresponding to lightly damped oscillations approaching the endemic equilibrium. Such behaviour would look like recurring epidemics. If the eigenvalues of the matrix of the linearization at an endemic equilibrium are $-u \pm iv$, where $i^2 = -1$, then the solutions of the linearization are of the form $Be^{-ut}\cos(vt+c)$, with decreasing "amplitude" Be^{-ut} and "period" $\frac{2\pi}{v}$.

For the model (4.1) we recall from (4.2) that at the endemic equilibrium we have

$$\beta I_\infty + \mu = \mu R_0, \beta S_\infty = \mu + \gamma + \alpha$$

and from (4.3) the matrix of the linearization is

$$\begin{bmatrix} -\mu R_0 & -(\mu+\gamma+\alpha) \\ \mu(R_0 - 1) & 0 \end{bmatrix}.$$

The eigenvalues are the roots of the quadratic equation

$$\lambda^2 + \mu R_0 \lambda + \mu(R_0 - 1)(\mu+\gamma+\alpha) = 0$$

which are

$$\lambda = \frac{-\mu R_0 \pm \sqrt{\mu^2 R_0^2 - 4\mu(R_0 - 1)(\mu+\gamma+\alpha)}}{2}.$$

If the mean infective period $\frac{1}{\gamma+\alpha}$ is much shorter than the mean life span $\frac{1}{\mu}$, we may neglect the terms which are quadratic in μ. Thus the eigenvalues are approximately

$$\frac{-\mu R_0 \pm \sqrt{-4\mu(R_0-1)(\gamma+\alpha)}}{2}$$

and these are complex with imaginary part $\sqrt{\mu(R_0-1)(\gamma+\alpha)}$. This indicates oscillations with period approximately

$$\frac{2\pi}{\sqrt{\mu(R_0-1)(\gamma+\alpha)}} .$$

We use the relation $\mu(R_0-1) = \mu\frac{L}{A}$ and the mean infective period $\tau = \frac{1}{\gamma+\alpha}$ to see that the inter-epidemic period T is approximately $2\pi\sqrt{A\tau}$. Thus, for example, for recurring outbreaks of measles with an infective period of 2 weeks or 1/26 years in a population with a life expectancy of 70 years, if R_0 is estimated as 15, we would expect outbreaks spaced 2.76 years apart. Also, as the "amplitude" is $e^{-\mu R_0 t}$, the amplitude is multiplied by a factor $e^{-(15)(2.76)/70} = 0.55$ over each cycle. In fact, many observations of measles outbreaks indicate less damping of the oscillations, suggesting that there may be additional influences which are not included in our simple model. To explain oscillations about the endemic equilibrium, a more complicated model is needed. One possible generalization would be to assume seasonal variations in the contact rate, not an unreasonable supposition for a childhood disease most commonly transmitted through school contacts, especially in winter in cold climates. Note, however, that data from observations are never as smooth as model predictions because models are inevitably gross simplifications of reality and can not account for random variations in the variables. It may be difficult to judge from experimental data whether an oscillation is damped or persistent.

"Epidemic" approach to endemic equilibrium. In the model (4.1), the demographic time scale described by the birth and natural death rates μK and μ and the epidemiological time scale described by the rate $(\alpha+\gamma)$ of departure from the infective class may differ substantially. Think, for example, of a natural death rate $\mu = \frac{1}{75}$, corresponding to a human life expectancy of 75 years, and epidemiological parameters $\alpha = 0$ and $\gamma = 25$, describing a disease from which all infectives recover after a mean infective period of $\frac{1}{25}$ year. Suppose we consider a carrying capacity $K = 1000$, and take $\beta = 0.1$, indicating that an average infective makes (0.1)(1000)= 100 contacts per year. Then $R_0 = 4.00$, and at the endemic equilibrium we have $S_\infty = 250.13$, $I_\infty = 0.40$, $R_\infty = 749.47$. This equilibrium is globally asymptotically stable and is approached from every initial state.

However, if we take $S(0) = 999$, $I(0) = 1$, $R(0) = 0$, simulating the introduction of a single infective into a susceptible population and solve the system numerically, we find that the number of infectives rises sharply to a maximum of 400 and then decreases to almost zero in a period of 0.4 years, or about 5 months. In this time interval, the susceptible population decreases to 22 and then begins to increase, while the removed (recovered and immune against re-infection) population increases to almost 1000 and then begins a gradual decrease. The size of this initial "epidemic" could not have been predicted from our qualitative analysis of the system (4.1). On the other hand, since μ is so small compared to the other parameters of the model, we might consider neglecting μ, replacing it by zero in the model. If we do this, the model reduces to the simple Kermack-McKendrick epidemic model (without births and deaths) of Section 2.

If we follow the model (4.1) over a longer time interval, we find that the susceptible population grows to 450 after 46 years, and then drops to 120 during a small epidemic with a maximum of 18 infectives, and exhibits widely spaced epidemics decreasing in size. It takes a very long time before the system remains close to the endemic equilibrium. The large initial epidemic conforms to what has often been observed in practice when an infection is introduced into a population with no immunity, such as the smallpox inflicted on the Aztecs by the invasion of Cortez.

If we use the model (4.1) with the same values of β, K and μ but take $\alpha = 25$, $\gamma = 0$ to describe a disease which is fatal to all infectives, we obtain very similar results. Now the total population is $S + I$, which decreases from its initial size of 1000 to a minimum of 22 and then gradually increases and eventually approaches its equilibrium size of 250.53. Thus the disease reduces the total population size to one fourth of its original value, suggesting that infectious diseases may have large effects on population size. This is true even for populations which would grow rapidly in the absence of infection, as we shall see in the next section.

The S-I-S model with births and deaths. In order to describe a model for a disease from which infectives recover with immunity against reinfection which includes births and deaths as in the model (4.1), we may modify the model (4.1) by removing the equation for R$'$ and moving the term γI describing the rate of recovery from infection to the equation for S'. This gives the model

$$
\begin{aligned}
S' &= -\beta SI + \mu(K - S) + \gamma I \\
I' &= \beta SI - \alpha I - \mu I - \gamma I
\end{aligned}
\tag{4.5}
$$

describing a population with a constant number of births μK in unit time, a proportional death rate μ in each class, and with a fraction α of infectives dying from infection and a fraction γ of infectives recovering with no immunity against re-infection. In this model, if $\alpha > 0$ the total population size is not constant and K represents a *carrying capacity*, or maximum possible population size, rather than a constant population size. The analysis of the model (4.5) is very similar to that of the S-I-R model (4.1), except that there is no equation for R' to be eliminated.

The only difference is the additional term γI in the equation for S', and this does not change any of the qualitative results. As in the S-I-R model we have a basic reproductive number

$$R_0 = \frac{\beta K}{\mu + \gamma + \alpha} = \frac{K}{S_\infty}$$

and if $R_0 < 1$, the disease-free equilibrium $S = K$, $I = 0$ is asymptotically stable while if $R_0 > 1$ there is an endemic equilibrium (S_∞, I_∞) with $\beta S_\infty = \mu + \gamma + \alpha$ and I_∞ given by (4.2) which is asymptotically stable. There are, however, differences which are not disclosed by the qualitative analysis. If the epidemiological and demographic time scales are very different, for the S-I-R model we observed that the approach to endemic equilibrium is like a rapid and severe epidemic. The same happens in the S-I-S model, especially if there is a significant number of deaths due to disease. If there are few disease deaths, the number of infectives at endemic equilibrium may be substantial, and there may be oscillations of large amplitude about the endemic equilibrium.

For both the S-I-R and S-I-S models, we may write the differential equation for I as

$$I' = I\big[\beta S - (\mu + \alpha + \gamma)\big] = \beta I[S - S_\infty]$$

which implies that whenever S exceeds its endemic equilibrium value, I is increasing and epidemic-like behavior is possible. If $R_0 < 1$ and $S < K$, it follows that $I' < 0$ and thus I is decreasing. Thus if $R_0 < 1$, I can not increase and no epidemic can occur.

5. Diseases as population controls. Many parts of the world experienced very rapid population growth in the 18th century. The population of Europe increased from 118 million in 1700 to 187 million in 1800. In the same time period the population of Great Britain increased from 5.8 million to 9.15 million, and the population of China increased from 150 million to 313 million [19]. The population of English colonies in North America grew much more rapidly, aided by substantial immigration from England, but the native population, which had been decimated by disease following the early encounters with Europeans and European diseases, grew even more rapidly. While some of these population increases may be explained by improvements in agriculture and food production, it appears that an even more important factor was the decrease in the death rate due to diseases. Disease death rates dropped sharply in the 18 th century, partly from better understanding of the links between illness and sanitation and partly because the recurring invasions of bubonic plague subsided, perhaps due to reduced susceptibility. One plausible explanation for these population increases is that the bubonic plague invasions served to control the population size and when this control was removed the population size increased rapidly.

In developing countries it is quite common to have high birth rates and high disease death rates. In fact, when disease death rates are reduced by improvements in health care and sanitation it is common for birth rates to decline as well, as families no longer need to have as many children to assure survival of enough to take care of the older generations. Again, it is plausible to assume that the population size would grow exponentially in the absence of disease but is controlled by disease mortality.

The S-I-R model with births and deaths of Kermack and McKendrick [17] includes births in the susceptible class proportional to population size and a natural death rate in each class proportional to the size of the class. Let us analyze a model of this type with birth rate r and a natural death rate $\mu < r$. For simplicity we assume the disease is fatal to all infectives with disease death rate α, so that there is no removed class and the total population size is $N = S + I$. Our model is

$$\begin{aligned} S' &= r(S+I) - \beta SI - \mu S \\ I' &= \beta SI - (\mu + \alpha)I \ . \end{aligned} \tag{5.1}$$

From the second equation we see that equilibria are given by $I = 0$ or $\beta S = \mu + \alpha$. If $I = 0$, the first equilibrium equation is $rS = \mu S$, which implies $S = 0$ since $r > \mu$. It is easy to see that the equilibrium (0, 0) is unstable. What actually would happen if $I = 0$ is that the susceptible population would grow exponentially with exponent $r - \mu > 0$. If $\beta S = \mu + \alpha$, the first equilibrium condition gives

$$r\frac{\mu+\alpha}{\beta} + rI - (\mu+\alpha)I - \frac{\mu(\mu+\alpha)}{\beta} = 0$$

which leads to

$$(\alpha + \mu - r)I = \frac{(r-\mu)(\mu+\alpha)}{\beta} \ .$$

Thus there is an endemic equilibrium provided $r < \alpha + \mu$, and it is possible to show by linearizing about this equilibrium that it is asymptotically stable (we shall not carry out this verification). On the other hand, if $r > \alpha + \mu$, there is no positive equilibrium value for I. In this case we may add the two differential equations of the model to give

$$N' = (r-\mu)N - \alpha I \geq (r-\mu)N - \alpha N = (r - \mu - \alpha)N$$

and from this we may deduce that N grows exponentially. For this model either we have an asymptotically stable endemic equilibrium or the population size grows exponentially. In the case of exponential population growth we may have either vanishing of the infection or an exponentially growing number of infectives.

If only susceptibles contribute to the birth rate, as may be expected if the disease is sufficiently debilitating, the behaviour of the model is quite different. Let us consider the model

$$\begin{aligned} S' &= rS - \beta SI - \mu S = S(r - \mu - \beta I) \\ I' &= \beta SI - (\mu + \alpha)I = I(\beta S - \mu - \alpha) \end{aligned} \tag{5.2}$$

which has the same form as the celebrated Lotka-Volterra predator-prey model of population dynamics. This system has two equilibria, obtained by setting the right sides of each of the equations equal to zero, namely (0, 0) and an endemic equilibrium $(\frac{\mu + \alpha}{\beta}, \frac{r - \mu}{\beta})$. It turns out that the qualitative analysis approach we have used for systems in the last two sections is not helpful as the equilibrium (0, 0) is unstable and the eigenvalues of the coefficient matrix at the endemic equilibrium are pure imaginary. In this case the behaviour of the linearization does not necessarily carry over to the full system. However, we can obtain information about the behaviour of the system by a method which begins with the elementary approach of separation of variables for first order differential equations. We begin by taking the quotient of the two differential equations and using the relation

$$\frac{I'}{S'} = \frac{dI}{dS}$$

to obtain the separable first order differential equation

$$\frac{dI}{dS} = \frac{I(\beta S - \mu - \alpha)}{S(r - \beta I)} .$$

Separation of variables gives

$$\int (\frac{r}{I} - \beta)\, dI = \int (\beta - \frac{\mu + \alpha}{S})\, dS .$$

Integration gives the relation

$$\beta(S + I) - r \log I - (\mu + \alpha) \log S = c$$

where c is a constant of integration. This relation shows that the quantity

$$V(S, I) = \beta(S + I) - r \log I - (\mu + \alpha) \log S$$

is constant on each orbit (path of a solution in the S-I plane). Each of these orbits is a closed curve, corresponding to a periodic solution.

This model is the same as the epidemic model of Section 2 except for the birth and death terms, and in many examples the time scale of the disease is much faster than the time scale of the demographic process. We may view the model as describing an epidemic initially, leaving a susceptible population small enough that infection can not establish itself. Then there is a steady population growth until the number of susceptibles is large enough for an epidemic to recur. During this growth stage, the infective population is very small and random effects may wipe out the infection, but the immigration of a small number of infectives will eventually restart the process. As a result, we would expect recurrent epidemics. In fact, bubonic plague epidemics did recur in Europe for several hundred years. If we modify the demographic part of the model to assume limited population growth rather than exponential growth in the absence of disease, the effect would be to give behaviour like that of the model studied in the previous section, with an endemic equilibrium which is approached slowly in an oscillatory manner if $R_0 > 1$.

EXAMPLE 3 (Fox rabies). Rabies is a viral infection to which many animals, especially foxes, coyotes, wolves, and rats are highly susceptible. While dogs are only moderately susceptible, they are the main source of rabies in humans. Although deaths of humans from rabies are few, the disease is still of concern because it is invariably fatal. However, the disease is endemic in animals in many parts of the world. A European epidemic of fox rabies thought to have begun in Poland in 1939 which spread through much of Europe has been modelled, and we present here a simplified version of a model due to R.M. Anderson and co-workers [2].

We begin with the demographic assumptions that foxes have a birth rate proportional to population size but that infected foxes do not produce offspring because the disease is highly debilitating, and that there is a natural death rate proportional to population size. Experimental data indicates a birth rate of approximately 1 per capita per year and a death rate of approximately 0.5 per capita per year, corresponding to a life expectancy of 2 years. The fox population is divided into susceptibles and infectives, and the epidemiological assumptions are that the rate of acquisition of infection is proportional to the number of encounters between susceptibles and infectives. We will assume a contact parameter $\beta = 80$, in rough agreement with observations of frequency of contact in regions where the fox density is approximately 1 fox km^2, and we assume that all infected foxes die with a mean infective period of approximately 5 days or $\frac{1}{73}$ years. These assumptions lead to the model

$$\begin{aligned} S' &= -\beta SI + rS - \mu S \\ I' &= \beta SI - (\mu{+}\alpha)I \end{aligned}$$

with $\beta = 80$, r= 1.0, $\mu = 0.5$, $\alpha = 73$. As this is of the form (5.2), we know that the orbits are closed curves in the S-I plane, and that both S and I are periodic functions of t. We illustrate with some simulations obtained using Maple (Figures 4, 5, 6). It should be noted from the graphs of I

in terms of t that the period of the oscillation depends on the amplitude, and thus on the initial conditions, with larger amplitudes corresponding to longer periods.

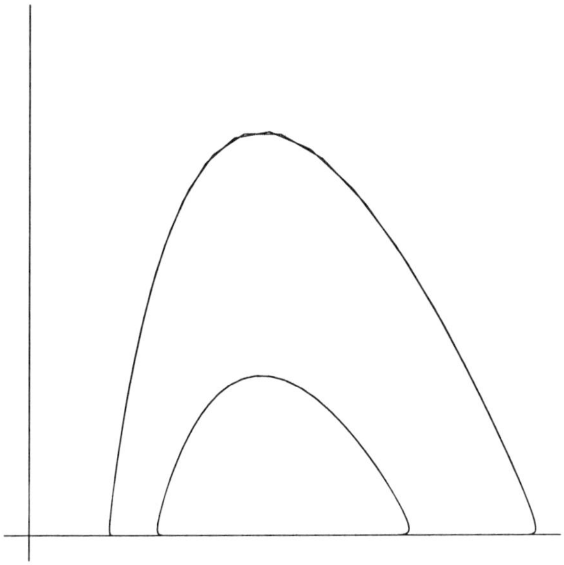

FIG. 4. *The S-I plane.*

Now let us modify the demographic assumptions by assuming that the birth rate decreases as population size increases. We replace the birth rate of r per susceptible per year by a birth rate of re^{-aS} per susceptible per year, with a a positive constant. Then in the absence of infection, the fox population is given by the first order differential equation

$$N' = N(re^{-aN} - \mu)$$

and equilibria of this equation are given by $N = 0$ and $re^{-aN} = \mu$, which reduces to $e^{aN} = \frac{\mu}{r}$, or

$$N = \frac{1}{a}\log\frac{r}{\mu}\ .$$

We shall omit the verification that the equilibrium $N = 0$ is unstable while the positive equilibrium $N = \frac{1}{a}\log\frac{r}{\mu}$ is asymptotically stable. Thus, much as for the logistic population model examined in Section 3, the population has a *carrying capacity* given by

$$K = \frac{1}{a}\log\frac{r}{\mu}$$

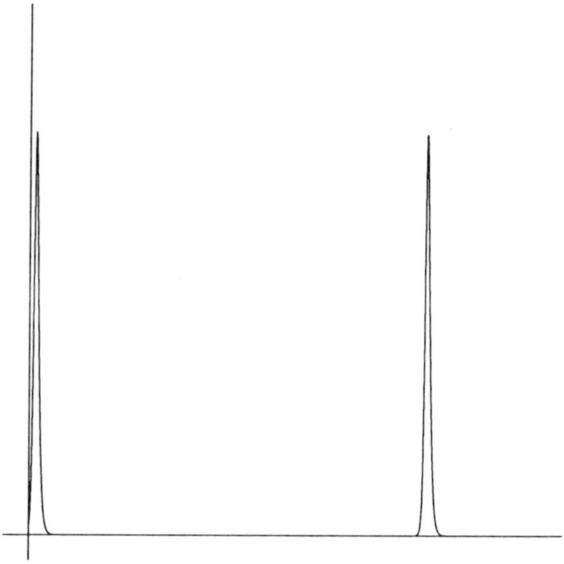

FIG. 5. *I as a function of t (larger amplitude).*

The model now becomes

$$S' = rSe^{-aS} - \beta SI - \mu S$$
$$I' = \beta SI - (\mu+\alpha)I$$

and we examine this by looking for equilibria and analyzing their stability. From the second equation, equilibria satisfy either $I = 0$ or $\beta S = \mu + \alpha$. If $I = 0$, the first equilibrium condition reduces to the same equation that determined the carrying capacity, and we have a disease-free equilibrium $S = K$, $I = 0$. If $\beta S = \mu + \alpha$, there is an endemic equilibrium with $\beta I + \mu = re^{-aS}$. A straightforward computation which we shall not carry out here shows that the disease-free equilibrium is asymptotically stable if $R_0 = \dfrac{\beta K}{\mu + \alpha} < 1$ and unstable if $R_0 > 1$, while the endemic equilibrium, which exists if and only if $R_0 > 1$, is always asymptotically stable. Another way to express the condition for an endemic equilibrium is to say that the fox population density must exceed a threshold level K_T given by

$$K_T = \frac{\mu + \alpha}{\beta} .$$

With the parameter values we have been using, this gives a threshold fox density of 0.92 foxes/km^2. If the fox density is below this threshold value, the fox population will approach its carrying capacity and the disease will

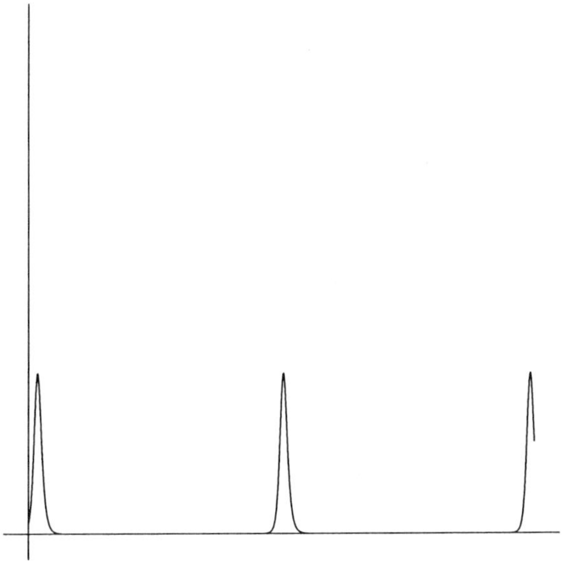

FIG. 6. *I as a function of t (smaller amplitude).*

die out. Above the threshold density, rabies will persist and will regulate the fox population to a level below its carrying capacity. This level may be approached in an oscillatory manner for large R_0.

6. Directions for generalization. We have been examining some general models for infectious diseases, looking for general classes of models rather than descriptions of specific diseases. As a result, the models we have been considering so far have been relatively simple. There are many effects of importance which we have not introduced yet. Detailed descriptions of the dynamics of many diseases may be found in such books as [3]. Here we list a few of the possible generalizations, some of which will be developed in later chapters. Some of the generalizations which we shall develop will make use of more advanced mathematical techniques than those used in this chapter.

1. **Models with more compartments.** One direction for generalization is the inclusion of more compartments in a compartmental model. For example, in most infectious diseases there is an exposed period after the transmission of infection from susceptible to potential infective members but before these potential infectives can re-transmit infection. If the exposed period is short, it is often neglected in modelling, but a longer exposed period could lead to significantly different model predictions. Fox rabies, for example, has an exposed period of about a month, considerably longer than the actual infective period. The inclusion of an exposed period

would mean an additional compartment in the model; thus we may speak of *S-E-I-S* or *S-E-I-R* models. Some diseases, such as malaria, provide a temporary immunity on recovery. This also would mean an additional compartment, giving an *S-I-R-S* model.

2. **Vertical transmission.** In many diseases, it is possible for some offspring of infected parents to be born infective. This effect, called vertical transmission, is significant in many diseases including AIDS, Chagas' disease, hepatitis B, and rinderpest (a cattle disease which may have been the plague of murrain inflicted on Egypt in the time of Moses). Vertical transmission may be incorporated into a model by including a fraction of the new-born members in the infective class. The book [6] describes many aspects of infectious disease models with vertical transmission.

3. **Vector transmission.** Malaria is one of many diseases which are not transmitted directly from human to human but are transmitted through a *vector.* Malaria is acquired by humans by being bitten by infected mosquitoes, and the mosquitoes become infective by biting infected humans. Thus the infection goes back and forth between mosquitoes and humans, and a model for vector transmission must include both species. The two species may have radically different demographic time scales, which may allow some simplification of the model, but in general a model for vector transmission requires twice as many compartments as a model for direct transmission. One of the earliest infectious disease models to be applied practically was the model of Sir R.A. Ross for malaria [22]. We have already described in the introductory section the triumph of mathematical epidemiology represented by Ross's work. Ross's relatively simple model is still the basis for malaria models, although many other factors such as temporary immunity, superinfection, and the development by mosquitoes of immunity against mosquito controls are important in malaria control. A good account of some of the specific features of malaria models may be found in the chapter on the population dynamics of malaria by J.L. Aron & R.M. May [4] in the book [1].

For sexually transmitted diseases which are transmitted by heterosexual contact, it is necessary to use models with separate compartments for males and females. These compartments may be of very different sizes. Gonorrhea has been modelled in this way, and the predictions of the models have been used to good effect for disease control. A good reference for such models is the book [15]. Two-sex models for sexually transmitted diseases have many properties in common with vector transmission models since the transmission of disease goes back and forth between the two groups.

4. **Non-homogeneous mixing.** We have confined ourselves to models in which the mixing of members of the population is homogeneous and the number of contacts per member in unit time is proportional to total population size. It may be more realistic to assume that the number of contacts per member in unit time grows less rapidly as population size increases. An

extreme case, which may be quite realistic for sexually transmitted disease models, would be a constant number of contacts per member in unit time. More generally, it may be appropriate to replace the proportionality constant β in our models by a non-negative, non-increasing function of total population size.

In sexually transmitted disease models, it is important to look closely at mixing patterns, as members may have very different levels of sexual activity and the mixing may include preferences for contacts with members having a specific activity level. A model which attempts to give a precise description of a sexually transmitted disease must incorporate an understanding of the sociological patterns in the population.

5. **Age-structured populations.** Populations are not necessarily homogeneous, and the mixing of members may be represented better if some structure is included in the populations by subdividing the basic compartments.One of the most obvious examples of non-homogeneity is age structure. For example, childhood diseases may be transmitted mainly between members of the population of the same age, and an age-structured population model with contact rates depending on age may be a better description than a simpler model. The classical "childhood" diseases, such as measles, chicken-pox, and rubella (German measles) are spread mainly by contacts between children of similar ages. To incorporate this into a model, one could consider an age-structured population with the rate of contact between members depending on the ages of the members. Such a model would be a system of partial differential equations whose independent variables are time and age, and whose dependent variables are the number of members of each class at a given time of a given age.

6. **Non-exponential distribution of time in compartments.** All the models we have examined so far have been ordinary differential equations or systems of ordinary differential equations. The reason for this is that we have assumed a rate of passage out of a compartment which are proportional to the number of members in the compartment, which is equivalent to assuming an exponential distribution of lengths of stay in the compartment. It may be more plausible to assume a fixed time in the compartment,which would lead to a differential-difference equation model. More generally, an arbitrary specified distribution of time of stay in a compartment, which would lead to a Volterra integral equation model, may be more realistic. In fact, exponential distributions, with a possibility of infinite time of stay, and fixed times, with an assumption of unreasonable precision, are quite implausible in real life. What have become known almost universally as the Kermack-McKendrick models are actually the special cases of the actual Kermack-McKendrick equations with exponentially distributed infective periods. The mathematical machinery available at the time could not cope with the full Kermack-McKendrick models.

7. **Distributions which are spatially non-uniform.** The history of bubonic plague describes the movement of the disease from place to place,

carried by rats. The course of an infection usually can not be modelled accurately without some attention to its spatial spread. To model this would require partial differential equations, possibly leading to descriptions of population waves, analogous to the waves of disease which have often been observed.

8. **Variable infectivity.** One of the important features of HIV/AIDS is that the infectivity of infective members depends on the time since becoming infected, sometimes called the infection age (as opposed to chronological age). Infected members are highly infective for a short period after having become infected and then have relatively low infectivity for a long period (possibly on the order of ten years) before again becoming highly infective shortly before developing full-blown AIDS. This would have to be incorporated into models to describe the spread of the disease.

9. **Macroparasitic infections.** We have been describing diseases caused by microparasites, including viruses and bacteria. The main feature of the models is that members of the population are either infective or not infective, and there is no distinction by level of infection. There are also infections caused by macroparasites, such as parasitic helminths and arthropods, where the number of infection agents in the host makes a difference. Often, the parasites tend to aggregate in a part of the host population. Such infections require different types of models which take account of the distribution of macroparasites in the hosts.

10. **Stochastic models.** Our models have been deterministic, with the progress of the disease determined entirely by the current state and possibly by the past history, but with no allowance for random effects. When population sizes are large, this is a reasonable approximation, but for small population sizes individual differences and random effects are important. Stochastic models are needed to describe such situations.

The idea of a threshold may be important in other disciplines as well. There are many phenomena where the rate at which individuals move from one compartment to another is proportional to the number of individuals who have already made the transition and to the number of individuals who have not yet moved. This is the term in the model equations which produces the threshold phenomenon. It has been suggested that some social problems are contagious in the same sense [7, 11]. Sociologists use the term tipping point for what we are calling the threshold; their models are descriptive rather than mathematical but there is some qualitative evidence to support the idea. The basic assumption is that social problems are spread through peer influence, so that rates of development of such problems as teen-age pregnancy and juvenile crime depend on the reservoir of potential victims and on the number of cases. One inference, if this idea is accepted, would be that if a level of preventive measures can be instituted in some neighbourhood which will reduce the basic reproductive number below 1, then maintenance of this state should be relatively easy. Thus it would make sense to target neighbourhoods which are experiencing such an epidemic or are at high risk.

REFERENCES

[1] R.M. Anderson (ed.), Population Dynamics of Infectious Diseases, Chapman & Hall (London), 1982.

[2] R.M. Anderson, H.C. Jackson, R.M. May, & A.M. Smith, Population dynamics of fox rabies in Europe, Nature (London) 289 (1981), 765–771.

[3] R.M. Anderson & R.M. May, Infectious Diseases of Humans, Oxford Science Publications (Oxford), 1991.

[4] J.L. Aron & R.M. May, The population dynamics of malaria, Population Dynamics of Infectious Diseases (R.M. Anderson, ed.), Chapman & Hall (London), 1982, pp. 139–179.

[5] F. Brauer & J.A. Nohel, The Qualitative Theory of Ordinary Differential Equations; An Introduction, Benjamin (New York), 1969; reprinted by Dover (New York), 1989.

[6] S. Busenberg & K.L. Cooke, Vertically Transmitted Diseases: Models and Dynamics, Biomathematics 23, Springer-Verlag (New York), 1993.

[7] J. Crane, The epidemic theory of ghettos and neighborhood effects on dropping out and teenage childbearing, Am. J. Sociology 96 (1991), 1226–1259.

[8] K. Dietz, Transmission and control of arbovirus diseases, Epidemiology (D. Ludwig and K.L. Cooke, eds.) Society for Industrial & Applied Mathematics, Philadelphia (1975), 104–121.

[9] S. Ellner, R. Gallant, & J. Theiler, Detecting nonlinearity and chaos in epidemic models, Epidemic Models: Their Structure and Relation to Data (D. Mollison, ed.), Cambridge University Press (Cambridge), 1995, pp. 229–247.

[10] A.S. Evans, Viral Infections of Humans, 2nd ed. Plenum Press (New York), 1982.

[11] M. Gladwell, The tipping point, The New Yorker, June 3, 1996, pp. 32–38.

[12] H.W. Hethcote, Qualitative analysis for communicable disease models, Math. Biosciences 28 (1976), 335–356.

[13] ———, An immunization model for a heterogeneous population, Theor. Pop. Biology 14 (1978), 338–349.

[14] ———, Three basic epidemiological models, Applied Mathematical Ecology (S.A. Levin, T.G. Hallan, & L.J. Gross eds.), Biomathematics 18, Springer-Verlag, (Berlin-Heidelberg), 1989, pp. 119–144.

[15] H.W. Hethcote & J.A. Yorke, Gonorrhea Transmission Dynamics and Control, Lecture Notes in Biomathematics 56, Springer-Verlag (Berlin-Heidelberg), 1984.

[16] W.O. Kermack & A.G. McKendrick, A contribution to the mathematical theory of epidemics, Proc. Royal Soc. London 115 (1927), 700–721.

[17] ———, Contributions to the mathematical theory of epidemics, Part II, Proc. Royal Soc. London 138 (1932), 55–83.

[18] W.H. McNeill, Plagues and Peoples, Doubleday (New York), 1976.

[19] ———, The Global Condition, Princeton University Press, (Princeton), 1992.

[20] R. Pearl & L.J. Reed, On the rate of growth of the population of the United States since 1790 and its mathematical representation, Proc. Nat. Acad. Sci. 6 (1920), 275–288.

[21] G.F. Raggett, Modelling the Eyam plague, IMA Journal 18 (1982), 221–226.

[22] R.A. Ross, The Prevention of Malaria, 2nd ed., Murray (London), 1911.

[23] H.E. Soper, Interpretation of periodicity in disease prevalence, J. Royal Statistical Soc. B 92 (1929), 34–73.

[24] P.F. Verhulst, Notice sur la loi que la population suit dans son acroissement, Corr. Math. et Phys. 10 (1838), 113–121.

EXTENSIONS OF THE BASIC MODELS

FRED BRAUER*

1. Exposed periods and temporary immunity. In Section 4 of Chapter I we described two basic elementary models for disease transmission, the S-I-R and S-I-S models with natural births and deaths and possibly deaths due to disease as well. In this chapter, we shall describe a variety of extensions of these basic models, beginning with two models of the same type with additional compartments, which will lead to systems of ordinary differential equations similar to those of Chapter I but of higher dimension.

In many diseases members do not pass directly from the susceptible to the infective class on becoming infected. There may be a latent or exposed stage. For example, in measles there is an incubation period of 11–14 days after infection before symptoms of the disease appear. For fox rabies, the incubation period is 28–30 days. For some diseases the incubation period may be short enough that neglecting it does not affect the model significantly; for example, the incubation period for influenza is 1–3 days.

Another possibility is that there may be a temporary immunity period on recovery from infection, so that there is a transition from the infective class to a removed class and then a later return to the susceptible class. This is true of many types of influenza and also of malaria.

We shall begin by considering the possibility of an exposed period, that is, an interval between the time when a susceptible is infected and the time this individual becomes infective and may pass the disease on to other individuals. To model this, we include an additional compartment in the model by letting $E(t)$ denote the number of members at time t who are exposed but not yet infected and assuming a transition rate ϵ, so that a fraction ϵ of the exposed members pass to the infective class in unit time, corresponding to a mean exposed period of $\frac{1}{\epsilon}$. We shall consider both S-E-I-S models, where infectives recover without immunity against reinfection, and S-E-I-R models, where recovered infectives have full immunity against reinfection.

We begin with the S-E-I-S model. The analogue of the S-I-S model (4.5) of Section 4 of chapter I is

$$\begin{aligned} S' &= \mu K - \beta S I - \mu S + \gamma I \\ E' &= \beta S I - \mu E - \epsilon E \\ I' &= \epsilon E - \mu I - \alpha I - \gamma I \ . \end{aligned} \tag{1.1}$$

*Department of Mathematics, University of British Columbia, Vancouver, B.C., V6T 1Z2, CANADA.

The analysis of this model is similar in principle to that of the S-I-S model but is technically more complicated because the dimension of the system has been raised by 1. An equilibrium is a constant solution (S, E, I) of the system (1.1). Equilibria are obtained by setting the right side of each of the three differential equations equal to zero, giving the algebraic system

$$\begin{aligned} \mu K &= \beta SI + \mu S \\ \beta SI &= \mu E + \epsilon E \\ \epsilon E &= \mu I + \alpha I + \gamma I \ . \end{aligned}$$

From the last of these equations we have

$$\epsilon E = I(\mu + \alpha + \gamma)$$

and substitution of this into the second equation give s

$$\beta SI = \frac{\mu + \epsilon}{\epsilon} \big(\mu + \alpha + \gamma\big) I \ .$$

From this we see that either $I = 0$ (disease-free equilibrium) or

$$\beta S = \frac{\mu + \epsilon}{\epsilon} \big(\mu + \alpha + \gamma\big)$$

(endemic equilibrium). If $I = 0$, it is easy to deduce that $S = K$, $E = 0$. The matrix of the linearization of the system (1.1) at an equilibrium (S, E, I), which is simply the matrix of partial derivatives with respect to the variables S, E, I of the right sides of the three equations in (1.1) is

$$\begin{bmatrix} -\beta I - \mu & 0 & -\beta S + \gamma \\ \beta I & -(\epsilon + \mu) & \beta S \\ 0 & \epsilon & -(\mu + \alpha + \gamma) \end{bmatrix} .$$

At the disease free equilibrium, this is

$$\begin{bmatrix} -\mu & 0 & -\beta K + \gamma \\ 0 & -(\epsilon + \mu) & \beta K \\ 0 & \epsilon & -(\mu + \alpha + \gamma) \end{bmatrix}$$

and because there is only one non-zero element in the first column we may reduce the question of whether the eigenvalues of this matrix have negative real part to the same question for the $2{\times}2$ matrix

$$\begin{bmatrix} -(\epsilon + \mu) & \beta K \\ \epsilon & -(\mu + \alpha + \gamma) \end{bmatrix} .$$

The trace of this matrix is clearly negative, and the condition that the determinant be positive is $(\epsilon + \mu)(\mu + \alpha + \gamma) - \beta K \epsilon > 0$, or

$$R_0 = \frac{\beta K \epsilon}{(\epsilon + \mu)(\mu + \alpha + \gamma)} < 1 \ .$$

Thus, as we would expect, the disease-free equilibrium is asymptotically stable if $R_0 < 1$. It is not difficult to show that this asymptotic stability is global, that is, that if $R_0 < 1$ every solution tends to the disease-free equilibrium regardless of the initial state.

The stability analysis at the endemic equilibrium is more difficult, because the matrix is now 3×3, and the stability condition for a 2×2 matrix that the trace must be negative and the determinant must be positive needs to be replaced by a more complicated condition. In general, the eigenvalues of a matrix A are the roots λ of the *characteristic equation* $\det[\lambda I - A] = 0$, where here I denotes the identity matrix with each diagonal entry 1 and all other entries zero. For an $n \times n$ matrix, this characteristic equation is a polynomial equation of degree n. There is a set of conditions, known as the *Routh-Hurwitz* conditions that all roots of a polynomial equation of degree n have negative real part. A derivation of this result may be found in books on matrix theory, for example [4, p. 194]. For a polynomial of degree 3,

$$\lambda^3 + a_1\lambda^2 + a_2\lambda + a_3 = 0$$

the conditions that all roots have negative real part are that

$$a_1 > 0,\ a_1 a_2 > a_3 > 0\ .$$

At the endemic equilibrium, the element in the second row, third column of the matrix is zero because of the equilibrium conditions. A complicated calculation which we omit gives

$$\begin{aligned}
a_1 &= (\mu + \beta I) + (\mu+\epsilon) + (\mu+\alpha+\gamma)\\
a_2 &= (\mu + \beta I)(\mu+\epsilon)+(\mu+\beta I)(\mu + \alpha + \gamma) + (\mu + \epsilon)(\mu + \alpha + \gamma)\\
a_3 &= (\mu + \beta I)(\mu+\epsilon)(\mu + \alpha + \gamma) + \beta I\epsilon(\mu + \alpha) + \beta I\mu(\mu+\alpha+\gamma)
\end{aligned}$$

and it is possible to verify that the Routh-Hurwitz conditions are satisfied. Thus it follows that the endemic equilibrium of the S-E-I-S model, which exists if $R_0 > 1$, is always asymptotically stable.

The S-E-I-R model is the analogue of the S-I-S model (4.1) of Section 4 of Chapter I, and is

$$\begin{aligned}
S' &= \mu K - \beta SI - \mu S\\
E' &= \beta SI - \mu E - \epsilon E\\
I' &= \epsilon E - \mu I - \alpha I - \gamma I\\
R' &= \gamma I - \mu R\ .
\end{aligned} \tag{1.2}$$

To analyze this model, we begin as in Chapter I by viewing the last equation as determining R once S, E, and I are known and considering the model as a three dimensional system. This system differs from the S-E-I-S system in an additional term γI in the equation for S', and the analysis is essentially the same as for the S-E-I-S model. Again, we find that the disease-free equilibrium is asymptotically stable if

$$R_0 = \frac{\beta K \epsilon}{(\epsilon + \mu)(\mu + \alpha + \gamma)} < 1$$

and the endemic equilibrium exists and is asymptotically stable if $R_0 > 1$.

The analysis of the models in this section is technically more complicated than that of the corresponding models without exposed stages because the dimension has been raised by 1. However, there is no essential change in the results other than the introduction of a factor $\dfrac{\epsilon}{\epsilon + \mu}$ in R_0.

We shall now modify the S-I-R model of Chapter I by allowing a period of temporary immunity on recovery from infection before return to the susceptible class. We let δ be the fraction of recovered members who return to the susceptible class in unit time. Then we obtain the model

$$\begin{aligned} S' &= \mu K - \beta S I - \mu S + \delta R \\ I' &= \beta S I - \mu I - \alpha I - \gamma I \\ R' &= \gamma I - \mu R - \delta R\ . \end{aligned} \tag{1.3}$$

The model (1.3) differs from the S-I-R model (4.1) of Chapter I only in the terms $\pm\delta R$ in the equations for S' and R'. The analysis of this model proceeds in exactly the same way as the analysis of the S-I-R model, and we obtain exactly the same results. The disease-free equilibrium is asymptotically stable if and only if

$$R_0 = \frac{\beta K}{\mu + \alpha + \gamma} < 1$$

and if $R_0 > 1$ there is an endemic equilibrium which is asymptotically stable.

We can construct more elaborate models such as S-E-I-R-S models and analyze them using the same approach. Another possibility, which in fact can exhibit instability of the endemic equilibrium and resulting sustained oscillations, is to examine models with more than one removed (immune) stage and transitions between these stages. Of course, an increase in the number of compartments in a model produces an increase in the dimension of the model and a more complicated analysis problem.

The incorporation of additional compartments carried out in this section is only one of the ways in which we shall extend the basic models of Chapter I. In the next section we shall generalize the rate of contacts between members of the population which was assumed in Chapter I to be proportional to the population size.

2. General contact rates. In Chapter I we assumed that an average infective makes contact sufficient to transmit infection with βN other members of the population in unit time, where N represents total population size. This assumption leads to an infection rate βSI in unit time. This term is sometimes described as *mass-action incidence.* For sexually transmitted diseases, it may be much more plausible to hypothesize that an average infective makes a constant number of contacts λ in unit time, and this would lead to an infection rate $\frac{\lambda SI}{N}$ in unit time, sometimes described as *standard incidence.* More generally, it may be reasonable to assume that the number of contacts made by an average infective in unit time tends to saturate, that is, for the number of contacts to grow less rapidly as population size increases. We shall assume in this section that the number of contacts sufficient to transmit infection in unit time per infective is a function $C(N)$ of the total population size N. Then the number of new infections in unit time is $C(N)SI/N$. It is convenient to define

$$\widehat{C}(N) = \frac{C(N)}{N} .$$

For example, a Michaelis-Menten type of interaction, often used to model handling times, would lead to an expression of the form

$$C(N) = \frac{aN}{1+bN} .$$

Another form based on a mechanistic derivation for pair formation [5] leads to an expression of the form

$$C(N) = \frac{aN}{1+bN+\sqrt{1+2bN}} .$$

Data for diseases transmitted by contact in cities of moderate size [7] suggests that the assumption of a form

$$C(N) = \lambda N^a$$

is fit quite well by data with $a = 0.05$. All of these forms satisfy the conditions

$$C'(N) \geq 0, \qquad \widehat{C}'(N) \leq 0 \tag{2.1}$$

and we shall assume in this section that the average number of contacts per infective in unit time is a function $C(N)$ of total population size is a function $C(N)$ which satisfies (2.1). Since the fraction of contacts which may produce a new infection is S/N, the number of new infectives in unit time is

$$\frac{C(N)SI}{N} = \widehat{C}(N)SI .$$

Thus the term βSI in the models formulated previously is replaced by a term $\widehat{C}(N)SI$. Because N enters the model in this term, it is often convenient to use N as one of the variables in the model. Thus in the S-I-S model we could use I and N as variables and replace S by $N - I$, and in the S-I-R model we could use I, R, and N as variables and replace S by $N - I - R$. The differential equation for N is obtained by adding the differential equations for S and I in the first case and the differential equations for S, I, and R in the second case to give $N' = \mu K - \mu I - \alpha I$.

The *S-I-S* model. The S-I-S model with density-dependent contact rate is

$$\begin{aligned} I' &= C(\widehat{N})I(N - I) - \mu I - \alpha I - \gamma I \\ N' &= \mu K - \mu N - \alpha I \end{aligned} \tag{2.2}$$

and we analyze this in the same way as for the original S-I-S model expressed in terms of S and I. The equilibrium conditions are

$$I[\widehat{C}(N)(N - I) - \mu - \gamma - \alpha] = 0, \qquad \mu K = \mu N + \alpha I$$

and the first of these gives $I = 0$ (disease-free equilibrium) or $\widehat{C}(N)(N - I) = \mu + \gamma + \alpha$ (endemic equilibrium). From the second equilibrium condition we see that at the disease-free equilibrium $N = K$. If $\alpha = 0$, so that there are no deaths due to disease, the second equilibrium condition implies that $N = K$ at each equilibrium. It is convenient to define

$$\beta = \widehat{C}(K)$$

and then if $\alpha = 0$ the endemic equilibrium is given by $\beta(N - I) = \mu + \gamma$, or $\beta I = \beta N - \mu - \gamma$ and $N = K$. If $\alpha > 0$, $N = K - \frac{\mu}{\alpha} < K$ and because of (2.1) $C(\widehat{N}) \geq \beta$. The matrix of the linearization of the system (2.2) at an equilibrium (I, N) is the matrix of partial derivatives with respect to I and N of the right sides of the two equations in (2.2), namely

$$\begin{bmatrix} NC(\widehat{N}) - 2IC(\widehat{N}) - \mu - \gamma - \alpha & I\{(N - I)\widehat{C}'(N) + C(\widehat{N})\} \\ -\alpha & -\mu \end{bmatrix}$$

and at the disease-free equilibrium, since $I = 0$, $N = K$, and $C(\widehat{N}) = \beta$, this reduces to

$$\begin{bmatrix} \beta K - \mu - \gamma - \alpha & 0 \\ -\alpha & -\mu \end{bmatrix}$$

and it is easy to see that the eigenvalues have negative real part if and only if

$$R_0 = \frac{\beta K}{\mu + \gamma + \alpha} < 1 .$$

This result, including the expression for R_0, is exactly the same as for the original S-I-S model of Chapter I. If $R_0 > 1$, there is an endemic equilibrium, and because of the equilibrium conditions, the matrix at this equilibrium is

$$\begin{bmatrix} -IC(\widehat{N}) & I\{(N-I)\widehat{C}'(N) + C(\widehat{N})\} \\ -\alpha & -\mu \end{bmatrix} .$$

It is obvious that the trace of this matrix is negative, and to show that its determinant is positive it would be sufficient to show that $(N-I)\widehat{C}'(N) + C(\widehat{N}) \geq 0$. To see this, we use $C'(N) \geq 0$, $\widehat{C}'(N) \leq 0$ to deduce that

$$(N-I)\widehat{C}'(N) + C(N) \geq N\widehat{C}'(N) + C(N) = [N\widehat{C}(N)]' = C'(N) \geq 0 .$$

Thus the endemic equilibrium, which exists if and only if $R_0 > 1$, is always asymptotically stable. Again, this is exactly the same as for the simple model of Chapter I.

The *S-I-R* model. The S-I-R model with density-dependent contact rate is

$$\begin{aligned} S' &= \mu K - \widehat{C}(N)SI - \mu S \\ I' &= \widehat{C}(N)SI - \mu I - \alpha I - \gamma \\ R' &= \gamma I - \mu R \ . \end{aligned}$$

We use N as a variable in place of R to give the model

$$\begin{aligned} S' &= \mu K - \widehat{C}(N)SI - \mu S \\ I' &= \widehat{C}(N)SI - \mu I - \alpha I - \gamma I \\ N' &= \mu K - \mu N - \alpha I \ . \end{aligned} \tag{2.3}$$

In Chapter I we were able to discard the equation for R and thus reduce the model to two dimensions with S and I as variables. Now we can not make such a reduction; there is no way to choose two differential equations out of the four equations for S, I, R, and N which can be expressed in terms of fewer than three variables. However, the analysis of the three-dimensional system (2.3) can be carried out with the aid of the Routh-Hurwitz conditions as in the models studied in Section 1. We find, as we might have expected, that there is a disease-free equilibrium which is asymptotically stable if and only if

$$R_0 = \frac{\beta K}{\mu + \gamma + \alpha} < 1$$

and if $R_0 > 1$ there is an endemic equilibrium which is asymptotically stable.

Although we have allowed the rate of contact between members of the population to depend on population size, we are still assuming that all members of the population are equivalent and that the mixing is homogeneous. Frequently the population is structured in some way which affects the mixing. For example, childhood diseases are often transmitted between members of the same age, and this may be modelled by including age structure in the population and assuming that mixing is age-dependent. For sexually transmitted diseases, different members of the population may have different numbers of partners and different levels of activity; this may be modelled by including activity levels in the structure of the population. We postpone until later the consideration of such models, but structured models and mixing questions are important factors in many infective diseases.

3. Infective periods of fixed length. Until now we have assumed that all rates of transition out of a compartment (except for the acquisition of infection) are proportional to the number of members in the compartment. This is equivalent,as we have seen in Section 4 of Chapter I, to an exponential distribution of times in the compartment. For example, the assumption that a fraction $(\mu + \gamma + \alpha)$ of members of a population leave the infective class in unit time is equivalent to the assumption that a fraction $e^{-(\mu+\gamma+\alpha)t}$ of the population remains in the infective class until (at least) time t, so that the mean stay in the infective class is $\dfrac{1}{\mu + \gamma + \alpha}$. It may be considerably more realistic to assume a different distribution of infective periods. For example, an infective period of fixed length may be much closer to the actual course of many diseases.

In this section, we shall describe how to formulate models for diseases with infective periods of fixed length. These models are more complicated mathematically than the systems of differential equations we have studied until now. While the analysis of these more complicated models is of mathematical interest, their epidemiological interest depends on the possibility of differences in qualitative behavior for different infective period distributions; there are some situations in which there are such differences.

A fixed infective period will lead to a differential-difference equation model. In the next section we shall examine models for diseases with a more general infective period distribution which will lead to Volterra integral equation models. The theory governing the analysis of differential-difference equation and Volterra integral equation models is considerably more complicated than for ordinary differential equation models. We will describe this theory in a form which exhibits the analysis of the qualitative behavior of systems of differential equations as a special case.

We begin by finding equilibria of the model, that is, constant solutions (just as in the ordinary differential equation case). We then linearize about an equilibrium by translating the equilibrium to the origin and expanding. The constant terms will always cancel at an equilibrium, and we retain all linear terms but discard all terms of higher order. In the ordinary differential equation case this gives a linear system of differential equations whose coefficient matrix is the matrix of partial derivatives of the right sides of the equations of the original system with respect to the variables, but in the more general situation it is necessary to carry out the expansion.

The characteristic equation at an equilibrium is the condition that the linearization at the equilibrium have a solution whose components are constant multiples of $e^{\lambda t}$. In the ordinary differential equation case this is just the equation which determines the eigenvalues of the coefficient matrix, a polynomial equation, but in the general case it is a transcendental equation. **The result on which our analysis depends is that an equilibrium is asymptotically stable if all roots of the characteristic equation have negative real part, or equivalently that the characteristic equation have no roots with real part greater than or equal to zero.** We will illustrate with some examples, concentrating on S-I-S models with an infective period of fixed length because these have fewer compartments than other models and are thus simpler to analyze.

The S-I-S model. We begin with the simple situation of an S-I-S model with no births or deaths and no disease-related deaths, making the following assumptions:

(i) An average infective makes contact sufficient to transmit infection with βN others in unit time, where N represents total population size.

(ii) The population size is a constant K; there are no births, deaths, or entrants into the population.

(iii) Infectives remain infective for a fixed time τ and then return to the susceptible class.

Because the total population size is a constant K, we have $S + I = K$ and we may formulate the model in terms of the single variable I, replacing S by $K - I$. The rate of new infections at time t is $\beta S(t)\,I(t) = \beta I(t)[K - I(t)]$, and the rate at which infectives recover and return to the susceptible class is $\beta S(t-\tau)I(t-\tau) = \beta I(t-\tau)[K - I(t-\tau)]$. As the only changes in the infective population size are the new infections and the recoveries, we have

$$I'(t) = \beta I(t)[K - I(t)] - \beta I(t-\tau)[K - I(t-\tau)] \; . \tag{3.1}$$

When we try to find equilibria of (3.1), we find that we have no condition to solve. The reason for this is that every constant value of I is a solution of (3.1). In other words, (3.1) is not a complete description and some additional condition must be imposed. To cope with this problem, we must incorporate initial data for $-\tau \le t \le 0$ into the model by writing it in the integrated form,

$$I(t) = \int_{t-\tau}^{t} \beta I(x)[K - I(x)]\,dx \tag{3.2}$$

describing $I(t)$ as the integral (sum) of members infected at time x between $t-\tau$ and t and therefore still infective. The equilibrium condition for (3.2) is

$$I = 0 \quad \text{or} \quad 1 = \beta\tau(K - I)$$

giving a disease-free equilibrium $I = 0$ and an endemic equilibrium $I = K - \frac{1}{\beta\tau}$. To linearize about an equilibrium I_∞, we substitute $I = I_\infty + u(t)$, giving

$$I_\infty + u(t) = \int_{t-\tau}^{t} \beta[I_\infty + u(x)][K - I_\infty - u(x)]\,dx$$

and neglect the quadratic term, giving the linearization

$$u(t) = \int_{t-\tau}^{t} \beta(K - 2I_\infty)u(x)\,dx\ .$$

The characteristic equation is the condition on λ that this linearization have a solution which is a constant multiple of $e^{\lambda t}$, namely

$$e^{\lambda t} = \int_{t-\tau}^{t} \beta(K - 2I_\infty)e^{\lambda x}\,dx = \frac{\beta(K - 2I_\infty)[e^{\lambda t} - e^{\lambda(t-\tau)}]}{\lambda}$$

or

$$\frac{\beta(K - 2I_\infty)[1 - e^{-\lambda\tau}]}{\lambda} = 1\ . \tag{3.3}$$

If we had linearized at an equilibrium using the differentiated form (3.1) of the model, we would have obtained as the characteristic equation the equation (3.3) multiplied through by λ. This would have $\lambda = 0$ as a root, but this root is extraneous, being caused by the use of a model for which every constant is a solution. At the disease-free equilibrium $I_\infty = 0$ and the characteristic equation (3.3) becomes

$$\frac{\beta K(1 - e^{-\lambda\tau})}{\lambda} = 1\ . \tag{3.4}$$

In order to establish asymptotic stability of the disease-free equilibrium we need to make use of the following fact, whose proof we delay because it is a special case of a result which we will need shortly in the study of *S-I-S* models with births and deaths:

LEMMA 3.1. *If* $\tau > 0$ *and* $\Re\lambda \geq 0$, *then*

$$\left|\frac{1 - e^{-\lambda\tau}}{\lambda}\right| \leq \tau\ .$$

It follows that if $\beta\tau K < 1$ then for $\Re\lambda \geq 0$ the absolute value of the left side of the equation (3.4) is no greater than 1 and thus there can be no root (except possibly the extraneous root $\lambda = 0$) of the equation (3.4) with $\Re\lambda \geq 0$ and thus that the disease-free equilibrium is asymptotically stable if

$$R_0 = \beta\tau K < 1 .$$

At the endemic equilibrium $I = K - \dfrac{1}{\beta\tau}$, $K - 2I = K - 2K + \dfrac{2}{\beta\tau} = \dfrac{2}{\beta\tau} - K$, and the characteristic equation (3.3) becomes

$$\beta\Big(\frac{2}{\beta\tau} - K\Big)\frac{1 - e^{-\lambda\tau}}{\lambda} = 1 .$$

If $\Re\lambda \geq 0$ the absolute value of the left side of this characteristic equation is at most $\beta(\dfrac{2}{\beta\tau} - K)\tau = 2 - R_0$. Thus if $R_0 > 1$ there is no root with $\Re\lambda \geq 0$ and the equilibrium is asymptotically stable. Qualitatively, the situation is exactly the same as for the S-I-S model with exponential transition rates studied in Section 3 of Chapter I: The disease-free equilibrium is asymptotically stable if and only if the basic reproductive number R_0 is less than 1 and the endemic equilibrium exists and is asymptotically stable if and only if the basic reproductive number exceeds 1.

The obvious next step is to incorporate births and deaths into the model as in Section 4 of Chapter I. Now the total population size is not necessarily constant and we need a two-dimensional model. While we could use S and I as variables, it is preferable to use I and N to facilitate an extension to models which incorporate a density-dependent contact rate. We begin with the assumption that there are no deaths due to disease; this implies that if the birth rate is μK and the death rate is μN, the differential equation for N is $N' = \mu K - \mu N$. In order to derive the differential equation for I, we use the facts that (i) the rate of new infections at time t is $\beta S(t)\, I(t) = \beta I(t)[\, N(t) - I(t)]$ and (ii), the rate of recoveries at time t is the rate of new infections $\beta S(t-\tau)\, I(t-\tau)$ at time $t - \tau$ multiplied by the fraction $e^{\mu\tau}$ of these new infectives who survive until time t. This gives the differential-difference equation

$$I'(t) = \beta I(t)[N(t) - I(t)] - e^{-\mu\tau}\beta I(t-\tau)[N(t-\tau) - I(t-\tau)]$$

and we now have the model

$$(3.5)\qquad \begin{aligned} I'(t) &= \beta I(t)[N(t) - I(t)] - e^{-\mu\tau}\beta I(t-\tau)[N(t-\tau) - I(t-\tau)] \\ N'(t) &= \mu K - \mu N(t) . \end{aligned}$$

We shall omit the details of the equilibrium analysis, which are analogous to the calculations we have made in the case $\mu = 0$ but slightly more complicated because we now have a two-dimensional system. On the other hand, since not all constants are solutions of the system we do not need to use an integrated form of the model in order to perform the equilibrium analysis. There is a disease-free equilibrium $I = 0,\ N = K$ and an endemic equilibrium $I = K - \dfrac{\mu}{\beta(1 - e^{-\mu\tau})},\ N = K$ which exists if

$$R_0 = \frac{\beta K(1 - e^{-\mu\tau})}{\mu} > 1 .$$

The characteristic equation at an equilibrium $I = I_\infty,\ N = K$ is

$$\frac{\beta(K - 2I_\infty)[1 - e^{-(\lambda+\mu)\tau}]}{\lambda + \mu} = 1 . \tag{3.6}$$

The analysis of this characteristic equation requires the following generalization of Lemma 1, which was used in the analysis of the S-I-S model without births and deaths.

LEMMA 3.2. *If* $\tau > 0$ *and* $\Re\lambda \geq 0$, *then*

$$\left|\frac{1 - e^{-(\lambda+\mu)\tau}}{\lambda + \mu}\right| \leq \frac{1 - e^{-\mu\tau}}{\mu} .$$

It follows that if

$$R_0 = \frac{\beta K(1 - e^{-\mu\tau})}{\mu} < 1$$

then for $\Re\lambda \geq 0$ the absolute value of the left side of the equation (3.6) with $I_\infty = 0$ is no greater than 1 and thus there can be no root of the equation (3.6) with $\Re\lambda \geq 0$ and thus that the disease-free equilibrium is asymptotically stable if $R_0 < 1$. At the endemic equilibrium,

$$\beta(K - 2I_\infty) = \frac{2\mu}{1 - e^{-\mu\tau}} - \beta K$$

and the absolute value of the left side of the equation (3.6) is no greater than $2 - R_0$, which is no greater than 1 since $R_0 > 1$. Again, there can be no root of the characteristic equation with $\Re\lambda \geq 0$ and thus the endemic equilibrium is asymptotically stable if $R_0 > 1$.

If we wish to incorporate deaths due to the disease into the model (3.5), we may assume that at the end of the fixed infective period, a fraction p of the infectives die while the remainder return to the susceptible class. Then the death rate from disease is

$$pe^{-\mu\tau}\beta I(t - \tau)[N(t - \tau) - I(t - \tau)]$$

and this term must be subtracted in the equation for $N'(t)$, giving a model

$$\begin{aligned} I'(t) &= \beta I(t)[N(t) - I(t)] - e^{-\mu\tau}\beta I(t-\tau)[N(t-\tau) - I(t-\tau)] - \mu I(t) \\ N'(t) &= \mu K - \mu N(t) - pe^{\mu\tau}\beta I(t - \tau)[N(t - \tau) - I(t - \tau)] . \end{aligned} \tag{3.7}$$

The analysis of this model leads to a characteristic equation

$$\frac{\beta[N_\infty - (2-p)I_\infty][1-e^{(\lambda+\mu)\tau}]}{\lambda+\mu} = 1 + \frac{p\beta I_\infty}{\lambda+\mu}\,. \tag{3.8}$$

It may be shown that the if $\Re\lambda \geq 0$ the real part of $\dfrac{p\beta I_\infty}{\lambda+\mu}$ is non-negative and thus that the right side of the equation (3.8) has absolute value greater than 1, while the left side has absolute value at most 1 if $I_\infty = 0$ and $R_0 < 1$ because $N_\infty \leq K$ and also at the endemic equilibrium if $R_0 > 1$ using $N_\infty - (2-p)I_\infty \leq N_\infty - I_\infty$. From this we may deduce that the disease-free equilibrium is asymptotically stable if and only if $R_0 < 1$ and the endemic equilibrium, which exists if and only if $R_0 > 1$, is asymptotically stable. This is true for all p, $0 \leq p \leq 1$.

To complete the analysis of S-I-S models, we must establish Lemma 2. (As Lemma 1 is the limiting case of Lemma 2 as $\mu \to 0$, we need not give a separate justification). Lemma 2 follows from the estimate, valid for $\mu > 0$ and $\Re\lambda \geq 0$,

$$\begin{aligned}\left|\int_0^\tau e^{-(\lambda+\mu)x}\,dx\right| &\leq \int_0^\tau |e^{-(\lambda+\mu)x}|\,dx = \int_0^\tau |e^{-\lambda x}|e^{-\mu x}\,dx \\ &\leq \int_0^\tau e^{-\mu x}dx = \frac{1-e^{-\mu\tau}}{\mu}\end{aligned}$$

and the integral expression

$$\int_0^\tau e^{-(\lambda+\mu)x}dx = \left.\frac{e^{-(\lambda+\mu)x}}{-(\lambda+\mu)}\right|_0^\tau = \frac{1-e^{-(\lambda+\mu)\tau}}{\lambda+\mu}\,.$$

The case $p = 1$ of (3.7), in which all infectives die from the disease at the end of the infective period, is equivalent to a universally fatal S-I-R model. We shall not carry out the formulation and analysis of S-I-R models for diseases from which some or all infectives recover with immunity, but the general ideas are similar to those for S-I-S models.

In this section we have examined some models in which the exponentially distributed infective periods and differential equation models studied in Chapter I are replaced by fixed infective periods and differential-difference equation models, but in all cases the qualitative behavior is the same. Essentially, the only difference is in the expression for the length of the infective period corrected for natural mortality, which is $\dfrac{1}{\mu+\gamma+\alpha}$ in the exponentially distributed case and $\dfrac{1-e^{-\mu\tau}}{\mu}$ in the fixed infective period case. If the behaviors were the same in all cases, the results would be of little epidemiological interest. However, in the next section we shall describe a model with a temporary immunity period of fixed length for which the endemic equilibrium is not necessarily asymptotically stable, and this is quite different from the analogous model with an exponentially distributed temporary immunity.

4. A model with a fixed period of temporary immunity. In the models of the first sections of this chapter we have generalized the models introduced in Chapter I but these generalizations have not affected the qualitative behavior of the models. There is some mathematical interest in some of the methods, but if every more general model behaves in the same way as the simple model that it is intended to replace there is little interest from an epidemiological view. In this section we shall consider an *S-I-R-S* model which differs from the *S-I-R-S* model (1.3) of Section 1 by assuming a constant period of temporary immunity following recovery from the infection in place of an exponentially distributed period of temporary immunity. It will turn out that the endemic equilibrium for this model may be unstable, thus giving an example of a generalization which leads to new possibilities for the behavior of a model. [6]

We shall assume, as in the models studied previously, a birth rate μK, a proportional death rate μ in each class, a rate of new infections βSI, a proportional recovery rate γ and a proportional disease death rate α in unit time. To these assumptions we add the assumption that there is a temporary immunity period of fixed length ω, after which recovered infectives revert to the susceptible class. The resulting model is described by the system

$$\begin{aligned} S'(t) &= \mu K - \mu S(t) - \beta S(t)I(t) + \gamma I(t-\omega)e^{-\mu(t-\omega)} \\ I'(t) &= \beta S(t)I(t) - (\mu+\gamma+\alpha)I(t) \\ R'(t) &= \gamma I(t) - \gamma I(t-\omega)e^{-\mu(t-\omega)} - \mu R(t) \ . \end{aligned}$$

For simplicity, we shall analyze only the special case $\mu = 0$, $\alpha = 0$ with no births, natural deaths, or disease deaths, but the general case could be analyzed in a similar way. Our special case is

$$\begin{aligned} S'(t) &= -\beta S(t)I(t) + \gamma I(t-\omega) \\ I'(t) &= \beta S(t)I(t) - (\gamma+\alpha)I(t) \\ R'(t) &= \gamma I(t) - \gamma I(t-\omega) \ . \end{aligned}$$

Since $S + I + R$ is constant, we may discard the equation for r and use a two-dimensional model

$$\begin{aligned} S'(t) &= -\beta S(t)I(t) + \gamma I(t-\omega) \\ I'(t) &= \beta S(t)I(t) - (\gamma+\alpha)I(t) \ . \end{aligned} \tag{4.1}$$

Equilibria are given by $I = 0$ or $\beta S = \gamma$. The characteristic equation at an equilibrium $(S_\infty,\ I_\infty)$ is obtained by the same approach used in the preceding section, and is

$$\beta\gamma I_\infty \frac{1 - e^{-\omega\lambda}}{\lambda} = -\lambda - (\gamma + \beta I_\infty - \beta S_\infty) \,. \tag{4.2}$$

At the disease-free equilibrium $S_\infty = K$, $I_\infty = 0$ this reduces to a linear equation with a single root $\lambda = \beta K - \gamma$ which is negative if and only if $R_0 = \frac{\beta}{\gamma} < 1$. In order to analyze the characteristic equation (4.2) at the endemic equilibrium, we need to solve for S_∞ and I_∞. In order to do this we need to use the equation for R which we have discarded because the two equations for S and I give only a single equilibrium condition. In addition, we must write the equation for R in the integrated form

$$R(t) = \int_{t-\omega}^{t} \gamma I(x)\, dx$$

to give $R_\infty = \omega\gamma I_\infty$. We also have $\beta S_\infty = \gamma$, and from $S_\infty + I_\infty + R_\infty = K$ we obtain

$$\beta K = \beta S_\infty + \beta(1 + \omega\gamma) I_\infty = \gamma + \beta(1 + \omega\gamma) I_\infty$$
$$\beta I_\infty = \frac{\beta K - \gamma}{1 + \omega\gamma} \,.$$

Now we may rewrite the characteristic equation (4.2) at the endemic equilibrium in terms of the parameters of the model as

$$\gamma \frac{\beta K - \gamma}{1 + \omega\gamma} \frac{1 - e^{-\omega\lambda}}{\lambda} = -\lambda \frac{\beta K - \gamma}{1 + \omega\gamma} \,. \tag{4.3}$$

We think of ω and K as fixed and consider β and γ as parameters. If $\gamma = 0$, the equation (4.3) is linear and its only root is $-\beta K < 0$. Thus there is a region in the (β, γ) parameter space which contains the β-axis for which all roots of (4.3) have negative real part. In order to find how large the stability region is, we make use of the fact that the roots of (4.3) depend continuously on β and γ. A root can move into the right half-plane only by passing through the value zero or by crossing the imaginary axis as β and γ vary. Thus the stability region contains the β-axis and extends into the plane until there is a root $\lambda = 0$ or until there is a pair of pure imaginary roots $\lambda = \pm iy$ with $y > 0$. Since the left side of (4.3) is positive and the right side of (4.3) is negative for real $\lambda \geq 0$, there can not be a root $\lambda = 0$.

The condition that there is a root $\lambda = iy$ is

$$\gamma \frac{\beta K - \gamma}{1 + \omega\gamma} \frac{1 - e^{-i\omega\gamma}}{iy} = -iy - \frac{\beta K - \gamma}{1 + \omega\gamma} \tag{4.4}$$

and separation into real and imaginary parts gives the pair of equations

$$\gamma \frac{\sin \omega y}{y} = -1, \qquad \gamma \frac{\beta K - \gamma}{1 + \omega\gamma} \frac{1 - \cos \omega y}{y} = y \,. \tag{4.5}$$

To satisfy the first condition it is necessary to have $\omega\gamma > 1$, since $|\sin \omega y| \leq |\omega y|$ for all y. This implies, in particular, that the endemic equilibrium is asymptotically stable if $\omega\gamma < 1$. In addition, it is necessary to have $\sin \omega y < 0$. There is an infinite sequence of intervals on which $\sin \omega y < 0$, the first being $\pi < \omega y < 2\pi$. For each of these intervals the equations (4.5) define a curve in the (β, γ) plane parametrically with y as parameter. The region in the plane below the first of these curves is the region of asymptotic stability, that is, the set of values of β and γ for which the endemic equilibrium is asymptotically stable. This curve is shown in Figure 1 for $\omega = 1$, $K = 1$.Since $R_0 = \dfrac{\beta}{\gamma} > 1$, only the portion of the parameter plane below the line γ=β is relevant.

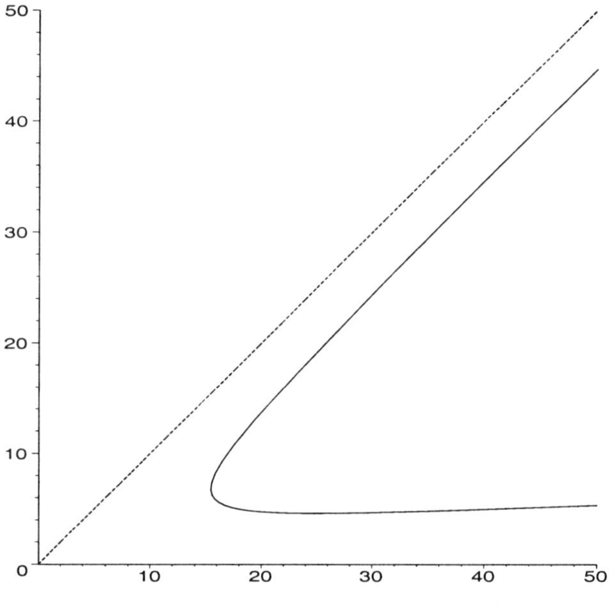

FIG. 1.

The new feature of the model of this section is that the endemic equilibrium is not asymptotically stable for all parameter values. What is the behavior of the model if the parameters are such that the endemic equilibrium is unstable? A plausible suggestion is that since the loss of stability corresponds to a root $\lambda = iy$ of the characteristic equation, there are solutions of the model behaving like the real part of e^{iyt}, that is, that there are periodic solutions. This is exactly what does happen, according to a very general result called the Hopf bifurcation theorem which says that when roots of the characteristic equation cross the imaginary axis a stable periodic orbit arises.

From an epidemiological point of view, periodic behavior is unpleasant. It implies fluctuations in the number of infectives which makes it difficult to allocate resources for treatment. It is also possible for oscillations to have a long period. This means that if data is measured over only a small time interval the actual behavior may not be displayed. Thus the identification of situations in which an endemic equilibrium is unstable is an important problem.

5. Arbitrarily distributed infective periods. The assumption of exponentially distributed infective periods which was made in Chapter I and the assumption of an infective period of fixed length introduced in Section 3 of this chapter are only two of many possibilities. In this section we shall describe the formulation and analysis of models under the assumption that there is a function $P(s)$ which represents the fraction of those infectives who became infective s time units in the past and are still alive who remain infective. The exponentially distributed case is given by $P(s) = e^{-(\alpha+\gamma)s}$ and the fixed infective period is given by

$$P(s) = \begin{cases} 1, & 0 \le s \le \tau \\ 0, & s > \tau \end{cases} .$$

Obviously, we must require that $P(s)$ be a non-negative, non-increasing function with $P(0) = 1$, and we shall also require that $\tau = \int_0^\infty P(s)\,ds$, the mean infective period, is finite. If we assume that there are no births or deaths, the equation for $I(t)$ is

$$\text{(5.1)} \qquad I(t) = \int_{-\infty}^{t} \beta S(x)I(x)P(t-x)\,dx = \int_0^\infty \beta S(t-u)I(t-u)P(u)\,du$$

and if we assume a proportional death rate μ in each class the equation for $I(t)$ is

$$I(t) = \int_{-\infty}^{t} \beta S(x)I(x)P(t-x)e^{-\mu(t-x)}\,dx = \int_0^\infty \beta S(t-u)I(t-u)P(u)e^{-\mu u}\,du.$$

The other equations in the model depend on the type of model. We shall consider only S-I-S models in this section in order to describe the methods with as little technical detail as possible. For an S-I-S model with no births or deaths either from natural causes or from disease, the total population size is a constant K and $S + I = K$. Thus the model is a single equation for I with S replaced by $K - I$, namely

$$\text{(5.2)} \qquad I(t) = \int_{-\infty}^{t} \beta I(x)[K - I(x)]P(t-x)\,dx\ .$$

Equilibria are given by

$$I = \beta I(K-I)\int_{-\infty}^{t} P(t-x)\,dx = \beta I(K-I)\int_0^\infty P(u)\,du = \beta I(K-I)\tau.$$

Thus there is a disease-free equilibrium $I = 0$ and an endemic equilibrium given by $\beta\tau(K-I) = 1$, or $I = K - \frac{1}{\beta\tau}$. The linearization at an equilibrium and the derivation of the characteristic equation follows the same pattern as for the $S-I-S$ model with no births or deaths and an infective period of fixed length except that instead of an integral of the kernel 1 over the interval $(t-\tau, t)$ we now have the integral of $P(t-x)$ from $-\infty$ to t, giving a characteristic equation

$$\beta(K-2I)\int_{-\infty}^{t} e^{-\lambda(t-x)}P(t-x)dx = \beta(K-2I)\int_{0}^{\infty} e^{-\lambda u}P(u)du = 1 \,. \tag{5.3}$$

The expression $\int_0^\infty e^{-\lambda u}\, P(u)\, du$ is called the Laplace transform of P. It is a function of the (complex) variable λ and is denoted by $\widehat{P}(\lambda)$. Thus

$$\widehat{P}(\lambda) = \int_{0}^{\infty} e^{-\lambda u}P(u)du \,. \tag{5.4}$$

The Laplace transform has the property that if $P(u)$ is a non-negative function and if $\Re\lambda \geq 0$, then

$$|\widehat{P}(\lambda)| \leq \int_{0}^{\infty} |e^{-\lambda u}|P(u)du \leq \int_{0}^{\infty} P(u)du = \widehat{P}(0) = \tau \,.$$

This property enables us to analyze the characteristic equation (5.3) easily. If $\Re\lambda \geq 0$ the absolute value of the left side of (5.3) is no greater than $\beta(K-2I)\tau$ and thus the roots of (5.3) all satisfy $\Re\lambda < 0$ if $\beta(K-2I)\tau < 1$. For the disease-free equilibrium $I = 0$, this condition is $\beta\tau K < 1$ and for the endemic equilibrium $I = K - \frac{1}{\beta\tau}$ this condition reduces to $\beta\tau K > 1$. Thus the disease-free equilibrium is asymptotically stable if and only if $R_0 = \beta\tau K < 1$ and the endemic equilibrium, which exists only if $R_0 > 1$, is asymptotically stable if $R_0 > 1$.

If we incorporate a birth rate μK and a natural proportional death rate μ in each class into an S-I-S model, the total population is no longer constant, and we must use two variables in the model. If we use S as one of the variables, the equation for S would have to include a recovery term obtained by differentiating the integral equation for I. This, as we shall see soon when we proceed to include disease deaths in the model, is complicated. It is more convenient to use I and N as variables, with S replaced by $N-I$, since N satisfies the differential equation $N' = \mu K - \mu N$. Thus we have the model

$$\begin{aligned} I(t) &= \int_{-\infty}^{t} \beta I(x)[N(x) - I(x)]P(t-x)e^{-\mu(t-x)}dx \\ N' &= \mu K - \mu N \,. \end{aligned} \tag{5.5}$$

For the analysis of this model it is convenient to define the function

$$P_\mu(u) = P(u)e^{-\mu u}$$

representing the fraction of infectives who remain alive and infective a time u after becoming infective.

The equilibrium conditions are $N = K$ and either $I = 0$ or $\beta I \int_0^\infty P_\mu(u)\,du = 1$. The same procedure that we have used frequently in this chapter leads to the characteristic equation

$$\det \begin{bmatrix} \beta(K-2I)\widehat{P}_\mu(\lambda) - 1 & \beta I \widehat{P}_\mu(\lambda) \\ 0 & -(\lambda+\mu) \end{bmatrix} = 0$$

and this reduces to

$$\beta(K-2I)\widehat{P}_\mu(\lambda) = 1$$

which is exactly the same as the characteristic equation obtained for the S-I-S model without births and deaths with $\widehat{P}(\lambda)$ replaced by $\widehat{P}_\mu(\lambda)$. Thus we again have asymptotic stability of the disease-free equilibrium if $R_0 < 1$ and asymptotic stability of the endemic equilibrium if $R_0 > 1$, with

$$R_0 = \beta K \int_0^\infty P_\mu(u)\,du\ .$$

The quantity $\tau_\mu = \int_0^\infty P_\mu(u)\,du$ represents the mean infective period corrected for natural mortality, that is the mean infective period averaged over all infectives, including those who die while still infective.

To model a universally fatal disease, with no recovered members returning to the susceptible class, we may use the above equation for I together with the differential equation $S' = \mu K - \mu S - \beta S I$, giving the model

$$\begin{aligned} S' &= \mu K - \mu S - \beta S I \\ I(t) &= \int_{-\infty}^{t} \beta S(x) I(x) P(t-x) e^{-\mu(t-x)}\,dx \end{aligned} \tag{5.6}$$

whose analysis is much the same as that of (5.5). The characteristic equation at an equilibrium (S, I) is

$$\det \begin{bmatrix} -(\lambda+\mu) - \beta I & -\beta S \\ \beta I\, \widehat{P}_\mu(\lambda) & \beta S\, \widehat{P}_\mu(\lambda) - 1 \end{bmatrix} = 0$$

which reduces to

$$\beta S\, \widehat{P}_\mu(\lambda) = 1 + \frac{\beta I}{\lambda + \mu}\ .$$

At the disease-free equilibrium $I = 0$ this is almost the same equation as the characteristic equation (5.3) analyzed earlier. We may infer that the disease-free equilibrium is asymptotically stable if and only if $R_0 = \beta\widehat{P}_\mu(\lambda)K < 1$. For the endemic equilibrium, we need only note that the absolute value of the left side is less than 1 if $\Re\lambda \geq 0$ since $|\beta S\,\widehat{P}_\mu(\lambda)| \leq \beta S\ \widehat{P}_\mu(0) = 1$, while the real part of the right side is greater than 1, as in the analysis of (3.8) in Section 3. Thus there can be no roots of the characteristic equation with $\Re\lambda \geq 0$, and the endemic equilibrium is asymptotically stable if it exists, that is, if $R_0 > 1$.

In order to consider an S-I-S model in which some but not all infectives die of disease, we must obtain an expression for the rate at which members leave the infective class. This requires the calculation of $I'(t)$, and in order to carry out this calculation we must differentiate an integral with respect to a variable which appears both in the limits of integration and in the integrand. There is a formula which may be found in most calculus texts on the differentiation of integrals which enables us to carry out this differentiation.

THEOREM 5.1. *If the function $F(t)$ is defined by the integral $F(t) = \int_a^t f(t,x)\,dx$, then its derivative is given by*

$$F'(t) = f(t,t) + \int_a^t \frac{\partial}{\partial t} f(t,x)\,dx\,.$$

When we apply this result to the integral

$$I(t) = \int_{-\infty}^{t} \beta I(x)[N(x) - I(x)]P(t-x)e^{-\mu(t-x)}\,dx$$

the term $\beta I(x)[N(x) - I(x)]$ acts as a constant factor in the partial differentiation while the term $P(t-x)e^{-\mu(t-x)}$ is a product of two functions, whose partial derivative is $P'(t-x)e^{-\mu(t-x)} - \mu P(t-x)e^{-\mu(t-x)}$. As a result, we obtain

$$\begin{aligned} I'(t) = {} & \beta I(t)[N(t) - I(t)] \\ & + \int_{-\infty}^{t} \beta I(x)[N(x) - I(x)]P'(t-x)e^{-\mu(t-x)}\,dx \\ & - \mu \int_{-\infty}^{t} \beta I(x)[N(x) - I(x)]P(t-x)e^{-\mu(t-x)}\,dx \qquad (5.7) \\ = {} & \beta I(t)[N(t) - I(t)] \\ & + \int_{-\infty}^{t} \beta I(x)[N(x) - I(x)]P'(t-x)e^{-\mu(t-x)}\,dx - \mu I(t). \end{aligned}$$

The first term on the right side of (5.7) represents the rate of new infections and the last term on the right side of (5.7) represents the rate of natural deaths. The integral term represents departure from the infective class due to recovery or death from disease.

We will consider an S-I-S model with a fraction of the infectives dying of disease. In order to conform to the notation of our elementary models, we let the fraction of infectives who recover be $\frac{\gamma}{\gamma+\alpha}$ and the fraction of infectives who die of the disease be $\frac{\alpha}{\gamma+\alpha}$. Then in terms of the variables S and I, since the rate of recoveries in unit time is

$$-\frac{\gamma}{\gamma+\alpha}\int_{-\infty}^{t}\beta S(x)I(x)P'(t-x)e^{-\mu(t-x)}\,dx$$

the S-I-S model with disease deaths is

$$\begin{aligned} S'(t) = {} & \mu K - \mu S(t) - \beta S(t)I(t) \\ & - \frac{\gamma}{\gamma+\alpha}\int_{-\infty}^{t}\beta S(x)I(x)P'(t-x)e^{-\mu(t-x)}\,dx \\ I(t) = {} & \int_{-\infty}^{t}\beta I(x)[N(x)-I(x)]P(t-x)e^{-\mu(t-x)}\,dx. \end{aligned} \tag{5.8}$$

In order to solve the equilibrium conditions, we need to integrate by parts to evaluate

$$\int_0^\infty P'(u)e^{-\mu u}du = P(u)e^{-\mu u}\Big|_0^\infty + \mu\int_0^\infty P(u)e^{-\mu u}du = -1+\mu\tau_\mu\ .$$

The equilibrium conditions are

$$\begin{aligned} \beta S I \tau_\mu &= I\ , \\ \mu K &= \mu S + \beta S I\left[\frac{\gamma}{\alpha+\gamma}(-1+\mu\tau_\mu)+1\right] = \mu S + \beta S I\left[\frac{\gamma\mu\tau_\mu}{\alpha+\gamma}+\frac{\alpha}{\alpha+\gamma}\right] \end{aligned}$$

which give a disease-free equilibrium $= 0$ and and an endemic equilibrium $\beta S\tau_\mu = 1$. By a rather complicated analysis, we may derive the characteristic equation at an equilibrium (S, I)

$$\beta\Big(S - \frac{\gamma}{\gamma+\alpha}I\Big)\widehat{P}_\mu(\lambda) = 1 + \frac{\alpha}{\gamma+\alpha}\frac{\beta I}{\lambda+\mu}$$

and deduce that $R_0 = \beta K\tau_\mu$, with the disease free equilibrium being asymptotically stable if and only if $R_0 < 1$ and the endemic equilibrium existing and being asymptotically stable if $R_0 > 1$.

Our way of including disease deaths in this model is consistent with the way used in Section 3 for models with an infective period of fixed length. An infective period of fixed length τ corresponds to the choice

$$P(s) = \begin{cases} 1, & 0 \le s \le \tau \\ 0, & s > \tau \end{cases}$$

for which $-P'(s) = \delta(s-\tau)$. Here $\delta(x)$ stands for the delta "function" originally introduced in quantum physics which has the value zero everywhere except at $x = 0$, where it is infinite in such a way that its integral is 1, and $\int_{-\infty}^{\infty} f(x)\delta(y-x)\,dx = f(y)$. With this interpretation, the number of recoveries in unit time is

$$\frac{\gamma}{\alpha+\gamma}\beta S(t-\tau)I(t-\tau)e^{-\mu\tau}$$

which is the same as the recovery term in Section 3 with $p = \dfrac{\gamma}{\gamma+\alpha}$.

The analysis of S-I-R models with arbitrary infective periods is more complicated because of the increased dimension, but the methods used in this section are easily adapted to the formulation of the models. There are no surprises in the results of the analysis; the disease-free equilibrium is asymptotically stable if and only if $R_0 < 1$ and the endemic equilibrium, which exists only if $R_0 > 1$ is asymptotically stable. However, as we shall see in the next section, a birth rate which is related to population size is one way to give a possibility of instability of the endemic equilibrium and resulting oscillatory behavior.

6. Nonlinear demographics. Until now, our demographic assumptions have been that there is a constant birth rate (except in Section 5 of Chapter I where we assumed a birth rate proportional to population size, allowing unbounded growth of the population size) and a natural death rate in each class which is proportional to the size of the class. We shall continue to retain this assumption about the death rate but now we assume a birth rate which may depend on population size in a non-linear way. In this section, we shall consider universally fatal diseases, which may be described as S-I-R models with R denoting permanent removal.

Let us consider a population in which the birth rate is a function of the number of susceptibles. This would be appropriate for a debilitating disease like rabies since infective members do not contribute to the birth rate. A model for fox rabies has been used to try to explain the prevalence of infection and population oscillations in regions where the density of foxes is high [1]. In this model it was assumed that foxes have a constant birth rate and a nonlinear death rate with a linear term and a quadratic term, with deaths divided proportionally among susceptible, exposed, and infective classes. The model is

$$\begin{aligned} S' &= aS - \mu S - cSN - \beta SI \\ E' &= \beta SI - (\mu + \epsilon + cN)E \\ I' &= \epsilon E - (\alpha + \mu + cN)I \end{aligned}$$

with $N = S + I$. In the absence of infection, the population obeys a logistic law with carrying capacity $K = \dfrac{a-\mu}{c}$. Here, a is a constant birth rate and μ is the death rate when population size is small and cN^2 represents increased mortality as the population density increases. The analysis of this model is somewhat complicated technically but straightforward in principle. There is a basic reproductive number

$$R_0 = \frac{\beta K \epsilon}{(a+\epsilon)(a+\alpha)} \tag{6.1}$$

and the disease-free equilibrium is asymptotically stable if and only if $R_0 < 1$. If $R_0 > 1$, there is an endemic equilibrium which is asymptotically stable for values of R_0 close to 1 but becomes unstable as R_0 becomes large, with oscillatory solutions. Thus the model is in qualitative agreement with observation. It is difficult to compare it with data because there is no good way to estimate the parameter c in the model, and the equilibrium values depend on c.

It is estimated that,with time measured in years, the parameter values for this model are approximately $a = 1$, $\mu = 0.5$ (corresponding to a life span of 2 years in uncrowded habitats), $\epsilon = 13$ (corresponding to a mean exposed period of 28 days or $\frac{1}{13}$ years), and $\alpha = 73$ (corresponding to a mean infective period of 5 days or $\frac{1}{73}$ years). The parameter which is most difficult to measure directly is the disease transmission coefficient β. Field studies for fox rabies in Europe indicate that there is a critical carrying capacity K_c of approximately 1.0 fox/km^2 below which rabies dies out and above which rabies is endemic. We may use the relation (6.1) above with $K = 1$ and $R_0 = 1$ to estimate $\beta = 80$. For high population densities, above 6 foxes/km^2, the solutions oscillate with a period (which depends on population density) of 3, 4 years. Actually, the oscillations depend on the density–dependent death rate; an analogous model with only susceptible and infective classes would also exhibit instability of the endemic equilibrium for high population densities.

Although there is some experimental evidence to suggest that the birth rate of foxes does not depend on the population density, let us try to construct and analyze a model with a proportional death rate μ as we have been assuming consistently and a nonlinear birth rate $g(S)$ which depends on the density of susceptible foxes. It is reasonable to assume that $g(0) = 0$ and that there is a carrying capacity K such that $g(S) > \mu S$ for $0 < S < K$ and $g(S) < \mu S$ for $S > K$. Then $g(K) = \mu K$, $g'(K) < \mu$. In most population models, we also have $\frac{g(S)}{S} > g'(S)$ and $\frac{g(S)}{S} > \mu$ for $0 < S < K$. The resulting model is

$$\begin{aligned} S' &= g(S) - \mu S - \beta S I \\ E' &= \beta S I - (\mu + \epsilon) I \\ I' &= \epsilon E - (\mu + \alpha) I \,. \end{aligned}$$

One equilibrium has $I = 0$, implying $S = K$, $E = 0$, and there is an endemic equilibrium with $\beta S = \frac{(\mu+\epsilon)(\mu+\alpha)}{\epsilon}$. The linearization matrix at an equilibrium (S, E, I) is

$$\begin{bmatrix} g'(S) - \mu - \beta I & 0 & -\beta S \\ \beta I & -(\mu+\epsilon) & \beta S \\ 0 & \epsilon & -(\mu+\alpha) \end{bmatrix}$$

At the disease-free equilibrium it is easy to see that the condition for stability is that the eigenvalues of the matrix

$$\begin{bmatrix} -(\mu+\epsilon) & \beta S \\ \epsilon & -(\mu+\alpha) \end{bmatrix}$$

have negative real part. As the trace of this matrix is obviously negative, the only requirement is that the determinant be positive, and the condition for this is

$$R_0 = \frac{\beta K \epsilon}{(\mu+\alpha)(\mu+\epsilon)} < 1 \ .$$

At the endemic equilibrium we have $\beta I + \mu = \frac{g(S)}{S}$, giving a matrix

$$\begin{bmatrix} g'(S) - \frac{g(S)}{S} & 0 & -\beta S \\ \beta I & -(\mu+\epsilon) & \beta S \\ 0 & \epsilon & -(\mu+\alpha) \end{bmatrix}$$

The characteristic equation is a cubic equation and the Routh-Hurwitz conditions may be used to determine the asymptotic stability of the endemic equilibrium. It turns out that if $g'(S) < \mu$, then the Routh-Hurwitz conditions are satisfied. Since $g(S) > \mu S$ for $0 < S < K$, and $g'(K) < \mu$, $g'(S) < \mu$ at least for sufficiently large S, but if the equilibrium value of S is small enough, instability is possible. It appears that this model also agrees qualitatively with the previous one. The two-dimensional analogue with no exposed period can not behave in the same way, as the endemic equilibrium is always asymptotically stable.

If we assume a proportional natural death rate μ as before, and a distribution $P(s)$ of infective periods as in the previous section, the S-I model is

$$\begin{aligned} S' &= g(S) - \beta SI - \mu S \\ I(t) &= \int_{-\infty}^{t} \beta S(x) I(x) P(t-x) e^{-\mu(t-x)} dx \ . \end{aligned} \tag{6.2}$$

Equilibria are given by $I = 0$ or $\beta S\tau_\mu = 1$ and $g(S) = \beta SI + \mu S$. The characteristic equation at an equilibrium (S, I) is

$$\det \begin{bmatrix} g'(S) - \beta I - (\lambda + \mu) & -\beta S \\ \beta I \widehat{P}_\mu(\lambda) & \beta S \widehat{P}_\mu(\lambda) - 1 \end{bmatrix} = 0$$

which reduces to

$$\beta S \widehat{P}_\mu(\lambda) = 1 + \frac{\beta I}{\lambda + \mu - g'(S)} .$$

At the disease-free equilibrium, $I = 0$ and $S = K$, the carrying capacity or limiting population size in the absence of disease given by $g(K) = \mu K$, $g'(K) < \mu$. The characteristic equation is $\beta K \widehat{P}_\mu(\lambda) = 1$ and as we have seen before all roots of this equation satisfy $\Re\lambda < 0$ if and only if $\beta K \widehat{P}_\mu(0) = \beta K \tau_\mu < 1$. Thus $R_0 = \beta K \widehat{P}_\mu(0) = \beta K \tau_\mu$. At the endemic equilibrium, since $\beta S \widehat{P}_\mu(0) = 1$, $\beta I = \dfrac{g(S)}{S} - \mu$, the characteristic equation is

$$\frac{P_\mu(\lambda)}{P_\mu(0)} = 1 + \frac{\dfrac{g(S)}{S} - \mu}{\lambda + \mu - g'(S)} .$$

The absolute value of the left side of this equation is no greater than 1 if $\Re\lambda \geq 0$, and by an argument we have used in the previous section we may show that the real part of the right side is greater than 1 if $g'(S) < \mu$. However, if I is sufficiently large and S is sufficiently small it is possible to have $g'(S) > \mu$. Again, there is a possibility of instability which may depend on the nature of the function $P(s)$. If $P(s) = e^{-\alpha s}$, the endemic equilibrium is always asymptotically stable. Note that instability is possible even without the assumption of an exposed period. At the endemic equilibrium we have $\beta S \tau_\mu = 1$, $\beta I + \mu = \dfrac{g(S)}{S}$, and from this it follows that

$$\beta N = \beta S + \beta I = \frac{1}{\tau_\mu} + \frac{g(S)}{S} - \mu . \tag{6.3}$$

If the birth rate has a logistic form, $g(S) = rS(1 - \dfrac{S}{A})$, we may calculate the carrying capacity of the population by solving the equation $g(K) = \mu K$, and we obtain $K = A(r - \mu)$, or $A = K/(r - \mu)$. Substituting for $g(S)$, we obtain

$$\frac{g(S)}{S} = r(1 - \frac{r - \mu}{\beta K \tau_\mu})$$

and this, combined with (6.3) gives

$$\beta N = \frac{1}{\tau_\mu} + r(1 - \frac{r-\mu}{\beta K \tau_\mu}) - \mu\ . \tag{6.4}$$

We think of the parameters β, r, μ, and τ_μ as fixed and allow the carrying capacity to grow large. From (6.4), we see that the population size remains bounded by the constant

$$\frac{1}{\beta\tau_\mu} + \frac{(r-\mu)}{\beta}\ .$$

Thus the population size becomes a very small fraction of the carrying capacity as the carrying capacity increases. This means that in regions of large fox density, the endemic equilibrium may have sufficiently small total population size that oscillations about the endemic equilibrium could wipe out the fox population. The tendency toward oscillations is increased by seasonal factors in both the reproduction of foxes and in disease transmission.

If we use an infective period of fixed length τ in the model (6.1), we obtain a differential-difference equation model. We could incorporate an exposed period of fixed length ω as well, to give the model

$$\begin{aligned} S' &= g(S) - \beta SI - \mu S \\ E' &= \beta S(t)I(t) - \beta S(t-\omega)I(t-\omega)e^{-\mu\omega} - \mu E \\ I' &= \beta S(t-\omega)I(t-\omega)e^{-\mu\omega} - \beta S(t-\omega-\tau)I(t-\omega-\tau)e^{-\mu(\omega+\tau)} \end{aligned} \tag{6.5}$$

which we may analyze in the usual way. It turns out that, if we assume that $g(S)$ is of logistic form, we have

$$R_0 = \beta\tau_\mu e^{\mu\omega} K\ .$$

If we use the values $r = 1$, $\mu = 0.5$, $\omega = \frac{1}{\epsilon} = \frac{1}{13}$, $\tau = \frac{1}{\alpha} = \frac{1}{73}$ corresponding to the values in the rabies model of Anderson et al., and use the observed data that $K = 1$ corresponds to $R_0 = 1$, we obtain the estimate $\beta = 70.5$, fairly close to the estimate from the earlier model.

If the birth rate is a function $g(S+I)$ of the total population size, the model analogous to (6.1) is

$$\begin{aligned} S' &= g(S+I) - \beta SI - \mu S \\ I(t) &= \int_{-\infty}^{t} \beta S(x)I(x)P(t-x)e^{-\mu(t-x)}\,dx \end{aligned} \tag{6.6}$$

and the resulting characteristic equation turns out to be

$$\beta S\widehat{P}_\mu(\lambda) = 1 + \frac{\beta I[1 - g'(S+I)P_\mu(\lambda)]}{\lambda + \mu - g'(S+I)}$$

and it is possible to show from this characteristic equation with the aid of the estimates

$$|P_\mu(\lambda)| \le \int_0^\infty e^{-\mu s}\,ds = \frac{1}{\mu}, \qquad g'(S+I) < \mu$$

that the endemic equilibrium is always asymptotically stable.

These results suggest that the reduction in birth rate caused by a debilitating illness can be a cause of instability and oscillations. The general question of the relations between demographic and epidemiological effects has many facets which have not yet been explored. There are many situations in which a time lag tends to promote instability, and we have seen in Section 4 that the time lag of a temporary immunity against reinfection may produce instability. An exposed period before becoming infective is another type of time lag, and we see in this section that it may produce instability in some ordinary differential equation models, but that models with other than exponential distributions of infective periods may be unstable even without an exposed period. This would suggest that exposed periods in themselves do not produce instability.

7. Well-posed problems. In our study so far, we have not dwelt on the theoretical mathematical background underlying the analysis of models. There are some important theoretical properties of which we should be aware, even though we will not give precise statements or proofs.

If a mathematical model is to be a plausible description of a natural phenomenon, there are some basic requirements which it must satisfy. For example, the model must have a solution or it can not hope to describe the behavior of a system. Also, the model must have only one solution; otherwise it could not be used to predict behavior. Since the initial data and parameter values in models are usually approximate and therefore subject to experimental error, a model should have the property that a small error in the data produces only a small error in the solution. These three properties are known respectively as *existence, uniqueness, and continuous dependence on initial data and parameters.* There are general theorems for differential equations [2] and more generally for functional differential equations, including integral and integral-differential equations [3,8] which guarantee that all the models we have formulated in these two chapters have these properties under very general assumptions on the functions in the problem. These references also contain proofs of the results we have used repeatedly on linearization at an equilibrium and asymptotic stability.

In addition, there are some properties that are needed for disease models in which all variables must remain non-negative. It is important to know that the total population size N remains bounded. In all the models we have considered in which there is a carrying capacity K, we have a differential equation for N which implies that $N' < 0$ if $N > K$. This implies that if $N \le K$ initially then $N(t) \le K$ for all $t \ge 0$. We also have a differential equation for S which implies that $S' < 0$ if $S > K$, implying that if $S \leq K$ initially then $S(t) \leq K$ for all $t \geq 0$. Likewise, in our models we have $S' \geq 0$ if $S = 0$, and this implies that S can not become negative. In some of our models we have $I' \geq 0$ if $I = 0$, so that I can not become negative. In other models the limit as $I \to 0$ of the quotient I'/I is finite, and this is enough to show that I behaves like an exponential function (with positive or negative exponent) when I is small and thus does not become negative. If $I(t)$ is given by an integral equation, we may easily see that if $I(x) \geq 0$ for $-\infty < x < t$ then the right side of the integral equation is non-negative and therefore $I(t) \geq 0$ for all t.

Another question we have avoided is the size of the region of asymptotic stability of an equilibrium. A linearization approach tells us only that solutions which begin close enough to an equilibrium approach that equilibrium but gives no information about how close the starting position must be in order that the solution will approach the equilibrium. Usually, it is not difficult to show that if $R_0 < 1$ the disease-free equilibrium is *globally asymptotically stable.* This means that every solution approaches the disease-free equilibrium if $R_0 < 1$. The proof involves making an estimate using the equation for I to show that if t is sufficiently large, then $I(t) < R_0\, I(t)$, and if $R_0 < 1$ this can happen only if $I(t) \to 0$. The details of the argument require some technical calculus machinery, namely the idea of the upper limit of a function.

The upper limit as $t \to \infty$ of a function $I(t)$, denoted by $\limsup I(t)$ is defined by the requirement that $\limsup I(t) = I^*$ if and only if for every $\epsilon > 0$ there is a number T such that $I(t) < I^* + \epsilon$ for all $t > T$ and $I(t) > I^* - \epsilon$ for some $t > T$. In other words, as $t \to \infty$ the function $I(t)$ is never much greater than I^* but comes close to I^*. In our models, we may always express $I(t)$ by an integral equation

$$\begin{aligned} I(t) &= \int_{-\infty}^{t} \beta S(x) I(x) P(t-x) e^{-\mu(t-x)}\, dx \\ &= \int_0^{\infty} \beta S(t-u) I(t-u) P(u) e^{-\mu u}\, du\ . \end{aligned}$$

If t is sufficiently large that $I(t-u) < I^* + \epsilon$, since $S(t-u) \leq K$ the integral is no greater than $\beta K(I^* + \epsilon) \int_0^\infty P(u)e^{-\mu u}\, du = R_0(I^* + \epsilon)$. This estimate is not quite right because we do not have $I(t-u) < I^* + \epsilon$ for large u, but for large u the contribution to the integral is small because $P(u)e^{-\mu u}$ is small]. Since $I(t) < I^* + \epsilon$ for large t, we see from the integral equation that $I^* + \epsilon < R_0(I^* + \epsilon)$ for arbitrarily small $\epsilon > 0$. If $R_0 < 1$, this can happen only if $I^* = 0$, and this implies the global asymptotic stability of the disease-free equilibrium if $R_0 < 1$.

For the endemic equilibrium, global asymptotic stability is largely an open problem. For two-dimensional models or models which can be reduced to two-dimensional models there are qualitative results which imply that every solution approaches either an equilibrium or a periodic orbit. There are also criteria which show that there can be no periodic orbits and this implies that a (locally) asymptotically stable equilibrium must be globally asymptotically stable. In higher dimensions, there are some results for specific models but there is no general theory.

We mention these theoretical questions because it is important to be aware that there is a sound mathematical basis for the analysis of models used in the study of other sciences. Even if one is concerned primarily with the applications to epidemiology, an understanding of what is true mathematically may help to avoid misinterpretations and incorrect conclusions. The results we have been using on the relation between the location of the roots of a characteristic equation and the stability of an equilibrium are elementary if the model is a system of ordinary differential equations and the characteristic equation is just the equation which determines the eigenvalues, but are very deep and quite difficult to establish in the more general situations we have introduced in this chapter.

REFERENCES

[1] R.M. Anderson, H.C. Jackson, R.M. May, & A.M. Smith, Population dynamics of fox rabies in Europe, Nature (London) 289 (1981), 765–771.

[2] E.A. Coddington & N. Levinson, Theory of Ordinary Differential Equations, McGraw-Hill (New York), 1955.

[3] O. Diekmann, S.A. van Gils, & S.M. Verduyn-Lunel, & H.O. Walther, Delay Equations: Functional-, Complex-, and Nonlinear Analysis, Springer Verlag (New York), 1995.

[4] F.R. Gantmacher, The Theory of Matrices, Vol. 2, Chelsea (New York), 1959.

[5] J.A.P. Heesterbeek & J.A.J. Metz, The saturating contact rate in marriage and epidemic models, J. Math. Biology 31 (1993), 529–539.

[6] H.W. Hethcote, H.W. Stech, & P. van den Driessche, Nonlinear oscillations in epidemic models, SIAM. J. App. Math. 40 (1981), 1–9.

[7] J. Mena-Lorca & H.W. Hethcote, Dynamic models of infectious diseases as regulators of population size, J. Math. Biology 30 (1992), 693–716.

[8] G.F. Webb, Theory of Nonlinear Age-dependent Population Dynamics, Marcel Dekker (New York), 1985.

NEW VACCINATION STRATEGIES FOR PERTUSSIS*

HERBERT W. HETHCOTE†

This paper is dedicated to Ken Cooke, a pioneer in mathematical epidemiology, an outstanding scientist, and a good friend.

Abstract. Both disease-acquired and vaccine-acquired immunity to pertussis (whooping cough) wane with time, so that several infections can occur in an individual's lifetime. The severity of a pertussis infection depends on how low the immunity has declined since the previous vaccination, infection, or exposure. In the United States five DTP or DTaP (diphtheria-tetanus-pertussis) vaccinations are recommended at ages 2, 4, 6, 15-18 months, and 4–6 years. The new acellular pertussis vaccine (aP) has fewer side effects, so that it is safe for adults. New strategies for reducing pertussis incidence include: 1) combining the aP vaccine with the current Td (tetanus-diphtheria) booster that is now recommended every ten years, 2) giving the aP vaccine to adolescents at age 12 years, 3) giving the aP vaccine to young adults at age 20 years, and 4) giving the aP vaccine to adults at age 50 years. The effects of these new vaccination strategies are analysed using an age-structured model.

Key words. Pertussis, vaccination, simulations, models.

1. Introduction. The infectious bacteria *Bordetella pertussis* is the agent for the disease called pertussis or whooping cough. In the prevaccine era pertussis was a common disease in infants and children with an average age of attack of about 5 years. Deaths from pertussis were frequent for infants under 6 months of age [12]. Pertussis vaccines were developed and were used in the early 1940s in the United States. In 1949 the whole-cell pertussis vaccine was combined with diphtheria and tetanus toxoids into the DTP vaccination [2]. The vaccination program for pertussis in the United States has greatly reduced its morbidity and mortality, but pertussis has remained endemic. Diphtheria, the other bacteria agent vaccine in the DTP combination, has almost disappeared in the United States [10]. This may be due to factors such as a more effective vaccine for diphtheria or the use of Td (tetanus-diphtheria) booster vaccinations every ten years for adults.

Since both infection-acquired and vaccine-induced immunity to pertussis wane with time, previously infected or vaccinated individuals slowly become more susceptible to pertussis [28, 27, 32]. An infected person with a typical case of pertussis has severe coughing and is ill for several weeks

*For presentation at the Workshop on Mathematical Approaches for Emerging and Reemerging Infectious Diseases, Institute for Mathematics and its Applications, Minneapolis, Minnesota, May 17–21, 1999.

†Department of Mathematics, University of Iowa, Iowa City, Iowa 52242, U.S.A. Email: hethcote@math.uiowa.edu.

[2]. Pertussis infections in older children and adults are often unrecognized, since pertussis infections after vaccination or previous infection are often atypical and usually have different, milder symptoms than an initial infection in a fully-susceptible person [37, 28]. Atypical pertussis cases still cough, but this symptom is often attributed to bronchitis or a respiratory infection. Atypical infections in adolescents and adults appear to be a major reservoir for the transmission of pertussis [3, 12, 30, 18, 29, 7, 22]. Fewer children now get pertussis, but their parents are now more frequently reported as the source of infection for those who are infected [14, 15, 23, 37].

Acellular pertussis vaccines (aP) consisting of pieces of the bacteria have recently been developed and tested. These aP vaccines cause fewer adverse reactions, but their vaccine efficacy may be lower than that of the killed whole-cell pertussis vaccines [19, 36, 21]. Vaccination for pertussis in the United States is now given in the form of DTaP or DTP vaccines, where aP is a new acellular pertussis vaccine. Vaccination is recommended at the ages of 2, 4, 6, and 15–18 months and before school entry at age 4–6 years [11]. Multiple vaccinations are given, because each additional dose of pertussis vaccine seems to provide additional temporary protection against severe pertussis disease and multiple doses can provide temporary protection against pertussis infection. The whole-cell pertussis vaccines are not recommended for adults, but the new acellular pertussis vaccines have fewer side effects, so that they can be used safely in adults [16]. Epidemiologists have suggested that acellular-vaccine booster doses be given to adolescents and adults [18, 28, 13–15, 27, 32, 17, 31]. Epidemiologists hope that the resulting reduction of the adult reservoir of pertussis infection would be great enough to significantly reduce the transmission to infants, who have high complication rates when infected [6].

The pertussis vaccination program in the United States led to a decrease in the reported incidence of pertussis by a factor of about 100 between the 1940s and the 1970s to a minimum of 1,010 cases in 1976 [12, 18]. After 1976, reported pertussis incidence continued to be cyclical with peaks every 3 or 4 years, but there has been a generally increasing trend with 6586 cases reported in 1993, 4617 in 1994, 4315 in 1995, 7796 in 1996, 5519 in 1997, and 6279 in 1998 [8–10]. Epidemiologists would like to know whether the general increase in reported cases of pertussis after 1976 corresponds to an actual upward trend in pertussis incidence in the United States or to some other factor such as an increase in the fraction of pertussis cases being reported. Epidemiologists would also like to understand the future effects of continuing the vaccination of children at the current level and of introducing new pertussis booster vaccination programs for adolescents and adults.

An age-structured epidemiologic model was developed for pertussis transmission and vaccination in the United States [24]. This model consisted of 12 epidemiological classes for individuals who were susceptible, infectious, immune, or vaccinated. Pertussis data were used to estimate parameter values in that model. Computer simulations using that mathematical model were used to study the current childhood pertussis vaccination program and various future pertussis vaccination scenarios. The sensitivities of the results to the parameter values were analyzed [24]. Related papers, including some on modeling of pertussis in the United Kingdom, were cited in [24].

The incidence of pertussis in the United States oscillated cyclically with peaks about every 4 years in the prevaccine era and this oscillation has continued as vaccination levels increased after 1940 [18, 29]. This irregular oscillatory behavior of pertussis incidence in the United States has been investigated using the mechanisms of seasonality and environmental stochasticity in an age-structured pertussis model [25]. Computer simulations of two different pertussis models have been used to obtain estimates of the potential effects of the addition of complete (100%) adult pertussis booster vaccinations every ten years on pertussis incidence in both adults and children [26]. The first model was the previously developed model [24] in which each pertussis booster moves the individual back up one vaccinated or removed class. The second model incorporated a more optimistic view of the effectiveness of pertussis booster vaccinations.

Here we continue to investigate new vaccination strategies for pertussis by considering four alternative additions to the current childhood vaccination program. These new strategies include some programs being considered by epidemiologists at the National Immunization Program at the National Centers for Disease Control and Prevention in Atlanta, Georgia. The first strategy combines the aP vaccine with the current Td (tetanus-diphtheria) booster that is now recommended every ten years. The next three strategies give the aP vaccine to adolescents at age 12 years, to young adults at age 20 years, or to adults at age 50 years. The first strategy has the advantages that it would be part of the tetanus-diphtheria booster vaccinations that are currently recommended every ten years and there would be no extra cost for administration of the combined TdaP vaccination instead of the current Td vaccination. For the single-dose pertussis booster vaccination strategies, age 12 years is chosen because many 12 year old adolescents would have lost their immunity from the last DTP vaccination at 4–6 years, and they are important spreaders since they are still in school where they have many contacts with other children. Age 20 years is chosen because many would have lost their immunity, and age 20 years is the start of the childbearing years for many young adults. Using pertussis vaccinations to increase the immunity among parents would decrease the likelihood that they would get pertussis and pass it on to their infants and young children, who have high complication rates when infected. Vaccination at age 50 years is chosen because many would not be immune at that age and because it allows comparison with vaccinations at younger ages.

Two alternative pertussis models were used in [26]. Because the incidences of typical pertussis cases using the second model are more consistent with estimates of clinical pertussis cases than those using the first model, the second pertussis model in [26] is used in the simulations here (see Section 3.1). After this model is presented in Section 2, previous simulation results are summarized in Section 3. The new vaccination strategies are investigated in Section 4, and the results are discussed in Section 5.

2. The age-structured pertussis model.

2.1. Formulation of the pertussis model. The pertussis model used here is the second model in [26]. The population is divided into sixteen distinct epidemiologic classes with four infectious classes, four removed classes, and seven vaccination classes as shown in Figure 1. When there is an adequate contact of a susceptible with an infective, transmission occurs and the susceptible becomes infected. Infected individuals enter the class $I_{highest}$ of highest-infectivity infectives at the rate λS, where S is the susceptible age distribution, and the force of infection λ is the total infectivity-weighted contact rate with infectives in all age groups. The latent period in which an individual is infected, but not yet infectious, is not included in the model, since it is only about one week for pertussis [2] [20, pp. 340–341].

Although not all infectives entering an infective class have the same symptoms and infectivities, it is convenient to describe those in each class by their average infectivity levels. It is assumed that those who had lower immunity have more severe disease symptoms and higher infectivity when they become infected. Because they come from the susceptible class where they had no immunity, most infectives in the highest-infectivity class have a severe-disease case of pertussis with a paroxysmal cough for at least 21 days and their average infectivity is highest [27]. Most infectives in the high-infectivity class have less severe pertussis and cough less, so their average infectivity is three-fourths of that of a highest-infectivity infective. Similarly, infectives in the medium- and low-infectivity classes cough even less and are less likely to infect a susceptible, so their average infectivities are only one-half and one-fourth, respectively, of that of a highest-infectivity infective. Hence the average levels of infectivity for the four infectious classes $I_{highest}$, I_{high}, I_{medium}, and I_{low} are 1, 0.75, 0.5, and 0.25, respectively. Because those in the highest-infectivity class $I_{highest}$ were fully susceptible before their infection, they usually have a classic pertussis case similar to the pertussis cases that everyone had in the prevaccine era. Hence they are called typical cases and those in the three other infectivity classes are called atypical.

In the model the fraction of vaccinated susceptibles that has increased immunity and enters the first vaccinated class V_1 is called the vaccine efficacy (VE). If some people in V_1 are given another vaccination, then the fraction VE of those vaccinated enter V_2. Similarly, when people in the vaccinated classes V_2 and V_3 are vaccinated, the fraction VE moves up to the class with the next higher immunity level as shown in Figure 1. For

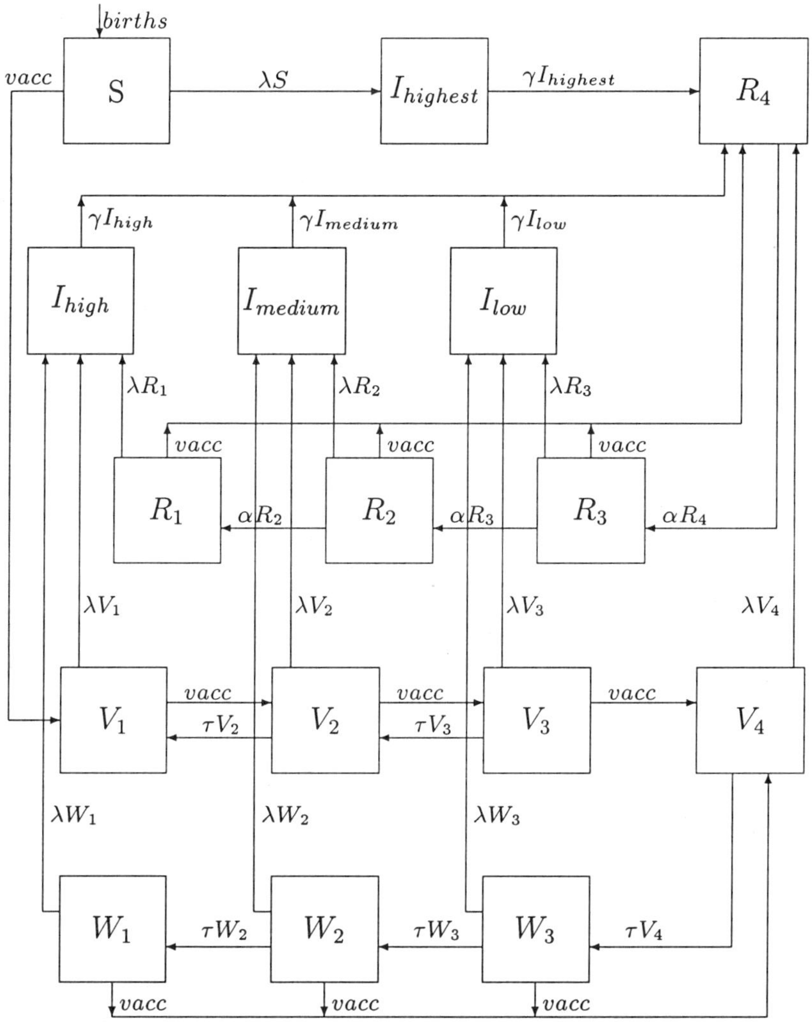

FIG. 1. *Transfer diagram for the pertussis model with vaccination.*

people who have had a previous pertussis infection or have had a series of at least 4 pertussis vaccinations, their immune system is already primed against the pertussis bacteria, so that a pertussis booster vaccination raises their immunity back up to the highest level. Thus when people in the removed classes R_1, R_2, and R_3 are vaccinated, the fraction VE moves up to R_4, the highest-immunity removed class. The vaccinated classes W_1, W_2, and W_3 correspond to those who have had at least 4 pertussis vaccinations, but now have lower immunity due to waning. When people in these vaccinated classes W_1, W_2, and W_3 are vaccinated, the fraction VE moves up to the V_4, the highest-immunity vaccinated class. People in V_4 or R_4 who are vaccinated do not change classes, since they already have very high immunity. Unlike the first model in [24, 26], people in the lowest immunity removed and vaccinated classes R_1, and W_1 never return to the fully susceptible class S due to the loss of all immunity.

Vaccination at age 2 months is incorporated by moving, to a higher removed or vaccination class, the appropriate fraction of those transferred due to aging between the 0–1 month and 2–3 month age groups. The transferred fraction is the product of the fraction vaccinated times the vaccine efficacy VE. The simulations of vaccinations at ages 4 months, 6 months, 1 year and 5 years, and of adolescent and adult booster doses are analogous. The waning of immunity is modeled by the movement down through the removed and vaccinated classes over time. As shown in Figure 1, the waning of infection-acquired or vaccine-induced immunity is modeled by moving recovered individuals through a sequence $R_4R_3R_2R_1$ of removed classes with decreasing immunity. As the vaccine-induced immunity wanes, people move down through the vaccinated classes $V_3V_2V_1$ or $V_4W_3W_2W_1$.

A pertussis infection provides immunity from infection for several years, but then an infection can occur and the severity of the disease depends on the time since the last infection or boosting exposure [13, 27, 32]. Individuals in the class R_4 can not be infected due to their high immunity. People in V_4 have very high vaccine-induced immunity, so if they have an adequate contact with an infective, they go directly to R_4, because they either are boosted without becoming infectious or have an asymptomatic infection with negligible infectivity. People in R_3, V_3, or W_3 have high immunity, but if they have an adequate contact with an infective, they can become infected, in which case they move to the low-infectivity class I_{low} and then go to R_4, the highest-immunity class. After adequate contact with an infective, people in R_2, V_2, or W_2 enter the medium-infectivity class I_{medium} and then go to R_4 when the infectious period ends. Those in R_1, V_1, or W_1 who are exposed enter the class I_{high} of high-infectivity people and then go to R_4 when they recover. The infection rates are always proportional to the age distributions in the classes with the same force of infection λ used for the transfer of susceptibles to the highest-infectivity class.

The demographic part of the model uses 1990 fertility and death rates in the United States to obtain a theoretical population whose total size is constant and whose age distribution has reached a steady state age distribution. The 32 age intervals in the model are 0–1 months, 2–3 months, 4–5 months, 6–11 months, years 1, 2, 3, ..., 18, 19, and the five or ten year intervals 20–24, 25–29, 30–39, 40–49, 50–59, 60–69, 70–79, 80–89, and over 90. Newborns enter the 0–1 month age group. In each age group there is a daily outflow corresponding to aging into the next age group and a daily death rate [24, 26].

The pertussis model is formulated first as a system of 16 first order partial differential equations as a function of age and time, but these are integrated over the 32 age intervals to get a system of ordinary differential equations with inflows due to births, transfers due to aging, and outflows due to deaths [26]. Thus the mathematical model corresponding to the transfer diagram in Figure 1 consists of 512 nonlinear differential equations giving the rates of daily transfers among the 16 epidemiologic classes and the 32 age groups. The computer simulations are the numerical solutions of these differential equations with vaccinations of specific age groups. The epidemiologic age distribution starts at a prevaccine steady state. Then after the childhood vaccination program starts in 1940, the epidemiologic age distribution changes in response to the vaccinations. More details about the epidemiologic model formulation are given in the related papers [24, 26].

2.2. Estimates of the parameters. As explained above, 1990 fertility and death rates are used to obtain a constant population size and a steady state age distribution. For pertussis the average infectious period is about 21 days [2] [20, pp. 340–341]; thus the rate constant γ is 1/21. The transfer rate constant $\alpha = 1/(5 * 365)$ corresponds to a five year average waiting period in classes R_4, R_3, and R_2. The waning in the vaccinated classes V_4, V_3, V_2, W_3, and W_2 is faster with a mean period of 2 years, so that $\tau = 1/(2 * 365)$. In [24] these estimates of the parameter values α and τ are shown to be consistent with recent pertussis studies [27, 32, 28, 15, 17, 31]. Forces of infection as a function of age for pertussis have been estimated in England and Wales in 1956 (before vaccination started there) from reported incidence data [1, p. 164]. The forces of infection in the pertussis model for the United States with 13 aggregated age intervals are based on the United Kingdom values. The contact matrix has been estimated using a proportionate mixing approach, so that the number of adequate contacts between the susceptibles in one age group and the infectives in another age group is assumed to be proportional to the mixing activity levels and sizes of the two groups. This proportionate mixing contact matrix is found from the forces of infection and the numbers of infectives. For the pertussis forces of infection, the activity level is highest for the 5–9 year old children [24].

A vaccine efficacy VE of 0.9 has been shown to be consistent with pertussis data [24]. Pertussis vaccination appears to have started around 1940 in the United States. The whole-cell pertussis vaccine was officially licensed in 1948 and the DTP combination was licensed in 1949 [4]. In the pertussis model the vaccination rates for the first three vaccinations increase linearly from zero in 1940 to the values 0.8, 0.78, and 0.76 in 1950. Then they increase linearly up to the values 0.96, 0.94, and 0.92 in 1995 and are constant after 1995. The vaccination rate at age 1 year increases linearly from zero in 1940 to 0.7 in 1960; then it increases linearly up to 0.86 in 1995 and is constant after 1995. For vaccination at age 5 years, the vaccination rate increases linearly from zero in 1940 to 0.6 in 1970; then it increases up to 0.8 in 1995 and is constant after 1995. These vaccination coverages have been shown to be consistent with immunization survey data. More details about the estimation of demographic, epidemiological, and vaccination parameters are given in the related papers [24, 26].

3. Summary of previous pertussis simulation results.

3.1. Comparisons with pertussis data. Data on pertussis incidence have severe limitations. Before vaccination was available, nearly all children had pertussis infections by age 15, so that the actual highest-infectivity incidence in children was approximately equal to the birth rate [20]. However, the 183,866 reported cases in 1940 are about 10 percent of the 1940 births. Pertussis reporting in the late 1980s was estimated to be only about 11.6 percent of actual cases [35]. Hence reported cases of pertussis have probably been only about 10 percent of actual cases since 1940. Other limitations of pertussis data are the disproportionate representation of classic and severe cases, the bias towards reporting cases in children, and the lack of uniform reporting [8].

Reported pertussis incidence rates per person per year decreased by a factor of about 100 between the 1940s and the period since 1970 [12, 18]. Because the reported fraction is higher for people who have severe cases, this 100 factor decrease may correspond primarily to a decrease in typical cases. In the simulations with the current model the incidence between 1940 and 1995 decreases by a factor of about 300 for typical cases, but the atypical cases decrease only slightly. Thus the magnitudes of the average decreases in incidences in the simulations are consistent with the observed drop of 100 in reported incidence.

The average age of typical case incidence in children in the simulations is 5.0 years in 1940, which agrees with the reported average age of attack of 5 years in the prevaccine era [20]. The percentage of reported pertussis cases among those over 10 years of age increased from 15 percent during 1977–79 to 20 percent in 1980–89, 18 percent in 1989–91 and 28 percent during 1992–94 [6, 8]. These age shifts are consistent with the simulations as shown in Figure 9 in [26], where there are major shifts in the age distribution of highest-infectivity cases towards older age groups from 1940 to 1980 and then smaller shifts in the same direction after 1980.

A recent estimate of the attack rate in German adults was 0.00052 per person per year [32]. A study [28] of university students in the United States with cough lasting at least 6 days found that 26 percent had pertussis infections. Based on the size of the total student population, the minimum yearly incidence was estimated to be 0.00069. Among members of a Kaiser health plan in San Francisco, 12.4 percent of those with a chronic cough had pertussis [31]. By considering the total number of patients visiting the facility and the number who complained of a chronic cough, the yearly incidence was estimated to be at least 0.00176 per adult. In the simulations shown in Figures 9 and 10 in [26], the total incidence per adult per year of pertussis between 1940 and 2040 is between 0.0004 and 0.0008 per adult between ages 18 and 70. These values are consistent with the first two estimates above, but they are less than the third estimate.

It was estimated [35] that 46% of infected infants under 1 year of age were hospitalized for pertussis in 1985–88 and that 34% of the hospitalizations of those under age 1 year were reported. This implies that at least 16% of pertussis cases in infants under 1 year of age are reported. There were 2370 reported pertussis cases in infants under age 1 year in 1996. Because at least 16% are reported, there were at most 15,000 pertussis cases in infants under age 1 year in 1996. In the simulations in [26], the yearly incidence after 1995 in those under age 1 year is 6000 to 8000 severe, typical cases and about ten times as many less severe, atypical cases. The study [35] also found that severe cases, especially those with hospitalizations and complications, are more likely to be reported, so that the simulation results are compatible with the upper estimate of 15,000 pertussis cases in those under age 1 year.

Two studies [32, 27] of pertussis in German adults (less than 5 percent were vaccinated) found that 32% of exposed adults had evidence of pertussis infection, so at least this percentage are susceptible to a detectable pertussis infection. This value is consistent with the year 1940 simulations, in which 15% to 35% of adults in age groups between 18 and 70 years are in the susceptible class S or the removed class R_1, where a highest- or high-infectivity infection can occur. The percentages of adult age groups in the susceptible class S or the removed class R_1 are between 20% and 50% in the simulations for 1995. This range is consistent with the 1992 Massachusetts outbreak, in which 19 to 28 percent of the classes in a highly-vaccinated high school population had pertussis [5].

The United States population size is 265 million, so that the 1995 simulation values using the current pertussis model correspond to about 10,000 typical cases in those under age 10 years and about 1000 typical cases for those at least age 10 years. A 1985–88 study [35] estimated that from 30,000 to as many as 125,000 cases of clinical pertussis disease occur annually in the United States. Since clinical cases would include the typical (highest-infectivity) cases and some of the atypical cases in the simulations, the model simulation value here of about 11,000 typical cases is consistent with the estimated range of clinical cases in the study [35]. Note that the model used here is labeled as the second model in [26]. The first model in [26] has not been used in our current simulations, because the simulation value in the first model of 560,000 typical cases per year in those at least age 10 years is too high to be consistent with the study upper bound of 125,000 clinical cases per year.

3.2. Previous conceptual results: childhood vaccination. Two age-structured models have been developed to study pertussis transmission and vaccination in the United States. In the first model each pertussis booster vaccination moves the individual back up one vaccinated or removed class [24]. However, those who have had a sequence of at least 4 pertussis vaccinations or have had a previous pertussis infection may have developed an immunological memory, so that a pertussis booster would raise their immunity back up to the highest level. The second model incorporates this more optimistic view of the effectiveness of pertussis booster vaccinations [26]. Many components of this second pertussis model are the same as in the first model, but it has an extra class for infectives with low-infectivity and three new vaccination classes for those who have had at least 4 previous pertussis vaccinations.

Demographic, epidemiological, and vaccination parameter values for these models have been estimated from data [24]. Most aspects of the computer simulations using the mathematical models are consistent with pertussis data since 1940. However, in contrast to the slow upward trend since 1976 in reported pertussis cases, the pertussis incidence in simulations with these models decreases very slowly after 1976 [24, 26]. This suggests that the observed upward trend does not reflect an increase in actual cases, but is due to some other factor such as an increase in the fraction of cases being reported. When the current vaccination program is continued in these simulations, the pertussis incidence continues at about the current level. This suggests that significant future changes would not be expected if the current pertussis vaccination program in children is continued.

Using the model simulations, childhood vaccinations reduce typical (full-disease or highest-infectivity) pertussis cases in children under 10 years of age by at least 99% [26]. In the simulations the typical cases among young children decrease after 1940 as vaccination levels increase and are replaced after 1960 by less severe disease, atypical cases with lower infectivity occurring in the removed and vaccinated classes. Hence childhood vaccinations prevent many severe pertussis infections in the early years of life, when the rates of infection complications are highest. In the simulations for both models, there are very modest (6% to 11%) reductions in the atypical (lower-disease or lower-infectivity) pertussis cases. This occurs because childhood vaccination prevents the early, typical, severe cases, but these children have less severe, atypical cases later when the vaccine-induced immunity wanes. Childhood vaccination tends to delay a person's first pertussis case, so that this first case is less severe. The simulation results are consistent with the concept that although pertussis vaccination provides only short term protection from infection, it does reduce the disease severity of a pertussis infection [22, 14, 15, 17, 31].

The simulations have shown that vaccination programs lead to some reduction in the reservoir of pertussis infection in the community, but they do not lead to herd immunity. Thus a major benefit of pertussis vaccination is that it provides direct, temporary protection for vaccinated individuals against pertussis infections with more severe disease. In the 1940 to 2040 simulations, adults typically have several less severe-disease pertussis infections with lower infectivity during their lifetime. Thus an adult reservoir of infection occurs both before and after the childhood vaccination program starts. Since the childhood reservoir of infection decreases due to vaccination of children, the adult reservoir of infection becomes more important in the transmission of pertussis. This observation is consistent with the data showing that atypically infected mothers (or fathers) are now frequently the source of infections in their children [7, 14, 15, 23, 37]. In the simulations the pertussis vaccination program does not eliminate the community-exposure type of pertussis boosting. Because a pertussis infection with a less severe-disease case boosts the immunity of the person, a case with more severe-disease is less likely to occur.

3.3. Previous conceptual results: complete adult boosting. Computer simulations of both pertussis models have been used to obtain estimates of the potential effects of the addition of complete (100%) adult pertussis booster vaccinations every ten years starting at age ten years on pertussis incidence in both adults and children [26]. In simulations with both models, when complete adult boosting is suddenly added in the year 2000, the incidence drops down from being nearly at an equilibrium and has a damped oscillatory approach to a new lower equilibrium. With complete adult boosting in the current pertussis model (the second model in [26]), pertussis cases at the new equilibrium are 41% lower in those at least 10 years of age and are 20% lower in those under age 10 years. In the current model, people who have been vaccinated or have had pertussis never lose all of their immunity and become fully susceptible. Thus in the simulations with childhood vaccinations, typical, severe cases in adults are rare and nearly all cases are atypical with lower severity. The addition of complete adult boosting decreases the adult reservoir of infection, but it does not lead to herd immunity. In simulations with the current model, the percentage of cases due to adults over age 18 decreases from 43% with only vaccination of children to 33% with the addition of complete adult boosting every ten years, which is about the same as the 34% of cases due to adults in the prevaccine era.

The simulations suggest that adult boosting would be moderately successful in reducing the number or severity of atypical cases in adults (41% reduction). But the simulations warn that complete adult boosting may be relatively unsuccessful in reducing the pertussis incidence in infants and children (only 20% reduction). As noted in Section 4.2, achieving 100% compliance with a recommendation for adult pertussis booster vaccinations is unrealistically optimistic, so achieving the reductions above is very unlikely. It was hoped that adult booster doses would cause a large decrease in pertussis cases in young children, so the relatively small decreases in the simulations are somewhat disappointing. But the simulations have provided another example of the concept that when the vaccine used gives only temporary immunity, a vaccination program does not have much effect on transmission in the population. Thus a primary benefit of pertussis vaccination of children or adults is the direct, temporary protection of those who are vaccinated.

3.4. Sensitivity to changes in parameter values. The sensitivity to parameter value changes has also been evaluated for the current pertussis model [26]. The general patterns are not sensitive to changes in the demographic assumptions and parameters. The results are also insensitive to changes in most of the epidemiological parameters. For example, changes in the mean infectious period are balanced by compensating changes in the contact matrix, since the contact matrix is determined from the forces of infection. Changes in some parameters lead to quantitative changes, but the general patterns are similar. For example, if the waiting times in the removed classes are doubled from 5 to 10 years, then protection given by an infection lasts longer. In this case the average lifetime numbers of typical and atypical cases decrease by about 1/3, but the overall patterns are the same and the effects of childhood and adult booster vaccinations are similar to those using the 5 year waiting times. The results are quantitatively somewhat sensitive to changes in the relative infectivities and the forces of infection, but the qualitative patterns are not changed.

The results are sensitive to changes in some vaccination parameter values, but are insensitive to other changes. If the mean waiting times in the vaccinated classes are changed from 2 years to 4 years, then vaccination provides longer protection. In this case vaccination programs decrease both typical and atypical cases by about twice as much. In particular, adult boosting is more effective in reducing cases in both adults and children. If the frequency of adult boosting is changed from 10 to 5 years, then the effects of complete adult boosting are greater with lower incidences in adults, but there are still only modest decreases in cases in children. Of course, from a practical point of view, 100% adult boosting every five years is not achievable. Decreases in the fraction of adults boosted in an adult vaccination program lead to similar decreases in effectiveness. For example, if only 60% of adults are given booster vaccinations every ten years instead of the complete adult boosting considered in [26], then the decreases would be only about 60% as large. Adult boosting every ten years with 60% coverage is considered as the first new vaccination strategy in Section 4.2.

The fraction successfully immunized is the product of the vaccine efficacy and the vaccination coverage, so that changes in the vaccine efficacy have the same effects as the corresponding changes in the vaccination coverage. If the vaccine efficacy or the vaccination coverages for each of the five childhood vaccinations is decreased by 10 percent (for example, the vaccine efficacy could go from 0.9 down to 0.81), then in the simulations with the current model there are more highest-infectivity, typical cases in children and increases of about 4% in the total incidences in 2000. Because one might expect the vaccine efficacy or vaccination level to be very important, this relative insensitivity to changes in these vaccination-related parameters is surprising. One reason is that the lower-disease cases in adults serve as a reservoir of infection that guarantees the persistence of pertussis. Another reason is that the redundancy due to successive childhood vaccinations at five different ages makes the fraction immunized successfully at each age less important. The simulations would be more sensitive to these vaccination-related parameters if there were fewer childhood vaccinations. An increase of 3% in the childhood vaccination coverages at each of the five ages leads to slightly fewer typical, severe-disease cases in children, but has very little effect on the total incidences and the percentage changes. More details on sensitivity are given in [26].

3.5. Previous conceptual results: oscillatory incidence. Reported cases of pertussis in the United States have oscillated cyclically with a period of about 4 years since data was collected starting in 1922 [18, 29]. This irregular oscillatory behavior of pertussis incidence in the United States has been investigated using the mechanisms of seasonality and environmental stochasticity in an age-structured pertussis model [25]. The mathematical model and computer simulations of pertussis transmission were used to study subharmonic resonance and stochastic perturbations as possible sources of the oscillations in pertussis incidence. Because seasonal (i.e. one year period) contact rates in models for measles led to subharmonic oscillations with a period of two years, it was expected that a seasonal contact rate in the pertussis model would lead to similar multiple-year oscillations, but this did not occur since the resulting oscillations in incidences in the computer simulations always had a period of one year. But 2% yearly stochasticity in the contact rate in the pertussis simulation model did lead to irregular oscillations with a 4 year period and a magnitude consistent with the reported pertussis data [25]. Hence a yearly random contact rate factor in the interval [0.98,1.02] due to weather, imported cases, or other causes is a possible explanation for the observed oscillating pertussis incidence in the United States.

4. Simulations using the current pertussis model. The childhood vaccination program started in 1940 is simulated first, and then each of the four new vaccination strategies for adolescents and adults is added in the year 2000 in a separate computer simulation.

4.1. Simulations of the childhood vaccination program. Conceptual results related to childhood vaccination are presented in Section 3.2. Here some quantitative effects of childhood vaccination using the current pertussis simulation model are given in order to facilitate comparison with the three new vaccination strategies for adults. A computer simulation with the estimated parameter values has been used to approximate the spread of pertussis from 1940 to 2040 using the estimated vaccination coverage for children. The solid lines in Figure 2 show the total incidence per year, the incidences of atypical cases for those in the removed classes and in the vaccinated classes, and the severe, typical-case incidences of those in the susceptible class S. In 1940 the highest-infectivity, typical incidence in the susceptible class is 0.99 times the annual birth rate, so that almost every child has a serious pertussis infection. Moreover, the lower-infectivity (high, medium and low) cases are 5.06 times the annual birth rate, so that in the prevaccine era people have an average of about 5 milder, atypical cases of pertussis during their lifetime. The largest changes in incidences occur between 1940 and 1960 as the vaccination coverage increases rapidly. In 2000 there are about 0.003 typical, highest-infectivity cases and about 4.5 atypical, lower-infectivity cases per person during their lifetime.

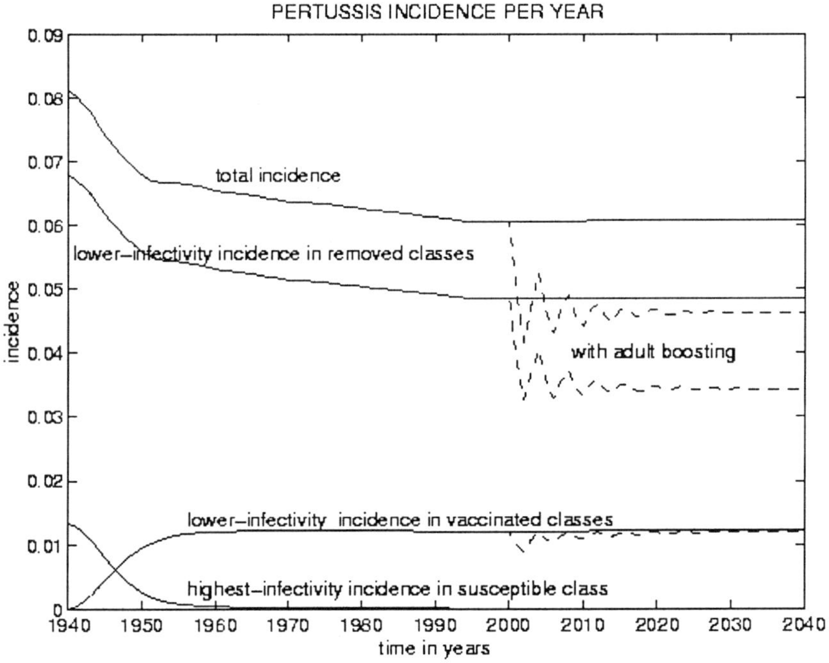

FIG. 2. *Pertussis incidences per year using the simulation model with the baseline parameter set (solid lines) and with the addition of 60% adult boosting (dashed lines). Incidences are given as a fraction of the total population.*

As the vaccination coverage increases, the total incidence decreases, and the atypical-disease, lower-infectivity incidence decreases in the removed classes R_1, R_2, and R_3 and increases in the vaccinated classes V_1, V_2, V_3, W_1, W_2, and W_3. The large decrease in the typical-disease, highest-infectivity cases is primarily due to the decrease in severe, typical cases in children. It is not surprising that the vaccination program would have the largest impact on children, because they are the group being given direct temporary protection by vaccination. Most of the children with typical cases in 1940 are replaced in 2000 by vaccinated children who have atypical cases, so that the total high-, medium- and low-infectivity, atypical cases in the removed and vaccinated classes decrease by only 11% between 1940 and 2000. The incidences remain almost constant after the year 2000 and rapidly approach an epidemiologic equilibrium, because the vaccination coverage does not change after 1995. At this equilibrium in 2040, the total incidence per year is 25% less than before vaccination. Although the total incidence has not changed drastically, the composition has changed, so that the typical-disease, highest-infectivity incidence is nearly zero, and nearly all cases are milder, atypical cases with lower infectivity.

The model used here is called the second pertussis model in [26]. More details about the simulations of the vaccination of children using this model are given in Sections 5 and 6 and in Figures 7–10 in [26]. Simulations with this model between the years 2000 and 2040 have been done with complete (100%) adult boosting every ten years starting at age 10 years. In contrast to the first model in [26], the current model does not have any removed or vaccinated people returning to the susceptible class, so that there are no older susceptibles who could get a highest-infectivity, typical case. Note that adult boosting has a larger impact in this model, because it uses a more optimistic mechanism for boosting than used in the first model considered in [26].

4.2. Simulations with the four new vaccination strategies. If adolescent and/or adult pertussis booster vaccinations were recommended, what fraction would follow the recommendations and obtain the pertussis booster vaccinations? Currently, a tetanus-diphtheria (Td) booster vaccination is recommended every ten years in the United States. National Health Interview Survey estimates of the percentages of adults in the age groups 18–64 and over 65 years, who received a tetanus-diphtheria (Td) booster within the past ten years, are 56% and 29% in 1991, 61% and 34% in 1993, and 56% and 28% in 1994 [34]. One goal of the Healthy People 2000 project is to have at least 62% of adults receive a Td booster within the last ten years. The data suggest that 100% compliance with recommendations for adult booster vaccinations is very unlikely. If the acellular pertussis booster vaccinations were combined with the Td boosters, then it seems that only about 60% of adults would receive these TdaP booster vaccinations. Indeed, the achievable vaccination levels using any vaccination program for adolescents and adults might be only about 60%. Hence 60% vaccination rates are used in the separate simulations for the four new adult vaccination strategies. The lifetime average number of cases per person and the percentage changes achieved by the simulations of these four vaccination strategies are presented in Table 1.

TABLE 1
The lifetime average number of cases per person from simulations of pertussis vaccination programs.

vaccination strategy	typ<10	atyp<10	tot<10	typ>10	atyp>10	tot>10	typ-all	atyp-all
no vaccination (1940)	0.92	0.56	1.48	0.07	4.50	4.57	0.99	5.06
year 2000 with childhood vaccination	0.0029	1.06	1.06	0.0003	3.46	3.46	0.0032	4.52
% change with childhood vaccination	-99.7%	+88.8%	-28.4%	-99.6%	-23.0%	-24.1%	-99.7%	-10.6%
year 2040 with 60% adult boosting	0.0024	0.93	0.93	0.00002	2.52	2.52	0.0024	3.45
% change with 60% adult boosting	-18.1%	-12.1%	-12.1%	-44.9%	-27.3%	-27.3%	-18.4%	-23.8%
year 2040 with 60% age 12 boosting	0.0028	1.03	1.04	0.00003	3.29	3.29	0.0028	4.32
% change with 60% age 12 boosting	-3.7%	-2.3%	-2.3%	-26.5%	-5.2%	-5.2%	-4.0%	-4.6%
year 2040 with 60% age 20 boosting	0.0028	1.03	1.03	0.00003	3.26	3.26	0.0028	4.29
% change with 60% age 20 boosting	-4.2%	-2.7%	-2.7%	-8.2%	-6.1%	-6.1%	-4.3%	-5.3%
year 2040 with 60% age 50 boosting	0.0028	1.04	1.04	0.00004	3.32	3.32	0.0029	4.36
% change with 60% age 50 boosting	-2.6%	-1.6%	-1.6%	+0.8%	-4.3%	-4.3%	-2.6%	-3.7%

Abbreviations: typ is typical cases (highest infectivity), atyp is atypical cases (high, medium, and low infectivity), tot is total cases, <10 is ages 1–9 years, >10 is ages 10 or more years, all means all ages.

The first new vaccination strategy is the addition of pertussis booster vaccinations every ten years starting at age 10 years. This simulation has an addition in the year 2000 of booster vaccinations with 60% vaccination coverage at the ages 10, 20, 30, ..., 90 years. Hereafter this is called 60% adult boosting. The results of the pertussis vaccination simulations with the first new vaccination strategy are presented as dashed lines in Figure 2. When 60% adult boosting every ten years is suddenly added in 2000, the incidences quickly move down from the 1999 incidences and have a damped oscillatory behavior with a period of about 4 years as they approach a new equilibrium. The childhood vaccination program has eliminated most typical pertussis cases, but 60% adult boosting between the years 2000 and 2040 causes an 18% decrease in typical cases under age 10 years and a 45% decrease in typical cases above age 10 years for an overall 18% decrease in typical cases from the level in the year 2000. The atypical cases decrease by 12% in those under age 10 years and by 27% in those above age 10 years for an overall 24% decrease in atypical cases from the level in the year 2000. These decreases are consistent with the direct protection of adults by vaccination. With 60% adult boosting, people in 2040 have a lifetime average of about 3.5 atypical pertussis infections, which is lower than the 4.5 atypical cases when only children are vaccinated.

The second new vaccination strategy involves the pertussis booster vaccination of 60% of adolescents at age 12 years. When this new vaccination strategy is introduced in the year 2000, the incidences drop down slightly and exhibit a damped oscillatory approach towards an equilibrium. The decreases due to this boosting of 60% of 12 year old adolescents are smaller than those for 60% adult boosting shown in Figure 2, but this is expected since only one booster dose is given instead of many booster doses. As listed in Table 1, in the year 2040 there is a 3.7% decrease in typical cases under age 10 years and a 26% decrease in typical cases above age 10 years for an overall 4.0% decrease below the level in the year 2000. Atypical cases decrease by 2.3% in those under age 10 years and by 5.2% in those above age 10 years for an overall 4.6% decrease from the level in the year 2000. With 60% boosting of 12 year old children, people in 2040 have a lifetime average of about 4.32 atypical pertussis infections, which is slightly lower than the 4.52 atypical cases when only children are vaccinated. Although the percentage decreases are relatively small, they are due to only one booster dose instead of the many booster doses used for the 60% adult boosting.

The third new vaccination strategy is 60% booster vaccinations for 20 year old adults. The results of adding this booster plan in the year 2000 are slightly larger, but similar to those when the boosting of 12 year old adolescents is added. In this case typical pertussis cases decrease by 4.2% in those under age 10 years and decrease by 8.2% in those above age 10 years for an overall 4.3% decrease in typical cases. There is a 2.7% decrease in atypical cases under age 10 years and a 6.1% decrease in atypical cases above age 10 years for an overall 5.3% decrease in atypical cases. With 60% boosting of 20 year old adults, there are a lifetime average of about 4.29 atypical pertussis infections, as compared with the 4.52 atypical cases with childhood vaccination.

The fourth new vaccination strategy is 60% booster vaccinations for 50 year old adults. The results of adding this booster plan in the year 2000 are smaller, but similar to those when the boosting of 12 year old adolescents or 20 year old young adults is added. In this case typical cases decrease by 2.6% in those under age 10 years and increase slightly in those above age 10 years for an overall 2.6% decrease from the level in the year 2000. There is a 1.6% decrease in atypical cases under age 10 years and a 4.3% decrease in atypical cases above age 10 years for an overall 3.7% decrease in typical cases below the level in the year 2000. With 60% boosting of 50 year old adults, there are a lifetime average of about 4.36 atypical pertussis infections, as compared with the 4.52 atypical cases when only children are vaccinated. Again the percentage decreases for this one booster dose strategy are relatively small.

5. Discussion of the four new vaccination strategies. The effects of childhood vaccination and the four additional vaccination strategies for adolescents and adults with 60% coverage are summarized in Table 1. Although the decreases in total cases in the age groups below and above 10 years due to childhood vaccinations are only 24% to 28%, the table shows very clearly that the childhood vaccination program has nearly eliminated the typical, severe-disease cases. As described in Section 3.2 on conceptual results, childhood vaccination seems to replace typical, severe-disease cases in children with later atypical, milder-symptom cases. Although the four new vaccination programs lead to percentage changes in typical cases between +0.8% and -44.9% in Table 1, the absolute changes in typical cases are small. Since typical cases are rare, it is better to judge the three new vaccination strategies by their effects on the atypical cases.

It may seem surprising that any adult vaccination could lead to an increase of 0.8% in typical cases in those at least 10 years of age, but this can be explained. Vaccination at age 50 years does give temporary immunity to some 50 year old adults, which would tend to lower the number of typical cases in those over age 10 years. But vaccination of 50 year old adults also decreases the forces of infection, which would increase the average age of infection and increase the number of typical cases in those at least 10 years old. With the 60% boosting at age 50 years, the latter factor dominates the former, so there is a slight 0.8% increase in typical cases in those at least 10 years of age.

In the simulations with single booster vaccinations given with 60% coverage as shown in Table 1, vaccinations of 20 year old adults are slightly more effective in reducing typical and atypical cases than vaccinations at age 12 years. This may seem counterintuitive. Because 12 year old adolescents have more contacts through their schools, preventing infections in this age group should have a greater impact. In the simulations 12 year old adolescents do have a higher contact activity level than 20 year old adults; the multiplying factors $l_j/D^{1/2}$ in the contact matrix are 0.5841 and 0.3505 for 12 and 20 year old people, respectively [26]. From these values it would seem that vaccinating 12 year old adolescents would be more effective in reducing incidences than vaccinating 20 year old adults. But the higher activity level of 12 year old adolescents implies that they have more contacts and more opportunities to have their immunity boosted by an infection than 20 year old adults. Thus in the simulation modeling with only childhood vaccination, the average immunity level is higher for those of age 12 years than those of age 20 years. Since the average immunity level is lower for 20 year old adults, vaccination would have a larger impact on those of age 20 years than those of age 12 years. Thus vaccination of 20 year old adults causes larger decreases in the community forces of infection and hence larger decreases in the incidences and lifetime average numbers of cases. Thus the originally surprising result that vaccinations are slightly more effective at age 20 years than at age 12 years is now understandable. The useful conceptual result here is that the effectiveness of vaccination in an age group depends on three factors: 1) the achievable coverage in that age group, 2) the contact activity level of that group, and 3) the average immunity level in that group. In the comparisons above with 60% coverage in the simulations, the average immunity level at age 20 is significantly lower than at age 12 years. Thus the third factor dominates the second factor, so that vaccination is more effective at age 20 years than at age 12 years. Of course, the vaccination coverage that is actually achievable at the two ages is also a factor. In the simulations, vaccination at age 12 years with a coverage above 70% is more effective in reducing pertussis incidences than vaccination at age 20 years with 60% coverage.

As shown in the comparisons with 60% coverage in Table 1, the vaccination of younger people at ages 12 or 20 years are both more effective than vaccination of 50 year old adults. This is plausible because the younger people have higher contact activity levels and larger contact matrix entries than people of age 50 years; in the simulations the multiplying factor $l_j/D^{1/2}$ in the contact matrix is 0.2336 for 50 year old people [26]. With 60% coverage for adult boosting every ten years starting at age 10 years, the lifetime average number of vaccinations per ten year old is 0.6×6.6, which is about 6.6 times the average number of vaccinations when one booster vaccination is given to 60% of 12 year old adolescents or 20 year old adults. But adult boosting every 10 years starting at age 10 years is only about 4 or 5 times as effective in reducing atypical cases as one booster vaccination at age 12 or 20 years. This is reasonable, because booster vaccinations for younger people with more contacts and larger contact matrix entries often cause larger decreases in the community forces of infection than booster vaccinations of older people with fewer contacts and lower contact matrix entries. In this case the second factor in the conceptual result in the previous paragraph dominates the third factor in the simulations. Thus the conceptual result is that booster vaccinations in adolescents and adults are generally more effective per vaccination when they are given to younger people who have more opportunities for transmission.

Based on a cost list distributed at a 1996 CDC Vaccine Economics Conference and inflation, the acellular pertussis vaccines would now cost about $20 per dose. The average cost for administering each vaccine dose would be about $10, so that the total cost of one acellular pertussis vaccination would be about $30. The number of people of ages 10, 20, 30, ... 90 years in the United States is about 23.8 million [33], so that vaccination of 60% of them at $30 per vaccination would cost about $428 million per year. The number of 12 year old adolescents, 20 year old adults and 50 year old adults are about 3.7 million, 3.8 million, and 2.7 million, respectively [33], so that vaccination with 60% coverage at these three ages would cost about $67 million, $68 million, and $49 million per year, respectively.

A crucial question is whether the reductions in typical and atypical cases using these four new vaccination programs would justify these significant annual expenditures for vaccinations. Using data on medical costs such as outpatient visits, emergency room visits, hospitalizations and deaths, and work-loss costs of the infectives or their parents, health economists could estimate the average cost per typical and atypical case in the age groups. These estimates could be combined with the simulation estimates of the reductions in typical and atypical cases for the four new vaccination strategies to compute the total savings for each of the new vaccination programs. Then the vaccination cost estimates in the previous paragraph could be compared with the dollar estimates of the savings due to prevented pertussis cases in a cost-benefit analysis of the four new vaccination strategies.

Acknowledgments. The author thanks Drs. Melinda Wharton, John Glasser, and Donald Ekwueme at the National Immunization Program, Centers for Disease Control for valuable information and discussions.

REFERENCES

[1] Anderson R.M. and May R.M. *Infectious Diseases of Humans: Dynamics and Control.* Oxford: Oxford University Press, 1991.

[2] Benenson, A.S. *Control of Communicable Diseases in Man, Sixteenth Edition.* Washington, D.C.: American Public Health Association, 1995.

[3] Biellik R.J., Patriarca P.A., Mullen J.R., et al. Risk factors for community- and household-acquired pertussis during a large-scale outbreak in central Wisconsin. *J Infect Dis* **157**:1134–41 (1988).

[4] Centers for Disease Control and Prevention. Pertussis surveillance-United States, 1989–1991, In: *CDC Surveillance Summaries,* December 11, 1992. *MMWR* **41**:11–20 (1992).

[5] Centers for Disease Control and Prevention, Pertussis outbreaks—Massachusetts and Maryland, 1992, *MMWR* **42**:197–200 (1993).
[6] Centers for Disease Control and Prevention. Resurgence of Pertussis-United States, 1993. *MMWR* **42**:952–960 (1993).
[7] Centers for Disease Control and Prevention. Transmission of Pertussis from Adult to Infant-Michigan, 1993. *MMWR* **44**:74–76 (1995).
[8] Centers for Disease Control and Prevention. Pertussis-United States, January 1992-June 1995. *MMWR* **44**:526–529 (1995).
[9] Centers for Disease Control and Prevention. Table II. Cases of selected notifiable diseases, United States. *MMWR* **45**:23–25 (1996).
[10] Centers for Disease Control and Prevention. Tables I and III. Provisional cases of selected notifiable diseases, United States. *MMWR* **46**:1262–1264 (1998).
[11] Centers for Disease Control and Prevention. Recommended Childhood Immunization Schedule-United States, 1998. *MMWR* **47**:8–12 (1998).
[12] Cherry J.D., Baraff L.J., and Hewlett E. The past, present and future of pertussis. *West. J. Med.* **150**:319–328 (1989).
[13] Cherry J.D. Acellular pertussis vaccines: A solution to the pertussis problem. *J. Inf. Dis.* **168**:21–24 (1993).
[14] Deen J.L., Mink C.A.M., Cherry J.D., et al. Household contact study of *Bordetella Pertussis* infections. *Clin. Inf. Dis.* **21**:1211–1219 (1995).
[15] Deville J.G., Cherry J.D., Christenson P.D., et al. Frequency of unrecognized *Bordetella Pertussis* infections in adults. *Clin. Inf. Dis.* **21**:639–642 (1995).
[16] Edwards K.M., Decker M.D., Graham B.S., et al. Adult immunization with acellular pertussis vaccine. *JAMA* **269**:53–56 (1993).
[17] Fackelmann K. 100-day cough. *Science News* **150**:46–47 (1996).
[18] Farizo K.M., Cochi S.L., Zell E.R., et al. Epidemiological features of pertussis in the United States, 1980–1989. *Clin. Infect. Dis.* **14**:708–719 (1992).
[19] Greco, M.D., Salmaso D., Mastrantonio P., et. al. A controlled trial of two acellular vaccines and one whole-cell vaccine against pertussis. *New Engl. J. Med.* **334**:341–348 (1996).
[20] Gordon J.E. and Hood R.I. Whooping cough and its epidemiological anomalies. *Am. J. Med. Sci.* **222**:333–361 (1951).
[21] Gustafsson L., Hallander H.O., Olin P. et al. A controlled trial of a two-component accellular, a five-component acellular, and a whole-cell pertussis vaccine. *New Engl. J. Med.* **334**:349–355 (1996).
[22] He Q., Viljanen M.K., Nikkari S., et al. Outcomes of bordetella pertussis infection in different age groups of an immunized population. *J. Infect. Dis.* **170**:873–877 (1994).
[23] Herwaldt L.A. Pertussis in adults: What physicians need to know. *Arch. Intern. Med.* **109**:1510–1512 (1991).
[24] Hethcote, H.W. An age-structured model for pertussis transmission. *Math. Biosci.* **145**:89–136 (1997).
[25] Hethcote, H.W. Oscillations in an endemic model for pertussis. *Canad. Appl. Math. Quart.* **6**:61–88 (1998).
[26] Hethcote, H.W. Simulations of pertussis epidemiology in the United States: Effects of adult booster vaccinations. *Math. Biosci.* **158**:47–73 (1999).
[27] von Konig C.H.W., Postels-Multani S., Bock H.L., et al. Pertussis in adults: Frequency of transmission after household exposure. *Lancet* **346**:1326–1329 (1995).
[28] Mink, C.A.M., Cherry J.D., Christenson P., et al. A search for *Bordetella pertussis* infection in university students. *Clin. Inf. Dis.* **14**:464–471 (1992).
[29] Mortimer E.A. Pertussis and pertussis vaccines: 15 years of change. *Sem. Pediatr. Infect. Dis.* **2**:82–90 (1991).
[30] Nelson J.D. The changing epidemiology of pertussis in young infants. *Am. J. Dis. Child.* **132**:371–373 (1978).

[31] NENNIG, M.E. ET AL. Prevalence and incidence of adult pertussis in an urban population. *JAMA* **275**:1672–1674 (1996).
[32] SCHMITT-GROHE S., CHERRY J.D., HEININGER U., ET AL. Pertussis in German adults. *Clin. Inf. Dis.* **21**:860–866 (1995).
[33] U.S. Bureau of the Census, Statistical Abstract of the United States, 1994, Government Printing Office, Washington, D.C., 1994.
[34] STRIKAS, R.A. Current vaccination levels in adults: The influenza and pneumococcal vaccines and tetanus toxoid. In 29th National Immunization Conference Proceedings, Centers for Disease Control, 67–71 (1995).
[35] SUTTER R.W. AND COCHI S.L. Pertussis hospitalizations and mortality in the United States, 1985–1988: Evaluation of the completeness of national reporting. *JAMA* **267**:386–391 (1992).
[36] TROLLFORS B., TARANGER J., LAGERGARD T., ET AL. A placebo-controlled trial of a pertussis-toxoid vaccine. *New Eng. J. Med.* **333**:1045–1050 (1995).
[37] WRIGHT S.W., EDWARDS K.M., DECKER M.D., ET AL. Pertussis infection in adults with persistent cough. *JAMA* **273**:1044–1046 (1995).

TIME DELAY IN EPIDEMIC MODELS

P. VAN DEN DRIESSCHE*

Abstract. Time delays are often used to model mechanisms (e.g., the infectious period) in the dynamics of epidemics. Such models can be formulated as functional differential and/or integral equations. A flavor of the modeling process and the mathematical tools used in the analysis is given. The ideas are illustrated by an SIS model in a variable size population with a constant delay corresponding to the infectious period.

1. Introduction. This paper, which is based on a tutorial lecture given at the IMA on May 14, 1999, aims to introduce the reader to ways in which time delays can be used in modeling the dynamics of epidemics. It relies heavily on the work of the author and collaborators, and focuses on the model considered in [16]. For basic terminology used in mathematical epidemiology, the reader is referred to [4].

For the epidemic models considered here, the population size is assumed to be large enough to be adequately described by a deterministic description and is divided into compartments (classes) based on the disease status of individuals. The number of compartments included depends on the disease being modeled. It always includes susceptible and infectious compartments, with numbers in each denoted as functions of continuous time by $S(t)$ and $I(t)$, respectively. It may also include other compartments; for example, exposed, recovered and vaccinated, with numbers denoted by $E(t)$, $R(t)$ and $V(t)$, respectively. The total population $N(t)$ is the sum of the numbers in all compartments. In most classical models $N(t)$ is assumed to be constant, but this is not realistic if disease deaths or population changes are significant. Thus many recent models assume variable demographic structure; for example, exponential or logistic demography.

A common assumption for models of a nonfatal disease is that the time in the infectious compartment is exponentially distributed. Thus the recovery rate is taken proportional to $I(t)$, and the SIS models are formulated as ordinary differential equations (odes). However, for some diseases, it may be more realistic to assume a constant infectious period, with all individuals becoming susceptible again after a fixed infectious period. Such an assumption introduces a time delay into the model. These two assumptions may be regarded as extreme cases, but an intermediate distribution may be more realistic (see, e.g., [1, p. 60], [5]).

Time delays can also be used to model a period of temporary immunity (in a model including R), a latent period (in a model including E), or a maturation period ([9]). When time delay is included, the models are formulated as functional differential and/or integral equations. For example,

*Department of Math. and Stats., University of Victoria, Victoria, British Columbia, V8W 3P4 Canada. Research supported in part by an NSERC Research grant. pvdd@math.uvic.ca.

Cooke and van den Driessche [8] considered an $SEIRS$ model with exponential demography and both constant latent and immune periods. They showed equivalent formulations as an integro-differential equation system and as a differential difference equation system with given initial and integral conditions [8, Theorem 2.1]. With time delay, the mathematical analysis becomes more difficult than that of the analogous ode system, and in certain cases the qualitative dynamics may be different. For example, Hethcote et al. [15] considered a constant population $SIRS$ model with a constant period of temporary immunity and showed that (in contrast to the analogous ode system) the endemic equilibrium can lose stability via a Hopf bifurcation to locally asymptotically stable periodic solutions. Such periodic behavior has been observed in data from several diseases, e.g., childhood diseases, influenza, and sexually transmitted diseases (see, e.g., [14]).

Hethcote and van den Driessche [16] formulated and analyzed an SIS epidemic model with variable population size and a constant infectious period (giving a delay). This model is used to illustrate the general ideas discussed here. For more mathematical details, the reader is referred to [16], and for a survey of some other epidemiological models with delays to [23].

2. Assumptions and model formulation. When constructing an epidemic model it is essential to focus on the characteristics of the disease being modeled. The ideal model should be biologically realistic and mathematically tractable. In reality, simplifications have to be made and the basic assumptions need to be clearly stated. A literature search must be conducted to guide in the formulation; for example, the citations in this paper constitute such a search for the model to be presented.

Here a very simple SIS model is constructed for a disease that confers no immunity and occurs in a population of varying size. The model is for an infectious disease caused by a bacterium or virus and spread by direct contact between a susceptible and an infective. Since the focus is on the effect of delay, vertical transmission of disease is ignored, as is age structure, seasonal and spatial variation, different strains etc. Some models including vertical transmission and delay are considered in [3] and [6, Chapter 4].

The incidence of the disease (number of new cases per unit time) must be specified. Two commonly used incidence functions are usually called *mass action* incidence (proportional to SI) and *standard incidence* (proportional to SI/N). The latter is more consistent with data on many diseases (see, e.g., [10]) and is assumed here. Thus individuals leave the susceptible compartment at a rate $\lambda SI/N$, where $\lambda > 0$ is the effective per capita contact rate constant of infectives, that is the product of the average number of contacts of an individual per unit time and the probability of transmitting the disease during one contact by an infective. Some models assume a density dependent contact rate, e.g., an incidence term $\lambda(N)SI/N$, as in [2, 7, 25]; or a contact rate that is dependent on I, e.g., $\lambda(I)SI$, as in [24].

Since the disease confers no immunity, surviving infectious individuals return to the susceptible compartment upon recovery. Let $P(t)$ be the fraction of individuals remaining infectious t time units after infection (this can be thought of as the probability that an individual remains infectious at least t units before becoming susceptible again). $P(t)$ is assumed to be nonnegative and nonincreasing with $P(0^+) = 1$. The expected time of leaving the infectious class is denoted by ω, where $\omega = \int_0^\infty P(t)dt$ is assumed to be positive and finite.

Assumptions must also be made on the demographic process. Here an exponential demographic structure is assumed, with a birth rate constant $b > 0$. All newborns are assumed to be susceptible (no vertical transmission). Thus the rate of entry into the susceptible compartment is bN. Natural death occurs in the whole population, with $d \geq 0$ as the natural death rate constant. In addition there is disease related death in the infectious class, with rate constant $\epsilon \geq 0$. Demographic structures used in other models include constant inflow into the susceptible compartment [7, 12, 17], generalized logistic structure [2, 17, 25], and birth functions nonlinear in N [9].

Based on the above disease transmission and demographic assumptions, the total population, $N = S + I$, changes according to the ode

$$N'(t) = (b - d)N(t) - \epsilon I(t). \tag{1}$$

Thus for $b \neq d$ or $\epsilon \neq 0$, the total population varies. In the absence of disease ($I = 0$), the population grows or decays exponentially for $b > d$ or $b < d$, respectively. For $t \geq 0$, $I(t)$ is given by the integral equation that sums the number of initial infectives that are still infectious at time t (denoted by $I_0(t)$), and those individuals who became infectious at time u and have neither recovered nor died (represented by an integral). This equation is:

$$I(t) = I_0(t) + \int_0^t \lambda \frac{S(u)I(u)}{N(u)} P(t-u) \exp\{-(d+\epsilon)(t-u)\}du. \tag{2}$$

For a discussion of the assumptions needed on $I_0(t)$ see [17].

Making the common assumption of a negative exponential for $P(t)$, namely $P(t) = \exp(-\gamma t)$ with $\gamma = 1/\omega$, and $I_0(t) = I(0)\exp\{-(\gamma+d+\epsilon)t\}$, equation (2) becomes

$$I(t) = I(0)\exp\{-(\gamma+d+\epsilon)t\} + \int_0^t \frac{\lambda S(u)I(u)}{N(u)} \exp\{-(\gamma+d+\epsilon)(t-u)\}du.$$

Differentiating this gives

$$I'(t) = \frac{\lambda S(t)I(t)}{N(t)} - (\gamma + d + \epsilon)I(t). \tag{3}$$

With $S(t)$ replaced by $N(t) - I(t)$, equations (1) and (3) comprise the ode system governing the dynamics of the disease for the case of a negative exponential $P(t)$. This is a special case of a more general SIS model analyzed in [25, Section 5]. Results for this ode model are proved globally, all solutions approach equilibria and there are never any periodic solutions.

Here we concentrate on the special case of the step function for $P(t)$, namely $P(t) = 1$ for $0 \leq t \leq \omega$, and $P(t) = 0$ for $t > \omega$, where ω is the constant infectious period. When $t \geq \omega$ all initial infectives must have recovered or died, so differentiating (2) gives

$$(4)\quad I'(t) = \lambda \frac{S(t)I(t)}{N(t)} - \lambda \frac{S(t-\omega)I(t-\omega)}{N(t-\omega)} \exp\{-(d+\epsilon)\omega\} - (d+\epsilon)I(t).$$

With S replaced by $N - I$, the system (1) and (4) governs the change of the total population and number of infectives. It is convenient to shift time so that (4) holds for $t > 0$ with given initial conditions $I(t) \geq 0$ and $N(t) > \max\{0, I(t)\}$ on $[-\omega, 0]$.

In some models with varying population size and standard incidence, it is convenient to work with proportions in each compartment. Defining $s = S/N$ and $i = I/N$ gives $s + i = 1$ and equation (1) becomes

$$(5)\qquad N' = (b - d - \epsilon i(t))N(t).$$

This can be integrated to

$$(6)\qquad N(t) = N(0)\exp\{(b-d)t - \epsilon \int_0^t i(p)dp\},$$

showing that N remains positive for $t \geq 0$. Using proportions, for $t \geq \omega$ (so that $i_0(t) = I_0(t)/N(t) = 0$) equation (2) gives

$$(7)\qquad i(t) = \int_{t-\omega}^{t} \lambda(1 - i(u))i(u)\exp\{-(b+\epsilon)(t-u) + \epsilon \int_u^t i(p)dp\}du,$$

where s has been replaced by $1 - i$ and N has been replaced by (6). Equations (6) and (7), which depends only on i, give an integral formulation of the model. Similarly, (4) gives

$$(8)\qquad \begin{aligned} i'(t) &= \lambda(1 - i(t))i(t) - (b+\epsilon)i(t) + \epsilon i^2(t) \\ &\quad -\lambda(1 - i(t-\omega))i(t-\omega)\exp\{-(b+\epsilon)\omega + \epsilon \int_{t-\omega}^{t} i(p)dp\}. \end{aligned}$$

This scalar delay integro-differential equation has been obtained from a very simple SIS model and illustrates the mathematical complexity introduced by a time delay. If the disease does not cause death ($\epsilon = 0$), then (8) reduces to a delay differential equation. Note that the natural death rate constant d does not occur in (7) or (8), rather it has been replaced by the birth rate constant b. The term $b+\epsilon$ can be regarded as giving a dilution of infectives.

To validate the model formulation, it is necessary to show that there exists a unique, continuous, nonnegative solution for all $t \geq 0$. For delay differential equations, this can usually be done by appealing to standard results, see, e.g., the book by Hale and Verduyn Lunel [13, Chapter 2]. For integral equations, results in the book by Miller [20, Chapter 2] can usually be used. For our illustrative SIS model, using (7), existence and uniqueness follow from results in [20]. Also it can be shown that if $1 > i_0(0) > 0$, then $1 > i(t) > 0$ for all finite $t \geq 0$. Thus solutions are biologically meaningful.

At this stage (or even earlier) it is also good to formulate some questions about the model. For example, what is the qualitative effect of the time delay, what is the interaction of the disease and the demographics, and is there a threshold parameter that is important in controlling the disease? More specifically, do all solutions approach constant values or are periodic solutions possible? If more complicated dynamics are possible, then do they occur for realistic parameter values? Most of these questions will be addressed for our illustrative SIS model.

3. Equilibria and threshold. To begin the analysis and address some of the questions posed, equilibria (i.e., constant solutions) are considered. For delay differential equations this means setting the derivatives to zero. The existence of positive equilibria is often governed by a threshold parameter such that there are no positive equilibria when this parameter is below a threshold value. In some models, multiple endemic equilibria can exist, leading to the possibility of backward bifurcation or hysteresis (see e.g., [24]).

For our SIS model, an important threshold parameter θ is defined as

$$\theta = \frac{\lambda(1-\exp\{-(b+\epsilon)\omega\})}{b+\epsilon}. \tag{9}$$

From (8) it follows that the disease free proportion equilibrium (DFE), namely $i=0$, is always a solution. Also for $i \neq 0$, an equilibrium of (8) satisfies

$$F(s) = 1 - \frac{\lambda s}{b+\epsilon s}(1-\exp\{-(b+\epsilon s)\omega\}) = 0. \tag{10}$$

Since $F'(s) < 0$, $F(s)$ is a decreasing function on $[0,1]$ with $F(0)=1$ and $F(1) = 1-\theta$. Thus there is a unique equilibrium with $0 < s^* < 1$ if and only if $\theta > 1$. The endemic equilibrium i value is then given by $i^* = 1 - s^*$ with $0 < i^* < 1$.

The threshold parameter θ is the product of the contact rate constant λ and the expected time in the i compartment during one passage. It is related to the usual basic reproduction number

$$R_0 = \frac{\lambda(1 - \exp\{-(d+\epsilon)\omega\})}{d+\epsilon}, \tag{11}$$

which is the average number of new infectives produced by one infective in the limiting situation of a fully susceptible population [1, p. 17]. Since in general $b \neq d$, it follows that $\theta \neq R_0$, so θ is referred to as a modified reproduction number. For ϵ positive, i^* cannot be evaluated explicitly; but for $\epsilon = 0$, $i^* = 1 - 1/\theta$. Note that i^* depends on the delay ω; when $\epsilon = 0$ this can be seen from (9).

4. Stability. Local asymptotic stability of an equilibrium is governed by linearization (assuming sufficient differentiability) of the model equations about this equilibrium. The zero solution of the nonlinear system is asymptotically stable if and only if the zero solution of the linear system is asymptotically stable. Assuming an exponential dependence on time, this linearization leads to a characteristic equation that is a quasipolynomial (cf. a polynomial equation that is obtained from an analogous ode model). Standard theory (see, e.g., [13, Appendix], [6, Section 4.7.2]) can sometimes be used to determine the signs of the real parts of roots of the characteristic equation. However, when coefficients in the characteristic equation depend on the delay, care must be taken in using standard results, and often new results must be developed (see, e.g., [16, Appendix]).

For example, in our *SIS* model, retaining only terms linear in i in (8) and assuming that i is proportional to $\exp(zt)$ gives the characteristic equation for the DFE as

$$z + b + \epsilon = \lambda(1 - \exp\{-(z+b+\epsilon)\omega\}). \tag{12}$$

If $\theta > 1$, then it can be seen geometrically that this equation has a positive root, thus the DFE is unstable. Assuming $\theta < 1$ and writing (12) in an equivalent integral form, it can be shown that all roots have negative real parts, thus the DFE is locally asymptotically stable.

Linearizing about i^* (the endemic equilibrium) results in a complicated characteristic equation of the form

$$Q_2(z) + Q_1(z)(1 - \exp\{-(z+q)\omega\}) = 0, \tag{13}$$

where $Q_j(z)$ is of degree j with coefficients depending on i^*, and q also depends on i^* ([16, (5.3)]). Recall that in general i^* is not known explicitly, and that it depends on the delay. When there is no disease related death ($\epsilon = 0$), a continuity argument is used to show that all roots of the characteristic equation (13) have negative real parts for $\theta > 1$. It thus appears that in the absence of disease related death there is a sharp threshold; if $\theta < 1$, then i tends to the DFE, if $\theta > 1$, then i tends to the endemic equilibrium with the disease persisiting in the population.

To verify the above statement, global stability results are needed. For delay differential equations, these are often difficult to find, and/or can be found only for a limited parameter range. For some models, Lyapunov type theorems or Razumikhim type theorems can be used; these are described in [13, Sections 5.3, 5.4] and [18, Sections 2.5, 2.6]. The former method was used to prove that below a threshold all solutions of an $SIRS$ model with exponential demographics and a constant immune period approach the disease free proportion equilibrium [8, Section 6], and the latter method was used to prove global asymptotic stability of the DFE of an $SEIRS$ model with recruitment-death demographics and both constant latent and immune periods [12, Theorem 2.3]. When the model can be transformed to a scalar intego-differential equation, a result of Londen [19] can sometimes be used to prove global convergence to the endemic equilibrium (for parameter values such that it exists). For example, Stech and Williams [21] used this result for a constant population $SIRS$ model. Following this work, the result was used for a variable population $SIRS$ model with a distributed length of the immune period and no disease fatality [7, Section 3.5], and for an $SIRS$ model including disease fatality [22].

For our SIS model, a difference equation argument can be used to show that if $\epsilon\omega \leq \theta \leq 1$, then the DFE is globally asymptotically stable ([16, Theorem 4.2]). As suggested by A. Ivanov, this result can be improved to give the following stronger result.

THEOREM 1. *If $\theta \leq 1$ and $\epsilon\omega \leq 1$, then the DFE of (7) is globally aymptotically stable.*

Proof. Consider the difference equation

$$r_{n+1} = \theta r_n(1 - r_n)\exp(\epsilon\omega r_n) = f(r_n) \tag{14}$$

for $r_n \in [0,1]$. Since $f(0) = 0$, there is an equilibrium at $r = 0$. For nonzero equilibria, consider

$$g(r_n) = \theta(1 - r_n)\exp(\epsilon\omega r_n) - 1, \tag{15}$$

for $r_n \in [0,1]$. Since $g(0) = \theta - 1 \leq 0$ for $\theta \leq 1$, $g'(0) = \theta(\epsilon\omega - 1) \leq 0$ and $g''(r_n) \leq 0$ for $\epsilon\omega \leq 1$, there are no nonzero equilibria. Thus $r = 0$ is the only equilibrium. From above $g(r_n) \leq 0$, implying that $r_{n+1} \leq r_n$ and thus $\lim_{n\to\infty} r_n = 0$. Now as in [16, Theorem 4.2], let $M = \max_{0\leq r\leq 1} f(r)$, then from (7)

$$i(t) \leq \frac{M}{\theta}\int_{t-\omega}^{t} \lambda \exp\{-(b+\epsilon)(t-u)\}du = M = r_1$$

for $t \geq \omega$. Continuation of this argument yields $i(t) \leq r_n$ for $t \geq n\omega$, showing that $\lim_{t\to\infty} i(t) = 0$. □

In the case of no disease related death the above result proves global asymptotic stability of the DFE for the full range $0 < \theta \leq 1$. Global stability of the endemic equlilibrium is an open problem.

For $\theta > 1$ and $\epsilon > 0$, examination of the characteristic equation (13) shows that there are no purely imaginary roots for $i^* < 2/3$ and such an endemic equilibrium is locally asymptotically stable. For $i^* > 2/3$, the possibility of roots of (13) crossing the imaginary axis cannot be ruled out. Thus the analysis leaves open the possibility that for certain parameter values a pair of pure imaginary roots can give rise to periodic solutions through Hopf bifurcation; but this has not been proved. For delay differential equation versions of the Hopf bifurcation theorem see, e.g., [6, Theorem 4.8], [13, p. 332] and [18, p. 60].

When $\theta > 1$ and i approaches the endemic equilibrium i^*, then (5) is asymptotically equivalent to $N' = (b - d - \epsilon i^*)N$; see [7]. Thus for $\epsilon = 0$, the population grows or decays for the growth rate constant $b-d$ positive or negative, respectively. For $\epsilon > 0$, the disease influences the demographics, with the population growing or decaying exponentially for $b-d-\epsilon i^*$ positive or negative, respectively. As suggested by H.W. Hethcote, the conditions can be written independently of i^* in terms of a parameter ψ, where ψ is defined as

$$\psi = \frac{b-d}{\epsilon} + \frac{1}{R_0}. \tag{16}$$

THEOREM 2. *When $\theta > 1$, $\epsilon > 0$ and solutions of (8) approach the endemic equilibrium i^*, then $N \to \infty$ if $b \geq d + \epsilon$ or if $\epsilon > b - d > 0$ and $\psi > 1$, and $N \to 0$ if $b \leq d$ or if $\epsilon > b - d > 0$ and $\psi < 1$.*

Proof. If $b \geq d+\epsilon$, then $b-d-\epsilon i^* > 0$ and so (by the statement above) $N \to \infty$. If $b \leq d$, then $b - d - \epsilon i* < 0$, and so $N \to 0$. The remaining range is $\epsilon > b - d > 0$. Consider $b - d - \epsilon i^* > 0$, which is equivalent to $s^* > 1-\frac{b-d}{\epsilon} > 0$. By the monotonicity of $F(s)$, which is defined in (10), this is in turn equivalent to $F(1-\frac{b-d}{\epsilon}) > 0$. Since $F(1-\frac{b-d}{\epsilon}) = 1-(1-\frac{b-d}{\epsilon})R_0$, see (11), this is equivalent to $\psi > 1$. Thus $\epsilon > b - d > 0$ and $\psi > 1$ imply that $N \to \infty$. The remaining case for $N \to 0$ follows similarly. □

A parameter ψ governs the growth or decay of the total population in the analogous ode model analyzed (globally) in [25, Section 5]. The first term in ψ is the ratio of the net growth rate constant $b-d$ and the disease related death rate constant ϵ. Thus the relationship between these quantities is important in determining whether the population grows or decays.

5. Numerics. As illustrated above, theoretical analyses of models with delay can be complicated, and so they are often complemented with numerical analyses. Sometimes a numerical solution of the steady state equations can help determine the number and location of endemic equilibria and aid in locating roots of the characteristic equations. If the model equations can be written as a delay system, then solutions can be obtained numerically using XPPAUT [11]. Such solutions are useful for verification or support in parameter ranges indicated by the theory.

In our SIS model, numerical investigation of the characteristic equation (13) indicates the existence of pure imaginary roots for a small set of parameter values. Defining $u(t) = \int_{t-\omega}^{t} i(p)dp$, equation (8) can be written as a two-dimensional delay system. Numerical solution with XPPAUT [11] of this system with initial values taken on $[-\omega, 0]$, confirms the presence of periodic solutions. For example, for a set of parameter values (see [16, Figure 1]), solutions oscillate about $i^* = 0.995$ with $\theta = 1.03 > 1$. These periodic solutions occur for a small set of (albeit unrealistic) parameter values as the population is rapidly dying out. Taking $\theta < 1$, numerical solutions suggest that the DFE is globally stable for all values of $\epsilon\omega$.

6. Conclusions. From a combination of analysis and numerics, the behavior of the model can now be summarized with particular reference to the questions posed in Section 2. Often there remain open analytical questions.

For our SIS model (as in [16]), a threshold parameter θ has been identified. This suggests a possible way of controlling the disease, namely forcing θ to be less than one, perhaps by reducing the contact rate constant λ. A combination of analytical and numerical techniques have been used to find periodic solutions for a small range of parameter values. Since in the analogous ode model [25] all solutions approach equilibria, it is apparent that the delay corresponding to a constant infectious period can change the qualitative behavior and give rise to periodic solutions. These occur only in the case of unrealistically high disease related death. Open theoretical problems remain regarding global stability and Hopf bifurcation.

If the population is assumed to be constant, then the number of infectives is given by the scalar integral equation (2) with constant N and $S = N - I$. Global stability of the DFE below the threshold ($R_0 = \lambda(1 - \exp(-b\omega))/b < 1$) and the endemic equilibrium above the threshold ($R_0 > 1$) can be proved; see [24] and references therein. However, in the case of a nonconstant population and disease related death, questions of global stability (especially of endemic equilibria) are more challenging. Global stability of the endemic equilibrium also remains an open problem in several of the models with variable population mentioned in Sections 1 and 2; for example, the $SEIS$ models in [8, 12].

Acknowledgements. Thanks to F. Brauer, K.L. Cooke, H.W. Hethcote and James Watmough for helpful comments and suggestions, and to A. Ivanov for suggesting the improvement given in Theorem 1.

REFERENCES

[1] R.M. Anderson and R.M. May, Infectious Diseases of Humans, Oxford University Press, 1991.

[2] F. Brauer, Some infectious disease models with population dynamics and general contact rates, Differential and Integral Equations (1990), **3**:827–836.

[3] F. Brauer, Models of diseases with vertical transmission and nonlinear population dynamics, Mathematical Biosciences (1995), **128**:13–24.

[4] F. Brauer, An introduction to mathematical epidemiology, IMA volume, preprint.

[5] F. Brauer and C. Castillo-Chavez, Basic models in epidemiology, In Ecological Time Series, Eds. T.M. Powell and J.H. Steele, Chapman and Hall, 1995, pp. 410–447.
[6] S. Busenberg and K.L. Cooke, Vertically Transmitted Diseases, Springer-Verlag, 1993.
[7] C. Castillo-Chavez and H.R. Thieme, Asymptotically autonomous epidemic models, In Mathematical Population Dynamics: Analysis of Heterogeneity, Volume One: Theory of Epidemics, Eds. O. Arino, D. Axelrod, M. Kimmel, and M. Langlais, Wuerz, 1995, pp. 33–50.
[8] K.L. Cooke and P. van den Driessche, Analysis of an SEIRS epidemic model with two delays, Journal of Mathematical Biology (1996), **35**:240–260.
[9] K. Cooke, P. van den Driessche, and X. Zou, Interaction of maturation delay and nonlinear birth in population and epidemic models, Journal of Mathematical Biology (1999), **39**:332–352.
[10] M.C.M. de Jong, O. Diekmann, and H. Hesterbeek, How does transmission of infection depend on population size? In Epidemic Models: Their Structure and Relation to Data, Ed. D. Mollison, Cambridge University Press, 1995, pp. 84–94.
[11] G.B. Ermentrout, XPPAUT 1.8 - The Differential Equations Tool, 1996.
[12] L. Genik and P. van den Driessche, An epidemic model with recruitment-death demographics and discrete delays, In Differential Equations with Applications to Biology, Eds. S. Ruan, G.S.K. Wolkowicz, and J. Wu, Fields Institute Communications (1999), **21**:237–249.
[13] J.K. Hale and S.M. Verduyn Lunel, Introduction to Functional Differential Equations, Springer-Verlag, 1993.
[14] H.W. Hethcote and S.A. Levin, Periodicity in epidemiological models, In Applied Mathematical Ecology, Eds. S.A. Levin, T.G. Hallam, and L.J. Gross, Springer-Verlag, 1989, pp. 193–211.
[15] H.W. Hethcote, H.W. Stech, and P. van den Driessche, Nonlinear oscillations in epidemic models, SIAM Journal of Applied Mathematics (1981), **40**:1–9.
[16] H.W. Hethcote and P. van den Driessche, An SIS epidemic model with variable population size and a delay, Journal of Mathematical Biology (1995), **34**: 177–194.
[17] H.W. Hethcote and P. van den Driessche, Two SIS epidemiologic models with delays, Journal of Mathematical Biology (2000), **40**:3–26.
[18] Y. Kuang, Delay Differential Equations with Applications in Population Dynamics, Academic Press, 1993.
[19] S.-O. Londen, On the variation of the solution of a nonlinear integral equation, J. Math. Anal. Appl. (1975), **52**:430–449.
[20] R.K. Miller, Nonlinear Volterra Integral Equations, Mathematics Lecture Note Series, W.A. Benjamin, 1971.
[21] H.W. Stech and M. Williams, Stability in a class of cyclic epidemic models with delay, Journal of Mathematical Biology (1981), **11**:95–103.
[22] H.R. Thieme and P. van den Driessche, Global stability in cyclic epidemic models with disease fatalities, In Differential Equations with Applications to Biology, Eds. S. Ruan, G.S.K. Wolkowicz, and J. Wu, Fields Institute Communications (1999), **21**:459–472.
[23] P. van den Driessche, Some epidemiological models with delays, In Differential Equations and Applications to Biology and to Industry, Eds. M. Martelli, K. Cooke, B. Tang, and H. Thieme, World Scientific, 1996, pp. 507–520.
[24] P. van den Driessche and James Watmough, A simple SIS epidemic model with a backward bifurcation. Journal of Mathematical Biology (2000), **40**:525–540.
[25] J. Zhou and H.W. Hethcote, Population size dependent incidence in models for diseases without immunity, Journal of Mathematical Biology, (1994), **32**: 809–834.

NONLOCAL RESPONSE IN A SIMPLE EPIDEMIOLOGICAL MODEL

K.R. HEIDERICH[†*], W. HUANG[†], AND C. CASTILLO-CHAVEZ[†‡]

Abstract. We use a simple epidemiological model to investigate the effects of a nonlocal feedback on the disease dynamics. We consider a context in which two groups can be identified: the population that is experiencing an epidemic and an "outside" population that acts primarily as a source and sink of uninfected individuals. The disease dynamics of the afflicted group is affected by immigration from the outside group, which, in turn, is affected by the state of the disease. The response to this type of feedback can be investigated using a model in which the net influx of susceptibles into the afflicted population is a function of the disease prevalence in that group. We extend and generalize the analysis of Blythe *et al.* (1997), Brauer et al. (1998) and Hadeler and Castillo-Chavez (1995) to include more general net immigration functions. Since the population does not respond instantaneously to the state of the epidemic we include a time delay in the immigration function. We find that state-dependent recruitment, which was found to be destabilizing by Blythe *et al.* and Brauer et al. (1998), can actually *stabilize* the dynamics when such a time delay is included. Furthermore, consistent over(under)-estimation of the disease prevalence reduces(increases) the size of the endemic equilibrium populations.

Key words. Epidemiological modelling – Nonlocal response – Behaviour-change – Time-delay.

1. Introduction.

The mathematical modelling of epidemics plays a crucial role in understanding the dynamics of many infectious diseases (for an introductory review, see, e.g., Hethcote (1989, 2000), Brauer and Castillo-Chavez (2001), and Brauer (2001a, 2001b; this volume). Models are particularly helpful as experimental tools with which to evaluate and compare control procedures and prevention strategies, and to investigate the relative effects of various sociological and biological factors on the spread of a disease. Recent advances have been made on many fronts. For example, models help us understand the consequences of the long and variable incubation and infectivity periods of the human immunodeficiency virus (HIV), which is believed to lead to acquired immunodeficiency syndrome (AIDS) [see, e.g., Castillo-Chavez *et al.* (1989a,b,c,d), and Thieme *et al.* (1989), (1993)]. Other models are helping to identify the role of nonhomogeneous mixing in populations, [see, e.g., Busenberg *et al.* (1991), Castillo-Chavez *et al.* (1991), Hyman and Stanley (1988), Hyman, Li, and Stanley (1994), Jacquez, et. al. (1988), Sattenspiel (1987a,b) and Sattenspiel *et al.* (1988)] and of the dynamical response of a population to an

*Department of Physics, Langara College, 100 West 49th Avenue, Vancouver, B.C., Canada, V5Y 2Z6.

†Department of Mathematical Sciences, University of Alabama in Huntsville, Huntsville, AL 23599, USA

‡Department of Biometrics, Statistics and Theoretical and Applied Mechanics, Cornell University, 432 Warren Hall, Ithaca, N. Y. 14853-7801, USA

epidemic [see, e.g., Blythe *et al.* (1993a,b, 1997), Brauer et al. (1998) and Hadeler and Castillo-Chavez 1995].

The responses of a population to the stresses of a disease are many fold, can occur at many levels, and can, in turn, significantly effect the disease dynamics. For example, governments may introduce prevention and control strategies such as vaccination schedules, education programs, and, even, mandatory quarantine [Perez-Stable (1991)]. At a more individual level, behavioural factors may come into play, which might change social interactions and the overall mixing structure, effect immigration patterns and migratory routes, and encourage more cautious and prevention-oriented behaviour. The type, degree, speed, and variety of responses depends on the particulars of both the population and the epidemic. Some factors which can influence the population's response include the severity of the epidemic, the lethality of the disease, the ease of contraction, educational awareness, public consciousness, availability of funds, and scientific knowledge. In attempts to control the disease, it is important to recognize which factors are involved and their potential impact on the disease dynamics.

When the time-scale of the epidemic is much shorter than the population's reaction time, one expects that the dynamical response of the population will have little effect on the current epidemic. However, when the time-scales are comparable, this feedback may be significant. For example, in the HIV/AIDS context, it has become clear that many behavioural changes are occurring at both the population and individual levels: the number of contacts and the number of partners are being reduced, the degree of interaction and the mixing structure is changing, [see, e.g., Centers for Disease Control (1985), Evans *et al.* (1989), Martin (1987), McKusick *et al.* (1985a,b), Griensven *et al.* (1989), Fineberg (1988), McClam, 2001]. Even if the effects of changing behaviour are not significant on the time-scale of individual epidemics, they may have significant consequences on an evolutionary time-scale [see, e.g., Ewald (1993)].

The dynamical consequences of some behavioural responses have been investigated by a number of researchers. For example, Blythe *et al.* (1991) investigate the effects of disease prevalence on incidence rates. Palmer *et al.* (1991) study the consequences of state-dependent mixing. Velasco-Hernandez and Hsieh (1994) analyze a model which takes into account a change in contact rate that results from individuals realizing that they are infected. Brauer et al. (1998) investigated the effects of the proportion versus the number of infected individuals on HIV dynamics. Velasco et al. (1996) and Hsieh and Cooke (2000) look at the impact of behaviour changes in populations where treatment is available

In these models, attention is essentially restricted to "local" population responses, i.e., only the behavioral response of the afflicted group is considered. Nonlocal effects may also be important. "Outside" groups can function as sources and sinks of individuals. For example, immigrants from a group which implements a different vaccination program could seriously undermine the vaccination strategy in the population being studied. In order to take into account such nonlocal effects in general, one must understand the structures that can exist in a population.

Structure in a population can occur at many levels: groups can be distinguished by age, sex, social interactions, geographical separation, contact levels, and so on. While it can be quite difficult to identify the relevant groupings, the particular choice can significantly affect the results of the analysis. Here we briefly consider two important historical modeling examples. Sattenspiel (1987a,b) and Sattenspiel and Simon (1988) discuss the 1979 hepatitis A outbreak in some regions of New Mexico among children attending day care. Within the set of daycare centers, most of the cases occurred in a small group of family owned centers. Mixing within this group of related centers was higher than mixing within the group composed of the remaining centers and higher than mixing between the two groups. In trying to understand the spread of the disease among the children, Sattenspiel and Simon argue that it is important to recognize this two-group structuring of the population. The dynamics were essentially driven by the group of family-owned centers while the role of the remaining centers was minimal. Hethcote and York (1984) postulate the existence of two distinct groups in their study of sexually transmitted diseases (STD): a "core-group", which constitutes the most sexually active group in the sexually-active population, and the "meta-population", which encompasses the rest of the sexually-active population. They found that most new cases of STD were generated by the core group. Again, the first-order dynamics were essentially driven by the core group and the effect of the meta-population was less important.

Theses examples motivate us to consider an epidemiological context in which essentially two groups can be identified: the core group and the outside population. The afflicted group can be regarded as driving the disease dynamics, while the coupling between groups, as well as the disease dynamics within the outside group, can be regarded as secondary. This type of division occurs naturally in many situations as illustrated by the preceding examples. The groupings are not static due to migration into and departure from each group, which most models have not taken into consideration [but see Scalia-Tomba (1991), Blythe *et al.* (1993b), Hadeler and Castillo-Chavez (1995)]. Net immigration between the outside population and the afflicted group may influence the dynamics of the epidemic. The immigration may, in turn, depend on the state of the disease in the "target" group (Fineberg (1988)). The consequences of some state-dependent recruitment scenarios have been investigated by Blythe *et al.* (1993b), Brauer et al. (1998), and Hadeler *et al.* (1995). Blythe *et al.* (1997) and Brauer et al. (1998) consider a simple two-variable (*SI*) epidemiological model. In that model, the equilibria are stable if the recruitment into the afflicted group is constant. However, if net immigration drops off as a function of the disease prevalence in the target population, then the endemic equilibrium can be destabilized. Brauer et al. (1998) considered the case where information on prevalence was available either in total numbers or as a fraction. Hadeler and Castillo-Chavez (1995) considered the role of education and the size of the non-core population (a dynamic variable). Hadeler and Castillo-Chavez' (1995) simple model is capable of supporting multiple endemic equilibria whenever R_0, the basic reproductive number, is less than one. This possibility had been previously illustrated by Castillo-Chavez et al. (1989b) and Huang et al. (1992) but in a more complex setting. It had been shown that the assumption of asymmetric probabilities of transmission between groups could generate multiple endemic equilibria via a backward bifurcation.

It is this "behavioural" response of the population at large to the population being studied that we investigate in detail using more realistic immigration functions in order to clarify the mechanisms relevant to the dynamics. In Blythe *et al.*'s or Brauer *et al.*'s models, the population is assumed to have instantaneous knowledge of the state of the epidemic. The response will be time-lagged, in general, due to the fact that it takes time to assess the state of the epidemic, time to publicize the information, and time for the population to react to the information. We will show that the inclusion of a discrete time delay in the immigration term can actually *stabilize* the dynamics.

We also deal explicitly with aspects of the fact that one never has exact knowledge of the state of the epidemic. Although exact knowledge is often assumed (e.g., Blythe *et al.* (1997); Brauer *et al.* (1998); Hadeler and Castillo-Chavez (1995)), there will always be a degree of inaccuracy and uncertainty. For example, the prevalence may be over- or under-reported, its severity over- or underestimated. It is the perceived state of the epidemic, not the actual state, to which the population will respond. If we suppose that the prevalence figures are consistently deflated or inflated by a constant fraction, or that the population, on average, consistently misinterprets the reports, then we find that if the figures are over-estimated then the size of the endemic equilibrium population is lower and, conversely, if they are under-estimated then the equilibrium size is higher. Although the parameter ranges for stability are slightly changed, the dynamics are qualitatively the same. This underscores the influence of the media and the value of educational programs.

In the next section, we investigate the dynamical consequences of a general state-dependent net immigration function on the disease dynamics of a simple epidemiological model. After discussing the model assumptions, we consider three functional dependencies of the immigration term, give the disease-free and endemic equilibria and their stability. In Section III, we study the effects of a time delay in the functional dependencies of the immigration term. Section IV contains a brief summary of our results.

2. State-dependent immigration model. As discussed in the introduction, we consider epidemiological contexts in which essentially two groups can be identified: the population which is experiencing an epidemic and the outside population. The outside population is weakly coupled to the afflicted group and its primary effect is as a source and as a sink of individuals to and from the afflicted population. The epidemic is driven by the outbreak in the afflicted group while the effect of the outside population is purely secondary and can be neglected as a higher order effect. Hence, in what follows, we consider the dynamics of only one group, namely the afflicted group. The number of healthy individuals in that group are called susceptibles and are denoted by $S(t)$, and the number of infected individuals, by $I(t)$, where t denotes time. To a first approximation, the progress of the disease can be modelled by two first-order ordinary differential equations,

$$\begin{aligned} \dot{S} &= g - \mu S - f \ , \\ \dot{I} &= f - \alpha I \ , \end{aligned} \tag{1}$$

where the recruitment function, $g = g(S, I)$, describes net immigration, μ is the (constant) natural mortality, the force of infection term, $f = f(S, I)$, describes the contact structure between infected and susceptible individuals, $\alpha = \sigma + \mu$, where σ is the constant migration out of the infected class due to death, recovery, emigration, etc., and the dot denotes derivative with respect to time. In this simple system there are four (or more) parameters (depending on the form of g and f). σ and μ have the dimensions of inverse time, and the functions g and f have the dimensions of number of individuals per unit time. To simplify the analysis, we do not include a recovered class. Thus, we implicitly assume that the disease is fatal, that all recovered individuals leave the afflicted group, or that the epidemic is short-lived relative to the length of illness and, therefore, that the recovered class does not contribute significantly to the dynamics. Since we are primarily interested in the effects of state-dependent net immigration, we do not include additional complications such as incubation periods. Given the context of interest, we do not include a birth term, although this would be straightforward to do. We also assume that immigrants are not yet infected [but see Hoover *et al.* (1991)].

The form of the force of infection, $f = f(S, I)$ depends on the particulars of the disease. Here we take the general form

$$f = c \frac{SI}{S + I} \ , \tag{2}$$

where c is a constant having the dimensions of inverse time. This term needs some justification (see also Busenberg and Cooke (1993)): suppose that a susceptible has x contacts per unit time. Assuming homogeneous mixing among susceptibles and infecteds, a fraction $I/(S + I)$ of these contacts are with infected individuals. (This assumes that all of the infecteds are intermingling as freely as those uninfected, i.e., that the disease is not sufficiently debilitating to restrict the movement of infecteds (which is a good approximation for some diseases such as gonorrhea and syphilis). More generally one could take into account the reduced mobility of infecteds by setting the fraction of contacts with infecteds to be $\rho I/(S+\rho I)$ where ρ represents the degree of non-homogeneity in the mixing (e.g., $\rho \ll 1$ for diseases which immobilize those infected and thereby significantly reduce the mixing of susceptibles with infecteds)). In the case of models for sexually-transmitted HIV, it is often assumed that individuals with AIDS are sexually-inactive (Castillo-Chavez et al. 1989a). Let the probability of contracting the disease per contact be p. Then the total number of contacts per unit time which lead to infection is given by Eq. (2) with $c = xp$. For some diseases it is reasonable to assume that the number of contacts per unit time, x, is a function of the total population size, $N = S + I$, i.e., $x = x(N)$. Additionally, one frequently assumes that $x(N)$ is directly proportional to N – this gives the so-called mass-action force of infection term $f = \beta SI$, where β is a constant. It is unlikely, however, in most epidemiological contexts that the number of contacts per unit time will increase indefinitely with population size. Therefore it is appropriate to introduce an upper threshold to the possible number of contacts per unit time. Then the force of infection term becomes $f = c(N)SI/(S+I)$, where $c(N)$ is an increasing function of population size assymptoting to the upper threshold at large N, e.g., $c(N) = c_0N/(1+N)$, (c.f. Holling's type II functional response, Holling (1959)). Since we take $c(N) = c =$ constant, we are therefore assuming that the changing size of the afflicted group does not significantly effect the contact rate. If we are considering a population that is distinguished by its (high) contact level (near the upper threshold, say, e.g., the "core" group in STD), then taking c to be a constant is appropriate: the group being modelled is near its contact threshold, in fact, it is defined by its contact level c. If the contact level of an individual changes so that the mixing is no longer described for that individual by the parameter c, then that individual is considered to have left the group. This is taken into account by the net immigration function, $g = g(S, I)$, and the emigration term, σ. Note, however, that since c is constant, we are assuming that the total population size in the afflicted group remains high enough to sustain the high contact level. Alternatively, if we are considering a population distinguished by, say, geographic location, the assumption that the parameter c is constant means that there is not much that this population does, or can do, to change their contact rate. Our prior work on HIV (Castillo-Chavez et al. 1989a) has shown that there is no qualitative difference between constant c and some realistic functional forms for $C(N)$.

There will generally be some mixing between the afflicted group and the outside population. We assume that this is a higher order effect that can be ignored. Explicitly, inter-group mixing could be included by taking the force of infection term to be, say,

$$f = \left(x_A \frac{I_A}{S_A + I_A} + x_B \frac{I_B}{S_B + I_B} \right) pS_B \ , \tag{3}$$

where the subscript A refers to the outside population which we call here group A, and the subscript B, refers to the afflicted population, here group B. A susceptible in group B will have x_B contacts per unit time with members of group B, and x_A contacts per unit time with members of group A. By assumption, there is little mixing between groups so that $x_B \gg x_A$. Further, we are interested in situations when an epidemic *is* occurring in group B and, although there are infections occurring in group A, the level of infection is such that $I_A/N_A \ll I_B/N_B$, where $N_A = S_A + I_A$, etc.. Combining inequalities, we have that $x_A I_A/N_A \ll x_B I_B/N_B$, and hence can neglect the second term in Eq. (3). Of course, I_B and S_B are dynamical quantities so that this condition should be satisfied throughout the course of the epidemic. In the absence of disease in group B we assume, of course, that there is no disease in group A.

It remains to discuss plausible forms for the immigration function $g = g(S, I)$. We assume that as the disease prevalence increases, net immigration into the susceptible population decreases. We further assume that the state of the epidemic is reported to the population in terms of either (i) the fraction of infecteds, $\eta = I/(S + I)$, so that $g = g(\eta)$, or (ii), the actual numbers of infected individuals, I, so that $g = g(I)$. Motivated by Blythe *et al.*, Brauer *et al.* and Hadeler and Castillo-Chavez (1995), we consider the following general class of decreasing functions:

$$g(\xi) = ae^{-b\xi^\gamma} \ , \tag{4}$$

where ξ is taken to be (i) η, or (ii) I, and where a, b and γ are real positive numbers. The dimensionless parameter γ is the shape parameter of the response function $\exp(-b\eta^\gamma)$ and describes the rate of reaction of the population: Small γ (< 0.5), describes a response curve that drops off sharply as a function of infection (i.e., $g(\eta)$ convex), while, larger γ (> 3), is appropriate to describe the response of a population that is more gradual (i.e., $g(\eta)$ concave). The parameter b is related to the scaling parameter, $b^{-1/\gamma}$, and describes the degree of the reaction: As b decreases in value, the reduction in net immigration will be less severe. The functional form given in Eq. (4) is quite general and describes a wide variety of plausible responses. Note that the function (4) is derived from the Weibull distribution and is often used to model survivorship curves in demographic models.

It would also make sense to consider other functional dependencies of $g = g(S, I)$. In the immigration function given by Eq. (4), we are assuming that the population is reacting to the precise state of the epidemic. However, assessments of the state of the epidemic will rarely be so accurate.

To get a rough first approximation of the effects of misinformation, we assume that the population consistently over- or under-estimates the disease prevalence by a constant proportion. This leads one to consider immigration functions that depend on, case (iii), $\tilde{\eta} = \chi I/(S + \chi I)$, where χ is a constant parameter approximating the degree of over- ($\chi > 1$) or under-estimation ($\chi < 1$) of the disease prevalence, (more generally, χ could be a random variable). Taking a recruitment function of the form given in Eq. (4) with functional dependence $g = g(\tilde{\eta})$, one finds qualitatively the same dynamics as in case (i). However, the parameter range of the various dynamics depends on χ. Additionally, it may be appropriate to take the immigration function g to be a decreasing function of the real or perceived virulence, $g = g(\nu)$. Such a model could be used to compare the relative importance of the recruitment term for different diseases which are distinguished by their virulence, however, we do not investigate this possibility here.

In summary, to model the disease dynamics (in the afflicted group), we take the system given by Eqs. (1) together with the form of the force of infection function, Eq. (2), and the form of the immigration function, Eq. (4), with functional dependencies (i) $g(\eta)$, (ii) $g(I)$, and (iii) $g(\tilde{\eta})$. For case (i), the system can be written, in dimensionless units, as follows

$$\begin{aligned} \dot{S} &= ae^{-b\eta^{\gamma}} - \mu S - \frac{IS}{(I+S)} \ , \\ \dot{I} &= \tfrac{IS}{I+S} - \alpha I \ , \end{aligned} \tag{5}$$

where we have non-dimensionalized by setting $S \to SK$, $I \to IK$, $ct \to t$, $a \to aKc$, $\mu \to \mu c$, $\sigma \to \sigma c$, and $c = 1$, where K is some constant reference population level. The parameter c has been eliminated and there are only four remaining (dimensionless) parameters μ, σ, a, and b.

First, let us consider case (i) where recruitment is taken to be a function of the fraction of infecteds, $g(\eta) = a\exp(-b\eta^{\gamma})$, Eq. (4). The disease-free equilibrium of the system (5) is

$$\bar{S}_0 = \frac{a}{\mu}, \qquad \bar{I}_0 = 0. \tag{6}$$

This equilibrium, $(\bar{S}_0, \bar{I}_0)$, is *globally* stable if $1 < \alpha$ (see Appendix A). If $1 > \alpha$, the endemic equilibrium of the system (5) is

$$S_0 = g_0 \frac{1}{1-\sigma} \ , \quad I_0 = S_0 \frac{1-\alpha}{\alpha} \ , \tag{7}$$

where $g_0 = g(\eta_0)$ and from Eqs. (5) one has that $\eta_0 = 1 - \alpha$. The size of the endemic equilibrium population (S_0, I_0) increases as γ increases: For larger γ, immigration will be relatively high at a given incidence level as compared to a population response that is described by smaller γ. The endemic equilibrium, (S_0, I_0), Eq. (7), is stable provided that

$$\partial_S g_0 < 1 - \sigma \ , \tag{8}$$

where $\partial_S = \partial/\partial S$ and $\partial_S g_0$ denotes $(\partial_S g)|_0 = (\partial_S g)|_{(S_0,I_0)}$. For the special case $\gamma = 1$, it can be shown that the equilibrium (7) is *globally* stable (Huang, personal communication), if (8) holds. At $\partial_S g_0 = 1 - \sigma$, the characteristic equation associated with the endemic equilibrium has a pair of purely imaginary roots and we have a Hopf bifurcation.

Substituting in $g(\eta) = a\exp(-b\eta^\gamma)$, the stability condition (8) can be written

$$b\gamma\alpha(1-\alpha)^\gamma < 1 \quad . \tag{9}$$

Figure 1 shows the regions of stability in terms of the parameters b and α. As γ increases, the boundary between the stable and unstable regions shifts towards smaller α. In other words, if the response of the population is gradual (large γ), the system will be stable for smaller values of σ, lower emigration. Conversely, for small γ, i.e., for a rapid response, the system will be unstable except for α large or small. Varying the parameter μ gives qualitatively similar curves as in Figure 1, however, the shape of the curves are modified

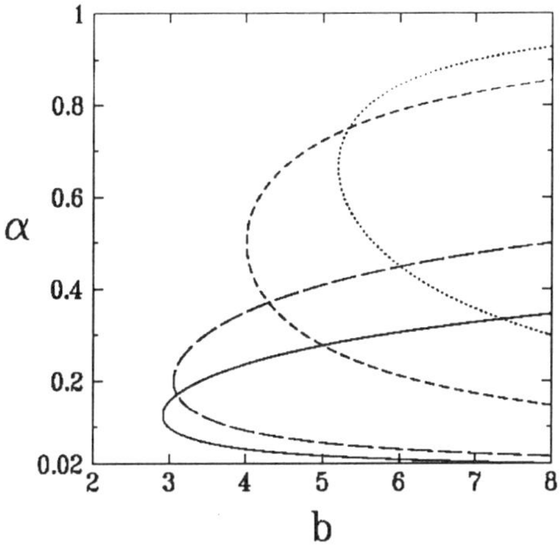

FIG. 1. *Stability regions of the endemic equilibrium (7) for the system (5) with* $g = a\exp(-b\eta^\gamma)$, *case (i), for four different* γ: $\gamma = 0.5$ *(dotted line),* $\gamma = 1.0$ *(short-dashed line),* $\gamma = 4.0$ *(long-dashed line), and* $\gamma = 7.0$ *(solid line). Each curve satisfies Eq. (9) with* $a = 0.02$ *and* $\mu = 0.02$. *To the left of each curve, the endemic equilibrium is stable, while to the right, it is unstable. We choose values of* a *and* μ *appropriate for gonorrhea (Hethcote and Yorke (1984)).*

For the case $\gamma = 1$, the equilibrium (7) is globally stable if $b\alpha(1-\alpha) < 1$. Thus, in terms of the parameters b and α, we have stability under the following conditions: if $b < 4$, for all α; if $b = 4$, except when $\alpha = 1/2$; if $b > 4$, for $\alpha > \alpha_+$ or $\alpha < \alpha_-$, where $\alpha_\pm$ are the roots of $b\alpha(1-\alpha) = 1$. Recall that the parameter b describes the degree of reaction of the population and the parameter $\alpha = \mu + \sigma$, where σ describes the migration out of the infected class. These results are essentially equivalent to those in Blythe *et al.*, where the model (5) is studied with $\gamma = 1$.

It will prove conceptually helpful in the next section to show how the local stability condition, $\partial_S g_0 < 1 - \sigma$, Eq. (8), arises from a second-order ordinary differential equation. Linearizing system (5) about the endemic equilibrium, (S_0, I_0), one gets two first-order ordinary differential equations for the linear perturbations S_1 and I_1, (i.e., $S = S_0 + \epsilon S_1$ and $I = I_0 + \epsilon I_1$, for ϵ small). Combining the equations for $\dot{S}_1$ and $\dot{I}_1$, one gets the second-order equation for S_1:

$$\ddot{S}_1 + (A - C)\dot{S}_1 + (B + D)S_1 = 0, \tag{10}$$

where

$$A = \partial_S f_0 + \mu + \alpha - \partial_I f_0, \tag{11}$$
$$B = \alpha\,(\partial_S f_0 + \mu) - \mu \partial_I f_0, \tag{12}$$
$$C = \partial_S g_0, \tag{13}$$
$$D = \partial_S g_0\,(\partial_I f_0 - \alpha) - \partial_I g_0 \partial_S f_0. \tag{14}$$

Equation (10) is the equation for a damped harmonic oscillator. Since linear oscillators are well understood, the conditions for stability can be read directly from Eq. (10): For negative restoring force and positive damping, $B + D > 0$, and $A - C > 0$ respectively, the system is damped so that the equilibrium is stable. On the other hand, if $A - C < 0$, the oscillations are unstable. This is (of course) precisely condition (8). For the recruitment function $g = a\exp(-b\eta^\gamma)$ and a force of infection term f given by Eq. (2), at the endemic equilibrium (7), we have $A = 1 - \sigma$, $B = A\alpha(1 - \alpha)$, $C = A\alpha b\gamma(1-\alpha)^\gamma$, and $D = 0$. Thus, one sees that the condition $A - C > 0$ is precisely the stability condition given by Eq. (9). (Of course, this is simply the Routh-Hurwitz criteria in two dimensions (see, e.g., Murray (1990)), where the determinant of the eigenvalue matrix of the linearized system is $B + D > 0$ and the trace, $-(A - C) < 0$. The harmonic oscillator analogy is, however, conceptually useful.)

These results are quite different than those obtained when the effect of the disease on net immigration is not taken into account. In this case, the recruitment is constant, which corresponds to taking $b = 0$ in Eq. (4) (giving $g(S, I) = a$). The disease-free and endemic equilibria are again given by Eqs. (6) and (7) respectively. However, for $b = 0$, the endemic equilibrium is always stable since the stability condition, $\partial_S g_0 = 0 < 1 - \sigma$, Eq. (8) always holds. On the other hand, if there is state-dependent immigration that is appropriately described by the function $g(\eta) = a\exp(-b\eta^\gamma)$, the system is unstable when $\partial_S g_0 > 1 - \sigma$. Further, due to the reduced net immigration as the epidemic spreads, the size of the endemic equilibrium population is smaller for nonzero b.

Now, we consider case (ii), where the immigration term is taken to be a function of the number of infecteds, $g(I) = a\exp(-bI^\gamma)$. The equilibria of the system (5) with this functional dependence of the recruitment function are the same as in case (i) and are given by Eqs. (6) and (7). However, in this case the endemic equilibrium, (S_0, I_0), is only defined implicitly by Eqs. (7) since $g_0 = a\exp[-(1-\alpha)^\gamma S_0^\gamma]$. The stability conditions are also as in case (i): the disease-free equilibrium is stable for $1 < \alpha$ and the endemic equilibrium is stable for $\partial_S g_0 < 1 - \sigma$, Eq. (8), i.e., $C < A$. For $g(I) = a\exp(-bI^\gamma)$, the coefficients A and B in (10) are as before. However, from (13) and (14) one finds that $C = \partial_S g_0 = 0$, and that $D = -\partial_I g_0(1-\alpha)^2$. Thus, the stability condition given by Eq. (8), $\partial_S g_0 = 0 < 1-\sigma$, is trivially satisfied, and the endemic equilibrium for system (5), with the recruitment function $g(I) = a\exp(-bI^\gamma)$, is always stable (in fact, globally stable, by the Bendixson-du Lac criterion, see, e.g., Clark (1990)). Consequently, if the state-dependent recruitment is best described as a function of I of the form (4), then, the equilibria are stable although the size of the equilibrium population is smaller than for constant recruitment.

As a final functional dependency of the immigration function, we consider case (iii), $g = g(\tilde{\eta})$, which crudely includes the effects of misinformation. Rather than taking recruitment to depend on the precise ratio of infecteds, suppose that the recruitment depends on $\tilde{\eta} = \chi I/(S+\chi I)$, where χ is a (dimensionless) positive real parameter that accounts for the fixed degree of over- or under-estimation of the disease prevalence on the part of the population. As one would expect, over-estimation, $\chi > 1$, leads to smaller endemic equilibrium populations, i.e., $\tilde{S}_0 < S_0$, while underestimation, $\chi < 1$, leads to higher equilibrium populations, i.e., $\tilde{S}_0 > S_0$, where $\tilde{S}_0$ is the equilibrium size of the susceptible population as determined from the recruitment function $g(\tilde{\eta})$, where $\tilde{g}_0 = g(\tilde{\eta}_0)$ with $\tilde{\eta}_0 = \chi(1-\alpha)/[\alpha+\chi(1-\alpha)]$, i.e., $\tilde{S}_0 = \tilde{g}_0/(1-\sigma)$, as in Eq. (7). For $g(\tilde{\eta})$, the coefficients A, B, D of the linearized system (10) are as for $g(\eta)$ and are given by Eqs. (11), (12), and (14). However, $C = \partial_S g_0$ is slightly modified by the parameter χ to

$$C = A\alpha b\gamma\chi^\gamma \frac{(1-\alpha)^\gamma}{(\alpha+\chi(1-\alpha))^{\gamma+1}}. \tag{15}$$

By inspection of the "harmonic oscillator" equation for S_1, Eq. (10), one sees that qualitatively, the dynamics of the system (5) will not be different than those with $\chi = 1$. Indeed, in the next section we combine cases (i) and (iii). Figure 2 shows how the boundary between stable and unstable regions, in terms of b and α, is modified by χ: Overestimation of the disease prevalence, i.e., $\chi > 1$, shifts the curve to higher α, while underestimation, shifts the curves to lower α. Figure 3 is a phase-plane diagram for a parameter choice where the endemic equilibrium is unstable. Note that the size of the population can change by almost an order of magnitude. Recall from Section 1, that since we take the contact rate, c, to be constant, we are assuming that the size of the population remains large enough to sustain this contact rate. Although we will not do so in this paper, one might also consider a contact rate that depends on the size of the population, N, e.g., $c(N) = c_0 N/(1+N)$, since N can change dramatically. In the next section, we will see how a time delay affects the results of this section.

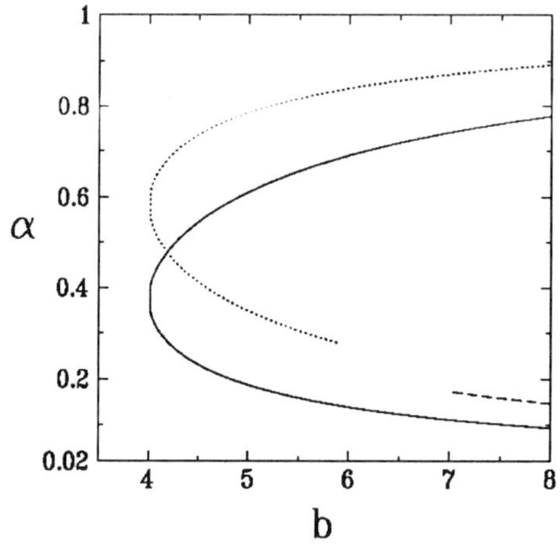

FIG. 2. *Stability regions of the endemic equilibrium (7) for the system (5) with* $g = a\exp(-b\tilde{\eta}^{\gamma})$, *case (iii), for three different* χ: $\chi = 0.6$ *(solid line),* $\chi = 1.0$ *(short-dashed line), and* $\chi = 1.4$ *(dotted line). The curves are* $A = C$, *where* $A = c - \sigma$, *and* C *is given by Eq. (15), with* $a = 0.02$, $\mu = 0.02$, $\gamma = 1.0$. *To the left of each curve, the endemic equilibrium is stable, while to the right, it is unstable.*

3. Time-delayed model. The results of the preceding section motivate consideration of more realistic forms for the recruitment function. Since the information of the state of the epidemic will not be instantaneously available, the population, is, in effect, responding to the state of the epidemic at some earlier time, $(t-\tau)$. This naturally leads one to consider the effects of a discrete time delay in the recruitment term. In this section we investigate the following time delayed modification of Eq. (5):

$$\begin{aligned} \dot{S} &= g\left(\eta(t-\tau)\right) - \mu S - f \ , \\ \dot{I} &= f - \alpha I \ , \end{aligned} \tag{16}$$

where τ is a discrete time delay, the force of infection term $f = f(S, I)$ is given by Eq. (2) and the functional form of $g = g(\xi(t-\tau))$ is given by Eq. (4). Recall that all quantities are dimensionless. We consider two cases: (i) net immigration is a function of the fraction of infecteds with $g(\tilde{\eta}(t-\tau)) = ae^{-b\tilde{\eta}(t-\tau)^{\gamma}}$, where $\tilde{\eta} = \chi I/(\chi I + S)$, and case (ii), recruitment is a function of the number of infecteds, $g(I(t-\tau)) = ae^{-bI(t-\tau)^{\gamma}}$. In case (i), we find that the time delay can stabilize the dynamics. Conversely, in case (ii), we find that the time delay can destabilize the dynamics.

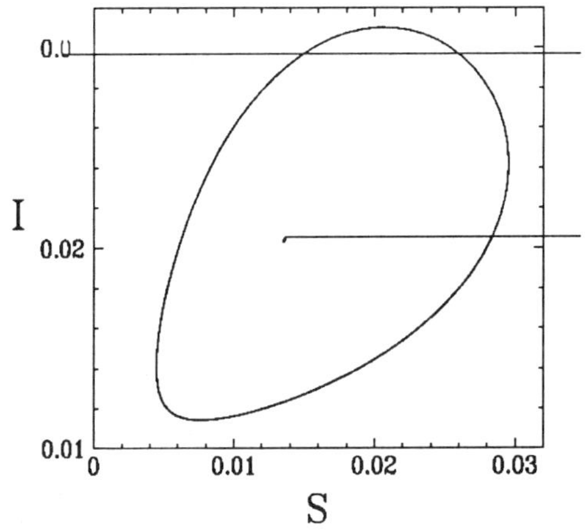

FIG. 3. *Phase-plane trajectories of system (16) for case (i),* $g(\tilde{\eta}(t-\tau))$. *The limit cycle (counter-clockwise flow) corresponds to* $\tau = 0$, *and the inward spiral corresponds to* $\tau = 5$. *The parameter values are* $\alpha = 0.4$, $b = 4$, $a = 0.02$, $\mu = 0.02$, $\gamma = 3.0$, $\chi = 1.0$, $\tau = 5$, *and are chosen to be in the range where a time delay is stabilizing. For this parameter range,* $S_0 = 0.0136$ *and* $I_0 = 0.0204$.

While the equilibria of (16) do not depend on τ, their stability does. We find that the disease-free equilibrium, $(\bar{S}_0, \bar{I}_0) = (a/\mu, 0)$, Eq. (6), is *globally* stable provided that $1 < \alpha$ (see Appendix A). The local stability of the endemic equilibrium, (S_0, I_0), of (16) can be determined from the sign of the real part of the eigenvalues, λ, of the characteristic equation:

$$0 = \lambda^2 + A\lambda + B + (-C\lambda + D)e^{-\lambda\tau} \quad , \tag{17}$$

where, A, B, C, D are as defined in Eqs. (11–14). For $\tau = 0$, the stability condition of the non-time-delayed equilibrium is recovered (stable if $A > C$, Eq. (8). For nonzero τ, there are infinitely many solutions $\lambda = \lambda(\tau)$ to Eq. (17). The endemic equilibrium (S_0, I_0) of system (16) is stable when none of these roots has a positive real part. See Appendix B for an outline of the analysis for the following results: If $A > C$, a time delay has no effect on the stability of the equilibria. Since in this parameter range, the endemic equilibrium is stable for $\tau = 0$, it is stable for all τ. The endemic equilibrium (S_0, I_0) of system (16) is said to be " absolutely stable" (Brauer (1987)) for $A > C$.

Since for $A < C$, the equilibrium is unstable for $\tau = 0$, a nonzero τ may actually stabilize the dynamics in this parameter range. The τ's for which the system is on the boundary between stable and unstable regions are defined by $\tau_1^{(n)} = (\theta_1 + 2\pi n)/\omega_1$, and $\tau_2^{(n)} = (\theta_2 + 2\pi n)/\omega_2$, where n is a natural number, $\theta_1 = \arcsin(A/C)$, $\theta_2 = 2\pi - \theta_1$, and $\omega_1 = \omega_-$, $\omega_2 = \omega_+$, with $\omega_\pm = \left(\pm\sqrt{C^2 - A^2} + \sqrt{C^2 - A^2 + 4B}\right)/2$, (see Appendix II for details). For τ between $\tau_1^{(0)}$ and $\tau_2^{(0)}$, the equilibrium is stable if $\tau_1^{(0)} < \tau_2^{(0)}$. Similarly, for τ between $\tau_1^{(1)}$ and $\tau_2^{(1)}$, the equilibrium is stable if $\tau_1^{(1)} < \tau_2^{(1)}$. These alternating regions of stability and instability (USU regions, i.e., Unstable-Stable-Unstable), will continue until $\tau_1^{(n+1)} > \tau_2^{(n+1)}$, for some n. In some parameter ranges, n can be quite large, (e.g., for $b = 12.8854$, $\alpha = 0.7$, $\mu = 0.02$, $\chi = 1.0$, and $\gamma = 1.0$, we find that $n = 338$). The time-delay which results in stable dynamics can also be quite large (e.g., for the parameters given above, we find that $\tau_2^{(338)} = 8.2 \times 10^3$, in dimensionless units. (To get the dimensionfull units, divide by the dimensionfull c. E.g., for the parameter range that is appropriate for gonorrhea (Hethcote and Yorke (1984)), $c = 0.05$ days^{-1} so that $\tau_2^{(228)} = 1.6 \times 10^4$ days).) Figure 3 shows the phase-plane trajectories of the system (16) with $\tau = 0$ and $\tau = 5$, where the parameter range is chosen so that the endemic equilibrium is unstable for $\tau = 0$ and asymptotically stable for $\tau = 5$. The regions where a time delay may give rise to stable equilibria are shown in Figure (4a) for a representative parameter range. The time delays associated with these regions of alternating stability and instability are shown in Figure (4b). Note that in certain parameter ranges, stability is very sensitive to time delays. Figure (4b) has the characteristic "pine-tree" shape (see MacDonald (1989)). The lower part of the "branches" correspond to the $\tau_1^{(n)}$'s while the upper part of the "branches" correspond to the $\tau_2^{(n)}$'s. The number of oscillations can exceed $n = 1599$, corresponding to time delays of over 2.6×10^4 ($b = 3.5007$, $\alpha = 3.98$, $a = 0.02$, $\mu = 0.02$, $\chi = 1.0$, and $\gamma = 1.0$). Our ability to detect high n is limited by the numerical mesh with which we look. Thus, while extremely high n and τ are possible, the parameter range in which they occur can be vanishingly small (see Figure (4a)).

It is interesting that a finite time delay can have a stabilizing effect on the dynamics. Some insight can be obtained by writing the linearized equations as in Eq. (10):

$$\ddot{S}_1 + A\dot{S}_1 + BS_1 - C\dot{S}_1(t-\tau) + DS_1(t-\tau) = 0 \quad . \tag{18}$$

For case (i), $D = 0$, so that the time delay only appears in the damping term ($C\dot{S}_1$). It is now intuitively plausible that if the damping is in phase with the oscillations, the system may be stabilized.

Now let us consider case (ii), where the recruitment is a function of I, $g = g(I(t-\tau))$. The first of the Eqs. (16) then becomes $\dot{S} = g(I(t-\tau)) - \mu S - f$. The disease-free equilibrium, $(\bar{S}_0, \bar{I}_0) = (a/\mu, 0)$, Eq. (6), is stable provided that $1 < \alpha$. For the endemic equilibrium, referring to (18), one sees that the time delay in this example appears in the restoring force, (DS_1), since for $g = g(I)$, $C = 0$, but $D \neq 0$. There are three possible stability consequences (see Appendix 2 for details): (a) If the restoring force is large enough, i.e., if $D > B$, the endemic equilibrium will be destabilized for large enough τ. In this parameter range, for $\tau < \tau_c =$

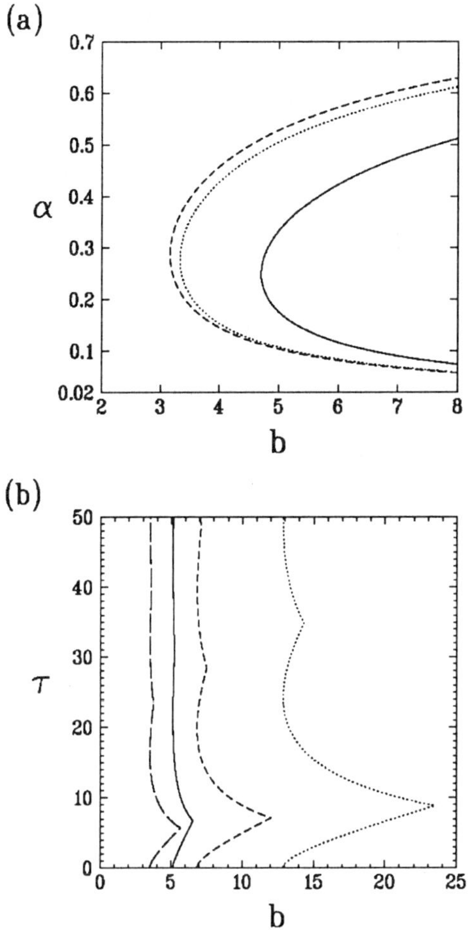

FIG. 4. *(a) Stability regions of the endemic equilibrium (7) for the system (16) with* $g = a\exp(-b\tilde{\eta}(t-\tau)^\gamma)$, *and* $a = 0.02$, $\mu = 0.02$, $\chi = 1.2$, *and* $\gamma = 3.0$. *The short-dashed curve corresponds to the stability boundary for the original* $\tau = 0$ *equations (5) (same as the short-dashed curves in Figures 1 and 2). The solid line is the boundary where* $\tau_1^{(0)} = \tau_2^{(0)}$ *so that to the left of this curve, the system (model0td) is stable for certain ranges of the parameter* τ *(see Figure 4b for the* τ *ranges). The dotted line is the boundary where* $\tau_1^{(1)} = \tau_2^{(1)}$ *so that in the region between the dashed and dotted curve, the system alternates at least twice between stability and instability as* τ *increases. (b) Stability regions of the endemic equilibrium (7) for the system (16) with* $g = g(\tilde{\eta}(t-\tau))$ *in the* $(\tau$ - $b)$*-plane for four different* α: $\alpha = 0.1$ *(solid line),* $\alpha = 0.4$ *(long-dashed line),* $\alpha = 0.6$ *(short-dashed line), and* $\alpha = 0.7$ *(dotted line). The parameters are* $a = 0.02$, $\mu = 0.02$, $\chi = 1.2$, *and* $\gamma = 3.0$. *To the left of each curve, the system is stable. For* $\tau = 0$, *model (5), the corresponding regions of stability are given approximately by:* $b < 3.513$ *for* $\alpha = 0.4$, $b < 5.13$ *for* $\alpha = 0.1$, $b < 6.53$ *for* $\alpha = 0.6$, *and* $b < 12.89$ *for* $\alpha = 0.7$.

$\arccos[(\omega^2 - B)/d]/\omega$, the endemic equilibrium will be stable. However, for $\tau > \tau_c$, the equilibrium will be unstable (*SU* regions, i.e., Stable-Unstable). Case (b): If the restoring force is of intermediate range, i.e., if $B > D$ and if $(A^2 - 2B)^2 - 4(B^2 - D^2) > 0$, one finds alternating regions of stability and instability provided that $2B > A^2$ (*SUS* regions). Case (c): if the restoring force is small, $B > D$ and $(A^2 - 2B)^2 - 4(B^2 - D^2) < 0$, or $2B < A^2$, there will be no stability change and the endemic equilibrium will be absolutely stable. These results are summarized in Figure (5a), which shows the regions in parameter space corresponding to the various stability regimes. The parameter range where the regions of stability and instability alternate (*SUS*) is very small and occurs for very large b and very small μ. (Of course, b, here, is dimensionless. Since the scaling parameter in Eq. (4) is actually $b^{-1/\gamma}$, the parameter b simply appears to be "unnaturally" large.) Figure (5b) shows the time delays that are associated with the various stability regions. For small b, instability occurs only for large τ (e.g., for $b = 4$, $\alpha = 0.15$, $a = 0.02$, $\mu = 0.001$, $\chi = 1.0$, and $\gamma = 1.0$, instability sets in when $\tau > 171$). On the other hand, for large b, instability can occur for quite small time delays (e.g., for $b = 100$, $\alpha = 0.4$, $\mu = 0.001$, $\chi = 1.0$, and $\gamma = 1.0$, instability sets in when $\tau > 6$). It might be interesting to compare these results with those obtained from a periodic forcing of the epidemiological model (1). Seasonal forcing, for example, often arises in childhood diseases due to cycles induced by the school year.

4. Conclusion. We consider a two-group *SI* model in which net immigration from a metapopulation into the core group depends on the status of the epidemic in the core group. Two different functional dependencies of a general state-dependent recruitment function $g(S, I) = g(\xi) = a\exp(-b\xi^\gamma)$ were investigated: (i) $g = g(\tilde{\eta})$ and (ii) $g = g(I)$. In case (i), if the recruitment is a decreasing function of the fraction of infecteds, $g(\eta)$, the endemic equilibrium can be destabilized. Furthermore, the effect of consistent over(under)-estimation of the disease prevalence lowers(raises) the size of the endemic equilibria population (see Figure 2). Similar results hold for the rate of response of the population (see Figure 1). In case (ii), if the recruitment is a function of the number of infecteds, $g(I)$, the stability of the equilibria does not change from that of constant recruitment, however, the size of the equilibrium population is effected. It would be interesting to see how these results compare to those obtained from queuing theory and stochastic balking models.

We find that a time delay in recruitment can significantly affect these results. In case (i), $g = g(\tilde{\eta}(t-\tau))$, we found that the time delay could have a stabilizing effect on the dynamics. There are significant regions in parameter space where the endemic equilibrium alternates between being stable and unstable as τ increases (see Figure 4). In case (ii), $g = g(I(t - \tau))$, we found that a time delay could destabilize the dynamics. Again, we found regions in parameter space where the endemic equilibrium alternates between

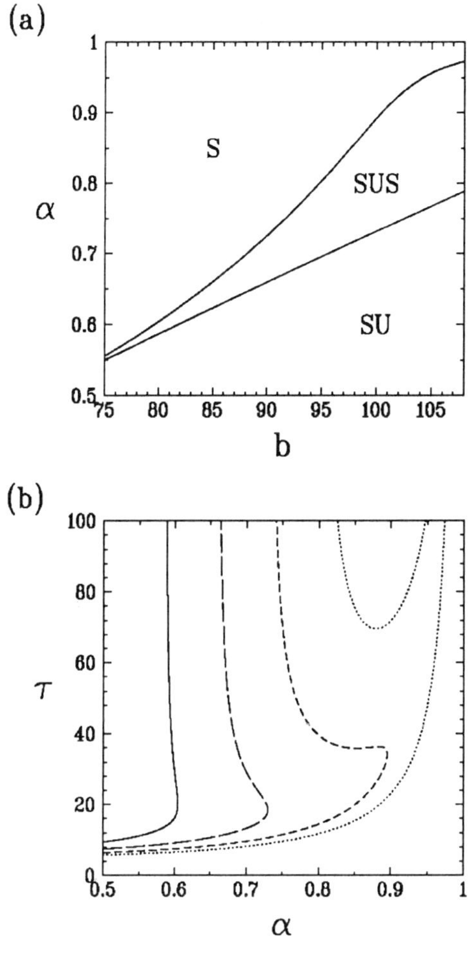

FIG. 5. *(a) Stability regions of the endemic equilibrium (7) for the system (model0td) with* $g = a\exp(-bI(t-\tau)^{\gamma})$, *and* $a = 0.02$, $\mu = 0.001$, $\chi = 1.0$, *and* $\gamma = 1.0$. *To the right of the lower curve, the SU region, the system is stable for small* τ, *and unstable for* $\tau > \tau_c$ *(see Figure 5b for the corresponding values of* τ_c*). In the region between the two curves, the SUS region, the system is stable for small* τ, *becomes unstable as* τ *exceeds* τ_1, *and stable as* τ *exceeds at* τ_2 *(see Figure 5b for the corresponding values of* τ*). To the left of both curves, the S region, the system is absolutely stable. (b) Stability regions of the endemic equilibrium (7) for the system (16) with* $g = g(I(t-\tau))$ *in the* (τ - α)*-plane for four different b:* $b = 80$ *(solid line),* $b = 90$ *(long-dashed line),* $b = 100$ *(short-dashed line), and* $b = 110$ *(dotted line). The parameters are* $a = 0.02$, $\mu = 0.001$, $\chi = 1.0$, *and* $\gamma = 1.0$. *To the right of each curve, the system is stable. The boundaries between the S and SUS regions are given approximately by:* $\alpha > 0.61$ *for* $b = 80$, $\alpha > 0.73$ *for* $b = 90$, $\alpha > 0.89$ *for* $b = 100$, *and* $\alpha > 0.98$ *for* $b = 110$ *(see Figure 5a). The boundary between the SU and SUS regions are approximately given by* $\alpha = 0.587$ *for* $b = 80$, $\alpha = 0.66$ *for* $b = 90$, $\alpha = 0.73$ *for* $b = 100$, *and* $\alpha = 0.81$ *for* $b = 110$ *(see Figure 5a).*

being stable and unstable as τ increases. However, these regions are small. We also found regions where, for large enough τ, the equilibrium becomes unstable (see Figure 5). Indeed, this occurs in some parameter ranges even for small time delays, indicating that the system is very sensitive to τ in these regions.

We have not investigated the effects of uncertainty about the particulars of the disease or the state of the epidemic. However, there are well-developed methods for dealing with decision making in the face of uncertainty. Very generally speaking, uncertainty tends to encourage cautiousness. Hence, it seems plausible that uncertainty will tend to reduce the immigration even further, resulting in even smaller endemic equilibrium populations.

We have investigated the consequences of state-dependent net immigration in only the simplest of epidemiological models. A key assumption is that the contact rate, c, is constant. Since we find that the size of the population can change by over an order of magnitude, it may be appropriate, in future modelling efforts, to consider a contact rate that depends on the size of the population. We have also made many other simplifying assumptions. It may be appropriate, in specific scenarios, to generalize the model further, by, say, incorporating long and variable incubation and infectivity periods, different vaccination scenarios, more general force of infection terms which take into account decreased mobility of infecteds, and so on. Furthermore, as it was shown in Hadeler and Castillo-Chavez (1995) the size of the noncore group can play an important role. Further detail will undoubtedly complicate the analysis considerably.

Acknowledgments. We are grateful to Fred Brauer and Jorge Velasco-Hernandez for helpful discussions. This research was partially supported by NSF and NSA grants to Castillo-Chavez. This work began several years ago and was recently revised while Castillo-Chavez was visting the IMA at the University of Minnesota Minneapolis.

APPENDIX

A. Proof of global stability of the disease-free equilibrium. In this appendix, the proof of global stability of the disease-free equilibrium of the systems (5) and (16) is given. First we consider system (5). Adding the two equations in Eqs. (5), one gets $\dot{N} = g(\xi) - \mu N - \sigma I$, where $N = S + I$, $S \geq 0$, $I \geq 0$. Since $g(\xi)$, where (i) $\xi = \tilde{\eta}$ or (ii) $\xi = I$, is a decreasing function, $\dot{N} < a - \mu N$. Thus, in the limit as $t \to \infty$, both N and S are bounded above by a/μ. From the second equation in (5), $\dot{I} < 0$ for $1 \leq \alpha$. Thus $\bar{I}_0 \geq 0$. To show that, in fact, $\bar{I}_0 = 0$, we suppose $\bar{I}_0 > 0$ and show that this leads to a contradiction. From the second equation of (5), we have

$$\dot{I} = -\left((\alpha-1)S + \alpha I\right)\frac{I}{S+I} \leq -\alpha I \frac{I}{S+I} \leq -\alpha \bar{I}_0 \frac{\bar{I}_0}{\bar{S}_0 + \bar{I}_0} < 0 \ .$$

Hence, in the limit as $t \to \infty$, $I(t) = I(0) + \int_0^t \dot{I}(r)dr \to -\infty$ which contradicts the supposition that $\bar{I}_0 > 0$ so that we must have $\bar{I}_0 = 0$. Further, since $g_0 = a$, integrating the first equation in (5), in the limit as $t \to \infty$, one gets that $\bar{S}_0 = a/\mu$. Since this analysis applies equally well for $g(\xi(t-\tau))$, for all $\tau > 0$, it follows that the disease-free equilibrium $(\bar{S}_0, \bar{I}_0) = (a/\mu, 0)$ is globally stable if $1 \geq \alpha$ for both (model0td) and (model0dim), for both (i) $\xi = \tilde{\eta}$ or (ii) $\xi = I$.

B. Linear stability analysis of the time-delayed system.

Case (i). In this appendix, we outline the linear stability analysis of the endemic equilibrium of system (16) with $g = g(\eta(t-\tau))$. The local stability of the endemic equilibrium of (16) is determined by the sign of the real part of the eigenvalues, $\lambda = \lambda(\tau)$, of the transcendental characteristic equation (17), which changes as τ increases. To find the τ's where changes in stability occur, we closely follow the analysis of MacDonald (1989) (and references therein), where the reader is referred to for details. It has been show that stability changes occur only at purely imaginary λ. For case (i), substituting $\lambda = i\omega$ into Eq. (17) one gets

$$e^{-i\omega\tau} = \frac{A}{C} + \frac{i}{C}\left(\omega - \frac{B}{\omega}\right) \ . \tag{19}$$

Plotting the two sides of (19) in the complex plane, one sees directly that if $A > C$, there are no solutions to (19). Consequently, for $A > C$, there will be no stability changes due to the time delay – equilibria that are stable for $\tau = 0$ will be stable for all τ. The equilibrium is said to be absolutely stable (Brauer (1987). However, if $A < C$, there are solutions, and changes in stability may occur. For $\tau = 0$, if $A < C$, the equilibrium is unstable. For finite τ, the system may be stabilized. We now find the ranges of τ where this occurs.

Consider first the interval where $0 < \omega\tau < 2\pi$, (when the RHS of Eq. (19), the unit circle, is traced out for the first time). Eq. (19) now has two solutions, $\theta_1 = \omega_1\tau_1$ and $\theta_2 = \omega_2\tau_2$, where $0 < \theta_1 < \pi/2$, and $3\pi/2 < \theta_2 < 2\pi$. Equating the real and imaginary parts of Eq. (19) and solving for ω one gets

$$\omega_{\pm} = \frac{1}{2}\left(\pm\sqrt{C^2 - A^2} + \sqrt{C^2 - A^2 + 4B}\right) \ , \tag{20}$$

with $\omega_2 > \omega_1$ (by inspection of plots of Eq. (19). Furthermore, $(d\mathrm{Re}(\lambda)/d\tau)|_{\lambda=i\omega_1} < 0$, and $(d\mathrm{Re}(\lambda)/d\tau)|_{i\omega_2} > 0$. Thus, if $\tau_1 < \tau_2$, an equilibrium that is unstable when $\tau < \tau_1$ becomes stable when $\tau > \tau_1$, and then, as τ exceeds τ_2, becomes unstable again provided that at $\tau = 0$ there is one pair of roots with positive real parts, all other roots have negative real parts.

This will be the case if $(C-A)^2 - 4B < 0$. Thus, in the parameter range where $A < C$, $(C-A)^2 - 4B < 0$, and $\tau_1 < \tau_2$, for $\tau_1 < \tau < \tau_2$, the system is stable. From (19) we have

$$\tau_1 = \frac{\theta_1}{\omega_1} \quad , \qquad \tau_2 = \frac{\theta_2}{\omega_2} \quad , \tag{21}$$

where $\theta_1 = \arccos(A/C)$, and $\theta_2 = 2\pi - \theta_1$. Thus, whether or not $\tau_1 < \tau_2$ depends on the parameters b, α, σ, χ, and γ. Numerically, we find that the parameter range where $(C-A)^2 - 4B < 0$ contains the parameter range for which $\tau_1 < \tau_2$. In the interval where $2\pi < \omega\tau < 4\pi$, when the unit circle (RHS of (19)) is traced out for the second time, there are again two points where there may be stability changes, namely $\omega_1\tau_1^{(1)} = \theta_1 + 2\pi$ and $\omega_2\tau_2^{(1)} = \theta_2 + 2\pi$. Again, if $\tau_1^{(1)} < \tau_2^{(1)}$, for $\tau_1^{(1)} < \tau < \tau_2^{(1)}$, the system will be stable. These alternating regions of stability and instability, as τ increases, will continue so long as $\tau_1^{(n)} < \tau_2^{(n)}$, where $\tau_1^{(n)} = (\theta_1 + 2\pi n)/\omega_1$, etc., with n a natural number. Since as τ increases, the stability of the equilibrium alternates between Unstable and Stable, these regions are denoted *USU*.

Case (ii). Proceeding as in case (i), we substitute $\lambda = i\omega$ into the characteristic equation (17). One gets

$$e^{-i\omega\tau} = \frac{1}{D}(\omega^2 - B) + i\omega\frac{A}{D} \quad . \tag{22}$$

This is precisely the equation discussed by MacDonald (1989), pp. 89–90. Briefly, equating the real and imaginary parts of (22), one finds that

$$\omega^2 = \frac{1}{2}\left(2B - A^2 \pm \sqrt{\left(A^2 - 2B\right)^2 - 4\left(B^2 - D^2\right)}\right) \quad . \tag{23}$$

For $0 < \omega\tau < 2\pi$, one finds the following cases: Case (a) $B < D$: Only the larger of the two ω's in (23), ω_+, will be real and positive. Since $(d\text{Re}(\lambda)/d\tau)|_{i\omega_+} > 0$, if $\tau < \tau_c = \arccos((\omega_+^2 - B)/D)/\omega_+$, the equilibrium is stable, however if $\tau > \tau_c$, it is unstable. If $D^2 > A^2B$ then $0 < \omega_+\tau < \pi/2$, whereas if $D^2 < A^2B$, one has $\pi/2 < \omega_+\tau < \pi$. Since the equilibrium is stable at $\tau = 0$ and then becomes unstable as τ exceeds τ_c, this region is denoted *SU*. Case (b) $B > D$: If the radical in (23) is positive, there will be two positive real roots with $\omega_1 > \omega_2$, provided that $2B > A^2$. Since $(d\text{Re}(\lambda)/d\tau)|_{i\omega_1} > 0$, and $(d\text{Re}(\lambda)/d\tau)|_{i\omega_2} < 0$, the system will become unstable at τ_1, as τ increases, and stable again at τ_2, provided that $\tau_1 < \tau_2$. As τ increases, the stability changes will continue to alternate until $\tau_1^{(n)} > \tau_2^{(n)}$, where $\tau_1^{(n)} = (\theta_1 + 2\pi n)/\omega_1$. Numerically, we have found only regions with one alternation. Since as τ increases, the equilibrium alternates between being stable and unstable, this region is denoted *SUS*. Case (c) $B > D$: If the radical in (23) is negative, or if $2B < A^2$, there will be no real positive solutions to (23), and, hence, there will be no stability change.

REFERENCES

BLYTHE, S.P., F. BRAUER AND C. CASTILLO-CHAVEZ Demographic Recruitment in Sexually Transmitted Disease Model. Proc. First World Congress on Computational Medicine, Public Health and Biotechnology Part II Austin, TX, 1994. Ed. Matthew Witten. Series in Mathematical Biology and Medicine **5**, 1438-1457, 1997.

BLYTHE, S.P., F. BRAUER, . CASTILLO-CHAVEZ AND J. X. VELASCO-HERNANDEZ Models for sexually transmitted diseases with recruitment. Biometrics Unit Technical Report BU-1193-M, Cornell University, 1993a.

BLYTHE, S.P., K. COOKE AND C. CASTILLO-CHAVEZ Autonomous risk-behavior change, and non-linear incidence rate, in models of sexually transmitted diseases. Biometrics Unit Technical Report BU-1048-M, Cornell University, 1993b.

BRAUER, F. Absolute stability in delay equations. J. Diff. Equations **69**, 185–191, 1987.

BRAUER, F. Basic Ideas of mathematical epidemiology. This volume.

BRAUER, F. Extensions of the basic models. This volume.

BRAUER, F., C. CASTILLO-CHAVEZ AND J.X. VELASCO-HERNANDEZ Recruitment into Core Group and its effect on the spread of a sexually transmitted disease. (1998). Advances in Mathematical Population Dynamics - Molecules, Cells, and Man (O. Arino, D. Axelrod, M. Kimmel, (eds), World Scientific Press, 477 - 486, 1998.

BRAUER, F., C. CASTILLO-CHAVEZ Mathematical Models in Population Biology and Epidemiology, Texts in Applied Mathematics, Volume 40. Springer-Verlag, New York, (2001), 416 pages.

BUSENBERG, S. AND C. CASTILLO-CHAVEZ A general solution of the problem of mixing subpopulations, and its applications to risk- and age-structured epidemic models for the spread of AIDS. IMA J. Math. Applied in Med. and Biol. **8**, 1–29, 1991.

CASTILLO-CHAVEZ, C. AND S. BUSENBERG On the solution of the two-sex mixing problem. In Proceedings of the international conference on differential equations and applications to biology and population dynamics, Busenberg, S., Martelli, M. (eds.). Lect. Notes in Biomath., Vol. **92**, pp. 80–98) Berlin Heidelberg New York, Springer 1991.

BUSENBERG, S. AND K.L. COOKE Vertically transmitted diseases: models and dynamics. Berlin New York: Springer 1993.

CASTILLO-CHAVEZ. C., K. COOKE, W. HUANG AND S.A. LEVIN On the role of long incubation periods in the dynamics of acquired immunodeficiency syndrome (AIDS), Part I: Single population models. J. Math. Biol. **27**, 373–398, 1989a.

CASTILLO-CHAVEZ. C., K. COOKE, W. HUANG AND S.A. LEVIN The role of long incubation periods in the dynamics HIV/AIDS. Applied Math. Letters **2**, 327–331, 1989b.

CASTILLO-CHAVEZ. C., K. COOKE, W. HUANG AND S.A. LEVIN The role of long periods of infectiousness in the dynamics of acquired immunodeficiency syndrome (AIDS). In Mathematical approaches to resource management and epidemiology, Castillo-Chavez, C., Levin, S.A., Shoemaker, C. (eds.). Lect. Notes in Biomath., pp. 177–189, New York, Springer 1989c.

CASTILLO-CHAVEZ. C., K. COOKE, W. HUANG AND S.A. LEVIN On the role of long incubation periods in the dynamics of HIV/AIDS. Part 2: Multiple group models. In Mathematical and statistical approaches to AIDS epidemiology, C. Castillo-Chavez (ed.), Lect. Notes in Biomath., pp. 200–217, New York, Springer 1989d.

CENTERS FOR DISEASE CONTROL Self-reported behavioral change among gay and bisexual men. San Fransicsco. MMWR **34**, 613–615 (1985).

CLARK, C.W. Mathematical Bioeconomics. New York: John Wiley & Sons 1990.

EVANS, B.A., K.A. MCLEAN AND S.G. DAWSON, *et al.* Trends in sexual behaviour and risk factors for HIV infection among homosexual men, 1984–1987. Br. Med. J. **198**, 215–218, 1989.

EWALD, P.W. Evolution of Virulence. Scientific American **268**, 86–93, 1993.

FINEBERG, H.F. Education to prevent AIDS: prospects and obstacles. Science **239**, 592–596, 1988, and references therein.

GRIENSVEN, VAN G.J.P., E.M.M. DE VROOME, J. GOUDSMIT AND R.A. COUTINO. Changes in sexual behavior and the fall in incidence of HIV infection among homosexual men. Br. Med. J. **298**, 298–221, 1989.

HADELER, K.P. AND C. CASTILLO-CHAVEZ A Core Group Model for Disease Transmission. Math Biosci. **128**, 41-55, 1995.

HETHCOTE, H.W. Three basic epidemiological models. In Applied Mathematical Ecology, Hallam, T., Gross, L., Levin, S.A. (eds.). Biomath., Vol.**18**, pp. 119–144, New York, Springer 1989.

HETHCOTE, H.W., The mathematics of infectious diseases , SIAM Review, **42**, 4, pp. 599–653.

HETHCOTE, H.W. AND YORKE, J.A. Gonorrhea: Transmisison dynamics and control. Lecture notes in Biomath., Vol. **56**, Berlin, Springer 1984.

HOLLING, C.S. Some characteristics of simple types of predation and parasitism. Can. Ent. **91**, 385–393, 1959.

HOOVER, D.R., A. MUNOZ, V. CAREY, N. ODAKA, J.M.G. TAYLOR, J.S. CHMIEL, J. ARMSTRONG AND S.H. VERMUND The unseen sample in cohort studies estimation of its size and effect. Statistics in Medicine **10**, 1993–2003, 1991.

HSIEH, Y. AND K. COOKE Behaviour change and treatment of core groups: its effect on the spread of HIV/AIDS. IMA J. of Math. Applied to Medicine and Biology **17**, 213–241, 2000.

HUANG, W. AND C. CASTILLO-CHAVEZ Age-structured Core Group Model and its impact on STD dynamics. This volume.

HUANG, W, K. L. COOKE, AND C. CASTILLO-CHAVEZ, Stability and bifurcation for a multiple-group model for the dynamics of HIV/AIDS transmission, SIAM J. Appl. Math., **52**, pp. 835–854, 1992.

HYMAN J. M. AND E. A. STANLEY, Using mathematical models to understand the AIDS epidemic, Math. Biosci., **90**, pp. 415–473, 1988.

HYMAN J. M. AND E. A. STANLEY, The effect of social mixing patterns on the spread of AIDS. In Mathematical Approaches to Problems in Resource Management and Epidemiology, C. Castillo-Chavez, S. A. Levin, and C. Shoemaker, eds., Lecture Notes in Biomathematics, vol. **81**, Springer-Verlag, New York, 1989.

HYMAN, J. M., LI, J. AND E. A. STANLEY, Threshold conditions for the spread of HIV infection in age-structured populations of homosexual men, J. Theor. Biol., **166**, pp. 9–31, 1994.

JACQUEZ J. A., C. P. SIMON, J.S. KOOPMAN, L. SATTENSPIEL, AND T. PERRY, Modeling and analyzing HIV transmission: The effect of contact patterns, Math. Biosci., **92**, pp. 119–199, 1988.

MACDONALD, N. Biological delay systems: linear stability theory. Cambridge: Cambridge University Press 1989.

MARTIN, J.L. The impact of AIDS in gay male sexual behavior patterns in New York City. Am. J. of Public Health **298**, 578–581, 1987.

MCCLAM, E. "Syphilis Outbreak alarms officials", Ithaca Journal, Section A., page 10A, February 23, 2001.

MCKUSICK, L., W. HORSTMAN AND T.L. COATES AIDS and sexual behavior reported by gay men in San Fransisco. Public Health Reports **75**, 493–496, 1985a.

MCKUSICK, L., J.A. WILEY, T.L. COATES, R. STALL, B. SAIKA, S. MORIN, K. CHARLES, W. HORSTMAN AND M.A. CONANT Reported changes in the sexual behavior of men at risk for AIDS. San Fransisco, 1983–1984: the AIDS behavioral research project, Public Health Reports **100**, 622–629, 1985b.

MURRAY, J.D. Mathematical Biology. (Biomath., Vol. **19**). Springer-Verlag, Berlin Heidelberg New York, 1990.

PALMER, J.S., C. CASTILLO-CHAVEZ AND S. P. BLYTHE State-dependent mixing and state-dependent contact rates in epidemiological models. Biometrics Unit Technical Report BU-1122-M, Cornell University, 1991.

PEREZ-STABLE, E. Cuba's response to the HIV epidemic. Americ. J. Public Health **8**, 5, 563–567, 1991.

PINDER, J.E., J.G. WIENER AND M.H. SMITH The Weibull distribution: a new method of summarizing survivorship data. Ecology **59**, 1, 175–179, 1978.

SATTENSPIEL, L. Population structure and the spread of disease. American Journal of Physical Anthropology **73**, 251–265, 1987a.

SATTENSPIEL, L. Epidemics in nonrandomly mixing populations. Human Biology **59**, 411–438, 1987b.

SATTENSPIEL, L. AND C. SIMON The spread and persitence of infectious diseases in structured populations. Math. Bios. **90**, 341–366, 1988.

SCALIA-TOMBA, G. The effect of structural behavior change on the spread of HIV. Math. Bios. **107**, 547–556, 1991.

THIEME, H.R. AND C. CASTILLO-CHAVEZ On the role of variable infectivity in the dynamics of the human immunodeficiency virus epidemic. In Mathematical and statistical approaches to AIDS epidemiology, Castillo-Chavez, C. (ed.). Lecture notes in Biomath., Vol. **83**, pp. 157–176. Berlin: Springer 1989.

THIEME, H.R. AND C. CASTILLO-CHAVEZ How May Infection-Age-Dependent Infectivity Affect the Dynamics of HIV/AIDS. (1993). SIAM J. Applied Math. **53**, No. 5, pp. 1447-79.

VELASCO-HERNANDEZ, J. X., F. BRAUER AND C. CASTILLO-CHAVEZ Effects of Treatment and Prevalence-dependent Recruitment on the Dynamics of a fatal disease. IMA Journal of Math. Medicine and Biology, **13** 3, 175-192, 1996.

VELASCO-HERNANDEZ J.X. AND Y. HSIEH Modelling the effect of treatment and behavioral change in HIV transmission dynamics. J. Math Biol. **32**, 233–249, 1994.

DISCRETE-TIME S-I-S MODELS WITH SIMPLE AND COMPLEX POPULATION DYNAMICS

CARLOS CASTILLO-CHAVEZ* AND ABDUL-AZIZ YAKUBU†

Abstract. The model for this study is an extension of a nonlinear discrete-time susceptible-infected-susceptible (S-I-S) epidemic model of Barrera *et al.* and Velazquez that includes populations exhibiting geometric, bounded or complex dynamics. Thresholds for disease persistence are computed and used to illustrate the analysis of the asymptotic global behavior of solutions. Extensions and results that include SIS models capable of supporting multiple attractors are discussed.

1. Introduction. Simple nonlinear discrete-time population models are capable of generating complex (chaotic) dynamics [4, 6, 9, 18, 21, 22]. A simple nonlinear discrete-time susceptible-infected-susceptible (S-I-S) epidemic model that assumes that the population is either asymptotically bounded, experiences geometric growth or is capable of generating complex dynamics is presented.

Theoretical studies of (S-I-S) epidemic models have been carried out in deterministic (discrete and continuous-time) and stochastic Markov chains for a long time (see Allen [1, 2]; Anderson *et al.* [3]; Bailey [5]; Castillo et al. [7–10]; Cooke and Yorke [11]; Hassell *et al.* [18] and Nåsell [23], to name a few). Barrera *et al.* [6]; Velazquez [27]; and Castillo-Chavez and Yakubu [9, 10] have developed models for the study of disease dynamics in populations with discrete generations and potentially complex (chaotic) disease-free dynamics. The models in this article overlap somewhat with (S-I-S) epidemic models found in the literature (see [6, 9, 10, 16, 27]).

2. Simple discrete-time epidemic models. Nonlinear discrete-time epidemic models are built under the assumption that the dynamics of the total population size in generation n, denoted by $T(n)$, are governed by an equation of the form $T(n+1) = f(T(n)) + \gamma T(n)$, where $0 \leq \gamma < 1$ denotes the constant probability of surviving per generation and f models the typically nonlinear birth or recruitment process. If f is not typical, that is, if f is a constant or a linear function of the total population then the population dynamics are rather simple. Specifically, if new recruits arrive at the constant per-capita rate μ or at the total constant rate Λ per generation then $f(T(n)) = \mu T(n)$ or $f(T(n)) = \Lambda$. An epidemic process is built on "top" of this demographic model that, by construction, has known disease-independent, and simple population dynamics for $T(n)$. Epidemics on simple demographic settings are the norm in the study of continuous-time epidemic models where the total population is typically assumed to be constant, asymptotically constant, or capable of supporting exponential

*Biometrics Department, Cornell University, Ithaca, New York 14853.
†Department of Mathematics, Howard University, Washington, DC 20059.

growth. This framework expands the range of complexity of the underlying population dynamics (see the next section for examples).

At generation n, $S(n)$ denotes the population of susceptibles; $I(n)$ denotes the population of infecteds, assumed infectious; $T(n) \equiv S(n) + I(n)$ denotes the total population size; and, $T_\infty \equiv \lim_{n\to\infty} T(n)$ denotes the demographic steady state for the total population whenever it exists. Individuals survive from one generation to the next with constant probability γ while infected, individuals recover with constant probability $1-\sigma$ per generation. Susceptible individuals (given that they had contacts with infectives) become infected with probability $1-G$ or, equivalently, remain susceptible with probability G per generation. $G : [0,\infty) \to [0,1]$ is a monotone concave function with $G(0) = 1; G^{'}(x) < 0$ and $G^{''}(x) \geq 0$ for all $x \in [0,\infty)$.

The population dynamics are fixed since it is assumed that the disease is not fatal. All recruits are susceptible, time is measured in generations, and recovery from the disease does not give permanent or temporary immunity. The modeling process implicitly assumes a sequential process: At the end of each generation, a fraction $(1-\gamma)$ of each class is removed (death); surviving susceptibles become infected with probability $(1-G)$; and, independently, surviving infectives recover with probability $(1-\sigma)$. It is important to note that this is a deterministic model and that *probabilistic lingo* is used *mainly* to facilitate understanding.

Our assumptions lead to the following discrete-time S-I-S epidemic model:

$$\left.\begin{aligned} S(n+1) &= f(T(n)) + \gamma S(n) G(\tfrac{\alpha I(n)}{T(n)}) + \gamma I(n)(1-\sigma), \\ I(n+1) &= \gamma(1 - G(\tfrac{\alpha I(n)}{T(n)}))S(n) + \gamma\sigma I(n), \end{aligned}\right\} \tag{1}$$

where $0 < \gamma, \sigma < 1$, and $T(n) > 0$. The constant α weighs the role of prevalence $(\frac{I(n)}{T(n)})$ on disease transmission. If α is large, then it is easier to become infected (see Figure 1). System (1), is an extension of the discrete-time (S-I-S) epidemic models of Barrera *et al.* and Velazquez [6, 27].

Since $T(n+1) \equiv S(n+1) + I(n+1)$, then

$$T(n+1) = f(T(n)) + \gamma T(n), \tag{2}$$

that is, Equation (2) models the dynamics (demography) of the total population.

3. Simple population dynamics and SIS epidemics. If $f(T(n)) = \mu T(n)$ then Equation (2), the demographic equation, reduces to the linear difference equation

$$T(n+1) = (\mu + \gamma) T(n), \tag{3}$$

and, consequently,

$$T(n) = (\mu + \gamma)^n T(0). \tag{4}$$

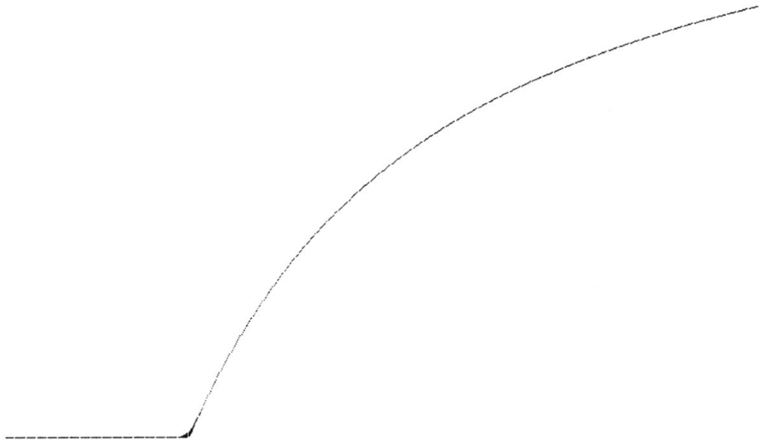

FIG. 1. *The size of infecteds increases from zero as α increases.*

The demographic basic reproductive number,

$$\Re_d = \frac{\mu}{1-\gamma},$$

is a dimensionless quantity. It gives the average number of descendants produced by a (typically) small pioneer population ($T(0)$) over its life-time. Hence, if $\Re_d > 1$, the population invades at a geometric rate and if $\Re_d < 1$ the population dies geometrically. The epidemic process constructed then lives in a population experiencing geometric dynamics.

If we let

$$x(n) = \frac{S(n)}{T(n)} \quad \text{and} \quad y(n) = \frac{I(n)}{T(n)}, \tag{5}$$

then System (1) with $f(T(n)) = \mu T(n)$ reduces to the one-dimensional autonomous "system" for $y(n)$:

$$y(n+1) = \frac{\gamma}{\gamma+\mu}\Big(1-y(n)\Big)\Big(1-G(\alpha y(n))\Big) + \frac{\gamma\sigma}{\gamma+\mu}y(n). \tag{6}$$

Since $x(n) + y(n) = 1$ for all n then all solutions live on the invariant line $\{(x,y) \in [0,\infty) \times [0,\infty) \mid x+y=1\}$.

$\Re_0$, the number of secondary infections generated by an infected (assumed infectious) individual over his or her lifetime in a population of susceptibles, determines whether or not the disease can invade. From Equation (6), we find that

$$\Re_0 = \frac{-\alpha\gamma G'(0)}{(1-\gamma)(\Re_d - 1) + (1-\gamma\sigma)},$$

after noticing that near the equilibrium point $(x_\infty, y_\infty) \equiv (1,0)$,

$$y(n+1) \approx \frac{\gamma}{\gamma+\mu}\Big(- \alpha G'(0) + \sigma\Big) y(n).$$

Whenever $\Re_d = 1$ (no demographic impact), the basic reproductive number, $\Re_0$, reduces to $\Re_0 = \frac{-\alpha\gamma G'(0)}{1-\gamma\sigma}$, where $\frac{1}{1-\gamma\sigma}$ denotes the average death-adjusted length of the infectious period in generations; γ is the proportion of surviving susceptibles who can be invaded by the disease; and, $-\alpha G'(0)$ is the maximum rate of infection per infective [9, 10]. Since $\frac{1}{(1-\gamma)(\Re_d-1)+(1-\gamma\sigma)}$ gives the demographic death-adjusted infectious period measured in generations then $\Re_0$ decreases with population growth $(\Re_d > 1)$ and increases with population decay $(0 < \Re_d < 1)$, that is, whenever $\Re_d \neq 1$ demography has an impact.

Result 1. *(a) Suppose that $\Re_d > 1$, that is, assume T is increasing at the geometric rate, $(\mu+\gamma)$. Then*

(i) $\Re_0 \leq 1$, implies that the proportion $\frac{I}{T}$ of infectives in the total population tends to 0 as $n \to \infty$. Hence, $(\frac{S}{T}, \frac{I}{T})$ tends to the disease-free equilibrium $(1,0)$, while S is increasing at the same geometric rate as T.

(ii) $\Re_0 > 1$, implies that the proportion $\frac{I}{T}$ of infectives in the total population tends to a positive number, $\overline{\frac{I}{T}}$ as $n \to \infty$. Hence, $(\frac{S}{T}, \frac{I}{T})$ tends to an endemic equilibrium while I, S and T are increasing at the same geometric rate.

(b) Suppose that $\Re_d < 1$, that is, assume T is decreasing at the geometric rate, $(\mu+\gamma)$. Then

(i) $\Re_0 \leq 1$, implies that the proportion $\frac{I}{T}$ of infectives in the total population tends to 0 as $n \to \infty$. Hence, $(\frac{S}{T}, \frac{I}{T})$ tends to the disease-free equilibrium $(1,0)$ while S is decreasing to zero at the same geometric rate as T.

(ii) $\Re_0 > 1$, implies that the proportion $\frac{I}{T}$ of infectives in the total population tends to a positive number $\overline{\frac{I}{T}}$ as $n \to \infty$. Hence, $(\frac{S}{T}, \frac{I}{T})$ tends to an endemic equilibrium while I, S and T are decreasing at the same geometric rate.

Proof. Define the reproduction function for the infected individuals of System (6), $h : [0,1] \to [0,1]$ by $h(y) = \frac{\gamma}{\gamma+\mu}(1-y)(1-G(\alpha y)) + \frac{\gamma\sigma}{\gamma+\mu}y$, where $h(0) = 0$ and $0 \leq y \leq 1$. The set of iterates of h is equivalent to the set of density sequence generated by the second equation in System (6). Differentiation with respect to y gives

$$\begin{aligned} h'(y) &= \tfrac{\gamma}{\gamma+\mu}(-1 + G(\alpha y) - \alpha(1-y)G'(\alpha y) + \sigma), \\ h''(y) &= \tfrac{\gamma}{\gamma+\mu}(2\alpha G'(\alpha y) - \alpha^2(1-y)G''(\alpha y)). \end{aligned}$$

$\Re_0 \leq 1$ implies that $h'(0) = \frac{\gamma}{\gamma+\mu}(-\alpha G'(0) + \sigma) \leq 1$. Therefore, the fixed point $\{0\}$ is locally stable under h-iteration. Since $G' < 0$ and $G'' \geq 0$

we have that, $h''(y) < 0$ for $y \in [0, 1]$. The monotonicity condition on h' and the fact that $h'(0) \leq 1$ imply that $h'(y) < 1$ or $h(y) < y$ for $y \in (0, 1]$. Hence, $\{y(n)\}_{n \geq 0}$, a strictly decreasing sequence bounded below by zero, converges to the only fixed point of h in the interval $[0, 1]$, $\{0\}$. If $\Re_0 \leq 1$, we have proved that $\frac{I}{T} \to 0$ as $n \to \infty$, while the proportion $\frac{S}{T} \to 1$ as $n \to \infty$.

$\Re_0 > 1$ implies that $h'(0) = \frac{\gamma}{\gamma+\mu}(-\alpha G'(0) + \sigma) > 1$ and, therefore, the fixed point $\{0\}$ is locally unstable under h-iteration. Let $\overline{y}$ denote the smallest positive fixed point of h in $[0, 1]$, and note that $h(1) = \frac{\gamma\sigma}{\gamma+\mu} < 1$. The Intermediate Value Theorem guarantees the existence of the positive fixed point $\overline{y} \in (0, 1)$ satisfying $h(\overline{y}) = \overline{y}$ and $h(y) > y$ for $y \in (0, \overline{y})$ and, consequently, $h'(\overline{y}) \leq 1$. Since $h''(y) < 0$ implies that $h'(y) < h'(\overline{y}) \leq 1$ for $y \in (\overline{y}, 1)$, then $\int_{\overline{y}}^{y} h'(u)du < \int_{\overline{y}}^{y} du$ and, we have $h(y) < y$ for $y > \overline{y}$. Hence, h has a unique positive fixed point $\overline{y} \in (0, 1)$. Furthermore, $h(y) > y$ for $y \in (0, \overline{y})$ and $h(y) < y$ for $y \in (\overline{y}, 1]$.

To establish the global stability of $\overline{y}$, we first prove the nonexistence of non-trivial two-cycles for h. Note that $1 + h'(y) = 1 + \frac{\gamma}{\gamma+\mu}(-1 + G(\alpha y) - \alpha(1-y)G'(\alpha y) + \sigma) \geq 1 - \frac{\gamma}{\gamma+\mu} + \frac{\gamma\sigma}{\gamma+\mu} > 0$. Hence, $1 + h'(y) \neq 0$ for $y \in [0, 1]$, that is, h has no non-trivial 2-cycles. Suppose h has a non-trivial 2-cycle $\{p, q\}$ where $p, q \in [0, 1]$, then $h(p) = q$ and $h(q) = p$ where $p \neq q$. The Mean Value Theorem guarantees the existence of a point ξ between p and q such that $h'(\xi) = \frac{h(p)-h(q)}{p-q} = -1$, and $1 + h'(\xi) = 0$, a contradiction. Hence, h has no non-trivial 2-cycles in $[0, 1]$. Sharkovskii's Theorem and $1 + h'(y) \neq 0$ imply the nonexistence of any $m - cycles$ for $m > 1$. From a result of Cull [12], the nonexistence of non-trivial 2-cycles for h implies global stability of the positive fixed point $\overline{y}$. Hence, $\Re_0 > 1$, implies that $\frac{I}{T} \to \overline{\frac{I}{T}} \in (0, 1)$ as $n \to \infty$, and $\frac{S}{T} \to \overline{\frac{S}{T}} \in (0, 1)$ as $n \to \infty$. □

A second simple example is provided with $f(T(n)) = \Lambda$. The demographic equation, reduces to the linear difference equation

$$T(n+1) = \Lambda + \gamma T(n) \tag{7}$$

and, hence

$$T(n) = (T(0) - \frac{\Lambda}{1-\gamma})\gamma^n + \frac{\Lambda}{1-\gamma}. \tag{8}$$

Since $0 < \gamma < 1$, the total population is asymptotically constant, that is, $T_\infty = \frac{\Lambda}{1-\gamma}$, that is, the demographic effects "eventually" disappear.

To study disease epidemics on (7), we assume that the total population $T(n) \equiv S(n) + I(n)$ has reached the positive steady state T_∞. If we redefine $S(n) = T_\infty - I(n)$ then from System (1) we obtain the following associated one-dimensional dynamically equivalent autonomous "system" for $I(n)$ [25, 28]:

$$
(9) \qquad \left.\begin{array}{rcl} S(n+1) & = & f(T_\infty) + c\gamma(T_\infty - I)G(\frac{\alpha I(n)}{T_\infty}) + \gamma I(n)(1-\sigma) \\ I(n+1) & = & \gamma(1 - G(\frac{\alpha I(n)}{T_\infty}))(T_\infty - I) + \gamma\sigma I(n). \end{array}\right\}
$$

Its basic reproductive number is

$$
\Re_0 = \frac{-\alpha\gamma G'(0)}{1-\gamma\sigma}
$$

and a simple application of earlier results gives the following the result [9, 10]:

Result 2. *Suppose* $f(T(n)) = \Lambda$ *in system (9)* then

(a) If $\Re_0 \leq 1$*, then all solutions* $(S(n), I(n))$ *approach the globally asymptotically stable disease free equilibrium,* $(\frac{\Lambda}{1-\gamma}, 0)$*, as* $n \to \infty$.

(b) If $\Re_0 > 1$*, then all solutions* $(S(n), I(n))$ *approach a unique positive and globally asymptotically stable endemic equilibrium,* $(\overline{S}, \overline{I}) \in (0, \infty) \times (0, \infty)$*, as* $n \to \infty$.

The proof of Result (2) is the same as that of Theorem (1) in [9].

Consider the following particular version of Model (1):

$$
(10) \qquad \left.\begin{array}{rcl} S(n+1) & = & f(T(n)) + e^{-d}S(n)e^{-\frac{\alpha I(n)}{T(n)}} + e^{-d}I(n)(1-e^{-\beta}), \\ I(n+1) & = & e^{-d}(1 - e^{-\frac{\alpha I(n)}{T(n)}})S(n) + e^{-d}e^{-\beta}I(n), \end{array}\right\}
$$

where α, β and d are positive constants. Here, we have taken $e^{-d} = \gamma$, $e^{-\frac{\alpha I(n)}{T(n)}} = G(\frac{\alpha I(n)}{T(n)})$ and $e^{-\beta} = \sigma$. $f(T(n)) = \mu T(n)$ implies that $T(n+1) = (e^{-d} + \mu)T(n)$ and $\Re_d = \frac{\mu}{1-e^{-d}}$. Using proportions reduces System (10) to the following system of equations (see, [6, 9, 10]):

$$
(11) \qquad \left.\begin{array}{rcl} x(n+1) & = & \frac{\mu}{e^{-d}+\mu} + \frac{e^{-d}}{e^{-d}+\mu}x(n)e^{-\alpha y(n)} + \frac{e^{-d}(1-e^{-\beta})}{e^{-d}+\mu}y(n), \\ y(n+1) & = & \frac{e^{-d}}{e^{-d}+\mu}x(n)(1-e^{-\alpha y(n)}) + \frac{e^{-d}e^{-\beta}}{e^{-d}+\mu}y(n). \end{array}\right\}
$$

The basic reproductive number,

$$
\Re_0 = \frac{\alpha^2}{1+\mu e^d - e^{-\beta}},
$$

determines the asymptotic behavior of System (11) [see Result 1].

We fix the constants $\beta = 0.1$, $d = \ln 2$ and $\mu = 0.1$ while we vary the transmission coefficient α. As we increase α, the basic reproductive number, $\Re_0$, increases from values less than 1 to numbers bigger than 1. A transcritical bifurcation occurs. The demographic basic reproductive number remains fixed at $\Re_d = \frac{\mu}{1-e^{-d}} = 0.25 < 1$. The system with proportions changes from a globally stable disease-free equilibrium to a globally stable endemic equilibrium while the total population is decreasing to zero at a geometric rate (see Figure 1). In particular, at $\alpha = 0.6$, $\Re_0 = 1.22 > 1$ and the system with proportions has a globally stable endemic equilibrium at $(0.5598, 0.4402)$.

4. Complex dynamics in S-I-S models. Equations (2) is capable of supporting complex (chaotic) dynamics. For example, if new recruits are governed by Smith-Slatkin model [11, 22],

$$f(T(n)) = \frac{aT(n)}{1 + (bT(n))^l},$$

where a, b and l are positive constants and $a > 1$ then

$$T(n+1) = \frac{aT(n)}{1 + (bT(n))^l} + \gamma T(n), \tag{12}$$

where a is maximal per-capita intrinsic growth rate of the population. The parameter l reflects the type and strength of intraspecific competition while the parameter b scales the carrying capacity of the population [13, 24]. Whenever $0 < l < \frac{2(a+\gamma)}{a+\gamma-1}$, the total population assumes a positive steady state at $T_\infty = \frac{(a+\gamma-1)^{\frac{1}{l}}}{b}$ and Result 2 applies. However, as l increases past $\frac{2(a+\gamma)}{a+\gamma-1}$, the positive equilibrium point undergoes period-doubling bifurcation resulting in a stable $2-$*cycle* (see Figure 2). This process of period doubling bifurcation continues indefinitely.

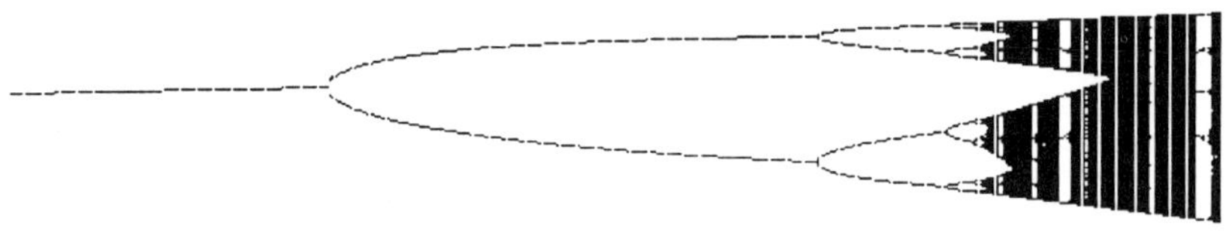

FIG. 2. *Period-doubling bifurcations route to chaos in the demographic equation under Smith-Slatkin model with* $a = 1.5$, $b = 1$, $\gamma = 0.1$ *and* $4.5 < l < 8.5$.

5. Backward bifurcations. Typically, epidemic models have a unique endemic equilibrium with the reproductive number of the disease serving as a threshold parameter (transcritical bifurcation). If the reproduction number is less than one, the disease dies out while if the reproduction number is bigger than one, the disease persists (a forward transcritical bifurcation). If the transmission rate $\alpha_i \equiv \alpha_i(\frac{I_i}{T_i})$ is non-constant but rather a function of the prevalence then multiple endemic equilibria for System (1) are possible even when the basic reproductive number is less than one (backward bifurcation).

Examples of epidemic models exhibiting this behavior were first established for continuous-time epidemic models by Castillo-Chavez *et al.* [7, 8, 14] and Huang *et al.* [19]. Recently, examples using simpler continuous-time models were constructed by Castillo-Chavez and Hadeler [17], Feng *et al.* [15], Kribs *et al.* [20] and P. van den Driessche *et al.* [26]. The results of Feng *et al.* [15], Huang *et al.* [19] and Castillo-Chavez and Hadeler [17] have far reaching implications for the implementation of effective public health policies for HIV and Tuberculosis. The results of P. van den Driessche and P. Watmough have important theoretical implications as they illustrate the possibility of backward bifurcations for simple epidemic processes (*S-I-S* epidemic models based on a Volterra integral equation [26]). Backward bifurcations are possible in classical discrete-time epidemic models, that is, when α is constant. An example using a classical (constant α) discrete-time susceptible-exposed-infective-susceptible (*S-E-I-S*) epidemic model has been recently developed [4].

To illustrate these results $\alpha(y) = y$, that is, $G(\alpha(y)y) = e^{-y^2}$. To make the example transparent, we use the approximation $e^{-y^2} \approx 1 - y^2$. Equation (6) becomes

$$y(n+1) = \frac{\gamma}{\gamma+\mu}(1 - y(n))y^2(n) + \frac{\gamma}{\gamma+\mu}\sigma y(n). \tag{13}$$

Since $\alpha(y) = y$ is a non-constant transmission rate, prior results do not apply. Linearization of Equation (13) near the disease-free equilibrium $(x_\infty, y_\infty) \equiv (1, 0)$ gives

$$y(n+1) \approx \frac{\gamma}{\gamma+\mu}(-\alpha G'(0) + \sigma)y(n).$$

Hence, $\Re_0 = \frac{\gamma\sigma}{(1-\Re_d)\gamma+\Re_d}$ where $\Re_d = \frac{\mu}{1-\gamma}$. A backward bifurcation using Equation (13) is illustrated numerically. We vary $\Re_0$ while the survival probability γ and the variable coefficient μ remain fixed at $\gamma = 0.98$ and $\mu = 0.01$. The following bifurcation curve (Figure 3) is generated:

The disease free equilibrium $(1, 0)$ is locally asymptotically stable for all values of the parameters. It is globally stable whenever $\Re_0 < 0.7525$. A backward bifurcation occurs at $\Re_0 \approx 0.7525$. When $\Re_0 \approx 0.7525$, an unstable endemic equilibrium appears, and for values of $\Re_0$ in the interval $(0.7525, 1)$ the system has 2 endemic equilibria coexisting with the disease free equilibrium (see Figure 3). Hence, the future of the disease depends on initial conditions, that is, the model supports multiple attractors.

6. Conclusions. Simple nonlinear discrete-time population models are capable of generating complex (chaotic) dynamics. Nonlinear discrete-time (*S-I-S*) epidemic models built on bounded or geometrically growing populations do not generate complex (chaotic) dynamics but could generate multiple attractors. We derived thresholds for the persistence of the disease and analyzed the global and local behavior of solutions. Extensions

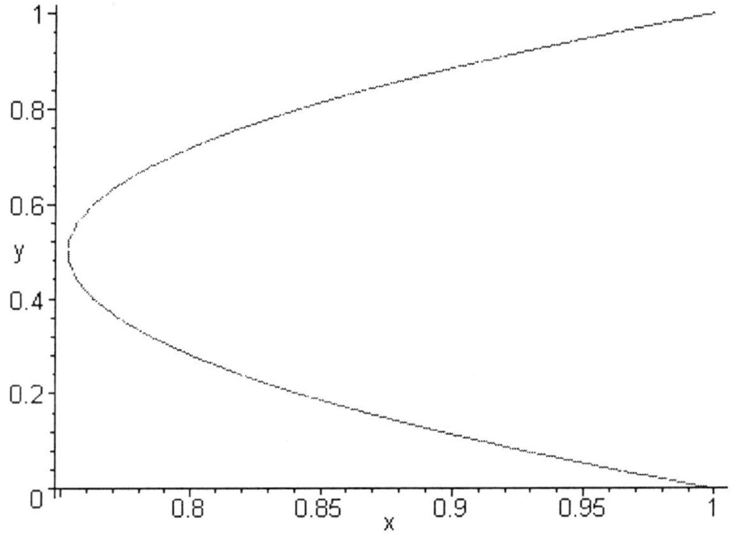

FIG. 3. *The relationship between the proportion of susceptibles and the basic reproductive number* $\Re_0$. *The horizontal axis,* $0.7 \leq \Re_0 \leq 1$, *and the vertical axis,* $0 \leq y_\infty \leq 1$.

to populations with complex population dynamics and multiple attractors were briefly discussed.

7. Acknowledgments. This study was partially supported by grants from National Science Foundation (NSF Grant DMS 9977919) and National Security Agency (NSA Grant MDA 9149710074). Abdul-Aziz Yakubu was supported in part by the NSF IGERT Program in Nonlinear Systems at Cornell University. This research was completed while Abdul-Aziz Yakubu was a Visiting Scientist at the Center for Applied Mathematics in Cornell University. We thank the office of the provost of Cornell University for its support and Intel Technology for Education 200 Equipment Grant. The examples that lead to this research were part of a summer research experience supported by the above grants. The related work of Barrera, J.H., Cintron-Arias, A., Davidenko, N., Denogean, L.R., Franco-Gonzalez, S.R. and Velazquez, J.P. (under our supervision) has been published as Biometrics Department Technical Reports (see references).

REFERENCES

[1] Allen, L. and Burgin, A.M. Comparison of deterministic and stochastic SIS and SIR models, *Dept. Math. & Statistics, Technical Report Series (Texas Tech. University)* (1999).

[2] Allen, L. Some discrete-time SI, SIR and SIS epidemic models. *Math. Biosci.*, **124**: 83–105 (1994).

[3] Anderson, R.M. and May, R.M. Infectious diseases of humans: *Dynamics and control.* Oxford University Press, Oxford (1992).

[4] Arreola, R., Crossa, A., and Velasco, M.C. Discrete-time S-E-I-S models with dispersal between two patches, *Biometric Department, MTBI Cornell University Technical Report* (2000).

[5] Bailey, N.T.J. The simple stochastic epidemic: a complete solution in terms of known functions. *Biometrika*, **50**: 235–240 (1963).

[6] Barrera, J.H., Cintron-Arias, A., Davidenko, N., Denogean, L.R., and Franco-Gonzalez, S.R. Dynamics of a two-dimensional discrete-time SIS model, *MTBI Cornell University Technical Report* (1999).

[7] Castillo-Chavez, C., Cooke, K., Huang, W., and Levin, S.A. The role of long periods of infectiousness in the dynamics of acquired immunodeficiency syndrome (AIDS), *J. Math. Biol.*, **27**: 373–398 (1988).

[8] Castillo-Chavez, C., Hethcote, H.W., Andreasen, V., Levin, S.A., and Liu, W.M. Cross immunity in the dynamics of homogeneous and heterogeneous populations. *Mathematical Ecology,* (ed. L.J. Cross, T.G. Hallam, and S.A. Levin), pp. 303–316 (1988).

[9] Castillo-Chavez, C. and Yakubu, A.A. Discrete-time *S-I-S* models with complex dynamics. Nonlinear Analysis T.M.A. (Accepted).

[10] Castillo-Chavez, C. and Yakubu, A.A. Dispersal, Disease and Life-History Evolution (Preprint).

[11] Cooke, K.L. and Yorke, J.A. Some equations modelling growth processes and gonorrhea epidemics, *Math. Biosci.*, **16**: 75–101 (1973).

[12] Cull, P. Local and global stability for population models. *Biol. Cybern.*, **54**: 141–149 (1986).

[13] Doebeli, M. and Ruxton, G.D. Evolution of dispersal rates in metapopulation models: Branching and cyclic dynamics in phenotype space. *Evolution,* **51**(6): 1730–1741 (1997).

[14] Dushoff, J., Huang, W., and Castillo-Chavez, C., Backwards bifurcations and catastrophe in simple models of fatal diseases. *J. Math. Bio.,* **36**: 227–248 (1998).

[15] Feng, Z., Castillo-Chavez, C., and Capurro, A. A model for Tuberculosis with Exogenous Reinfection, *Theor. Popln. Biol.*, **57**: 235–247 (2000).

[16] Gonzalez, P.A., Saenz, R. and Sanchez, B. The influence of dispersal between two patches on the dynamics of a disease. *Biometric Department, MTBI Cornell University Technical Report* (2000).

[17] Hadeler, K.P. and Castillo-Chavez, C. A core group model for disease transmission. *Math. Biosci.,* **128**: 41–55 (1995).

[18] Hassell, M.P., Anderson R.C., and Cohen, J.E., et al. Impact of diseases on host populations (group report). In population biology of infectious diseases, (ed. R.M. Anderson and R.M. May), Springer-Verlag, New York (1982).

[19] Huang, W., Cooke, K.L., and Castillo-Chavez, C. Stabilitiy and bifurcation for a multiple-group model for the dynamics of HIV/AIDS transmission. *SIAM J. Appl. Math.*, **52**(3): 835–854 (1992).

[20] Kribs-Zaleta, C.M. and Velasco-Hernández, J.X. A simple vaccination model with a backward bifurcation, *Math. Biosci.,* **164**(2): 183–201 (2000).

[21] May, R.M. Simple mathematical models with very complicated dynamics, *Nature,* **261**: 459–469 (1977).

[22] May, R.M. Stability and complexity in model ecosystems, *Princeton University Press* (1974).

[23] Nåsell, I. The quasi-stationary distribution of the closed endemic SIS model. *Adv. Appl. Prob.*, **28**: 895–932 (1996).

[24] Smith, M. and Slatkin, M. The stability of predator-prey systems. *Ecology,* **54**: 384–391 (1973).

[25] Thieme, H.R. Convergence results and a Poincaré-Bendixson trichotomy for asymptotically autonomous differential equations, *J. Math. Biol.*, **30**: 755–763 (1992).

[26] van den Driessche, P. and Watmough, J. A simple SIS model with a backward bifurcation, *J. Math. Biol.*, **40**: 525–540 (2000).

[27] Velazquez, J.P. SIS nonlinear discrete-time models with two competing strains, *MTBI Cornell University Technical Report* (1999).

[28] Zhao, X.-Q. Asymptotic behavior for asymptotically periodic semiflows with applications. Comm. Appl. Nonl. Anal., **3**: 43–66 (1996).

INTRASPECIFIC COMPETITION, DISPERSAL AND DISEASE DYNAMICS IN DISCRETE-TIME PATCHY ENVIRONMENTS

CARLOS CASTILLO-CHAVEZ* AND ABDUL-AZIZ YAKUBU†

Abstract. In this article, a simple framework for the study of the effects of dispersal and disease on the dynamics of a population experiencing density dependent discrete-time intraspecific competition in several patches is provided. The population dynamics in each patch are modeled by nonlinear functions of the densities and, therefore, capable of generating complex (chaotic) dynamics. The role of dispersal on the local patch dynamics is first studied under various competition regimes. Ways of incorporating disease dynamics on an illustrative two-patch system are presented. Suggestions on possible approaches to the study of the effects of dispersal on disease persistence and re-emergence are briefly discussed.

1. Introduction. The effect of incorporating both dispersal and complex local dynamics in simple discrete-time models was carried out by Hastings [16]. Hastings used discrete-time logistic maps to model local dynamics and allowed constant per-capita dispersion between (two) patches. He showed that the interaction between local dynamics and dispersal could lead to the elimination of chaotic dynamics and the creation of multiple attractors with fractal basin boundaries. Here, the effects of different intraspecific competitive regimes in discrete-time patchy environments connected by constant per-capita dispersion are explored. The exploration of the effects of disease (epidemics) in systems with dispersal is briefly discussed in the last two sections.

Scramble and contest competition are two extreme forms of intraspecific competition for resources [14, 15, 23]. Systems under scramble competition try to support all individuals including those who are non-reproductive. In scramble competition, the resources are equally divided among individuals, so that, beyond a threshold density, none can get enough of a share of the resource to survive and reproduce. The logistic model and the more biologically sound Ricker's model provide two examples of systems where new recruits face scramble competition [14, 23, 24]. In contest competition, some individuals get a big enough share of the resource to survive and reproduce at the expense of the rest. The Verhulst model is an example where new recruits face contest competition [14, 23].

The local dynamics in each patch are modeled by a discrete-time model while dispersal between patches is assumed to be proportional to the local densities. We show that, independent of initial population densities, the aggregate dynamics of the full multi-patch system is qualitatively the same as the local patch dynamics under contest or pseudo-contest competition [Theorem 3 and Theorem 4]. However, when the local dynamics are driven

*Biometrics Department, Cornell University, Ithaca, New York 14853.
†Department of Mathematics, Howard University, Washington, DC 20059.

by scramble competition (in the oscillatory regime with cycles) then the aggregate dynamics of the full system are complex [Examples 1 and 2], that is, the qualitative dynamics of the full system are different from local patch dynamics. In other words, the patch system does not have the same dynamics of the patch components. Models with mixed competitive local dynamics (contest versus scramble competition [Example 2]) also generate complex dynamics. Their aggregate dynamics cannot be (in general) identified with that of a single-patch system.

If the initial conditions are identical on each patch, then we say that the patches are in-phase otherwise, the patches are out-of-phase. If the local population dynamics are identical in each patch, we obtain that, for in-phase initial conditions, the full system behaves as a single patch system [Lemma 4]. We use Ricker's model of scramble competition [Example 1] to show that the system is sensitive to initial conditions even when the local dynamics are identical in each patch, for out-of-phase initial conditions. Example 1 illustrates a system with two coexisting attractors and fractal basin boundaries. Hastings studied similar fractal basin boundaries using the logistic map for the local dynamics [13, 16]. The number of attractors seem to depend strongly on specific local dynamics (results are different for the logistic map, see [9, 16]). Hence, from our numerical simulations [8], we see that the geometric shapes and sizes of the basins of attraction depend on the exact form of the local dynamics.

In the absence of dispersion, multi-patch systems with local contest competition regimes allow for the possibility of population extinction on some patches. Example 3 illustrates a case of total persistence, that is, populations survive in all patches, thanks to dispersion. In other words, in this example, the removal of dispersion leads to some local extinctions.

2. Model equations. Let $x_i(t)$ be the population size in Patch $i \in \{1, 2, ..., N\}$ at time t, and let $\widetilde{x}_i(t)$ denote the population size, local dynamics, before the dispersal phase. Thus, the equations for the local dynamics in each Patch $i \in \{1, 2, ..., N\}$ at time t have the following general form:

$$\widetilde{x}_i(t) = x_i(t) g_i(x_i(t)), \qquad (i = 1, 2, ..., N) \tag{1}$$

where the per-capita growth functions, $g_i : [0, \infty) \to (0, \infty)$, are assumed to be strictly decreasing, positive and twice differentiable(C^2 on $[0, \infty)$). These functions may take on values greater than 1 and less than 1 but $\lim_{x_i \to \infty} g_i(x_i) = 0$. System (1) is a Kolmogorov-type, discrete-time single-species population model with N (uncoupled) patches. It describes the population dynamics of pioneer species without dispersion between patches [10–12] (species that thrive at very small population densities when left to their own natural devices with no interference are *pioneer species*).

Scramble competition involves equal partitioning of the resource and hence an equal division of the effects of competition between competitors.

In scramble competition, $\lim_{x_i(t)\to\infty} \widetilde{x}_i(t) = 0$. For example, Ricker's model, $\widetilde{x}_i(t) = x_i(t)\exp(r_i - k_i x_i(t))$ [r_i and k_i positive constants] has been used to model the net effects of scramble competition on a population's rate of change in numbers [14, 15, 20–26].

Contest competition differs from scramble in that resources are unequally partitioned. Some individuals get all they require while others do not get enough resources to guarantee their survival or reproduction. Contest competition supports a constant population size when resources are fixed. In contest competition, $\lim_{x_i(t)\to\infty} \widetilde{x}_i(t) > 0$. Verhulst equation, $\widetilde{x}_i(t) = r_i x_i(t)/(x_i(t) + k_i)$ [r_i and k_i positive constants with $r_i > k_i$] is the typical example of a model of a population under contest competition [14, 15, 20–26].

The N patches in System (1) are now coupled by dispersion that is proportional to local densities. Each d_{ij} (assumed constant) denotes the fraction of the population that disperses from Patch i to j, where $i \neq j \in \{1, 2, ..., N\}$. These assumptions lead to the following system of N nonlinear coupled difference equations:

$$(2) \qquad x_i(t+1) = \Big(1 - \sum_{\substack{j=1 \\ j\neq i}}^{N} d_{ij}\Big)\widetilde{x}_i(t) + \sum_{\substack{j=1 \\ j\neq i}}^{N} d_{ji}\widetilde{x}_j(t), \qquad (i = 1, 2, ..., N)$$

where $d_{ij} = d_{ji}$, $0 < d_{ij} < 1$ and $0 < \sum_{\substack{j=1 \\ j\neq i}}^{N} d_{ij} < 1$.

System (2) is a generalization of the model of Hastings [16] to a multipatch system. Others have studied continuous-time versions of System (2) [1, 18, 19].

3. Notation and preliminaries. To write System (2) as a map, we denote the vector of population densities $x(t) = (x_1(t), x_2(t), ..., x_N(t))$ by $x = (x_1, x_2, ..., x_N)$ and define the map $F : \mathbb{R}_+^N \to \mathbb{R}_+^N$ by $F(x(t)) = x(t+1)$. Thus, for each $i \in \{1, 2, ..., N\}$, $F_i(x) = (1 - \sum_{\substack{j=1 \\ j\neq i}}^{N} d_{ij}) x_i g_i(x_i) + \sum_{\substack{j=1 \\ j\neq i}}^{N} d_{ji} x_j g_j(x_j)$. F^t is the map F composed with itself t times, and $F_j^t(x)$ is the jth component of F^t evaluated at the point x in $\mathbb{R}_+^N$. Therefore, F^t gives the population densities in generation t. The set of iterates of the map F is equivalent to the set of all density sequences generated by System (2).

For each $i \in \{1, 2, ..., N\}$, we define the map $f_i : \mathbb{R}_+ \to \mathbb{R}_+$ by $f_i(x_i) = x_i g_i(x_i)$. If all patches are empty, except Patch i, and there is no dispersion between patches ($d_{ij} = 0$), then the set of iterates of the map f_i is equivalent to the set of all density sequences generated by System (2). Thus, f_i describes the local dynamics in Patch i.

For each $i \in \{1, 2, ..., N\}$, the growth function $g_i : [0, \infty) \to (0, \infty)$ is a strictly decreasing smooth function that takes on positive values bigger than 1 and less than 1. As a result, the equation $g_i(x_i) = 1$ has a unique positive solution, denoted by X_i in $(0, \infty)$. Hence, X_i is the unique positive fixed point of the map f_i.

Since g_i is a strictly decreasing continuous function, $f_i(x_i) > x_i$ whenever $0 < x_i < X_i$ and $f_i(x_i) < x_i$ whenever $x_i > X_i$. Consequently, under f_i iterations, $I_i \equiv f_i([0, X_i])$ is a compact invariant interval in $\mathbb{R}_+$. Every point either eventually enters I_i and stays or just reaches a limit in it. Thus, $I_i \equiv f_i([0, X_i])$ is a global attractor under f_i iterations.

For Ricker's model (scramble competition), $f_i(x_i) = x_i \exp(r_i - k_i x_i)$, there exists a unique positive equilibrium point, $X_i = \frac{r_i}{k_i}$, that is globally stable in $(0, \infty)$,whenever $0 < r_i < 2$. As the parameter r_i increases past 2, the positive equilibrium point, $X_i = \frac{r_i}{k_i}$, undergoes period doubling bifurcations in its route to chaos [see Figure 1, [20–21]].

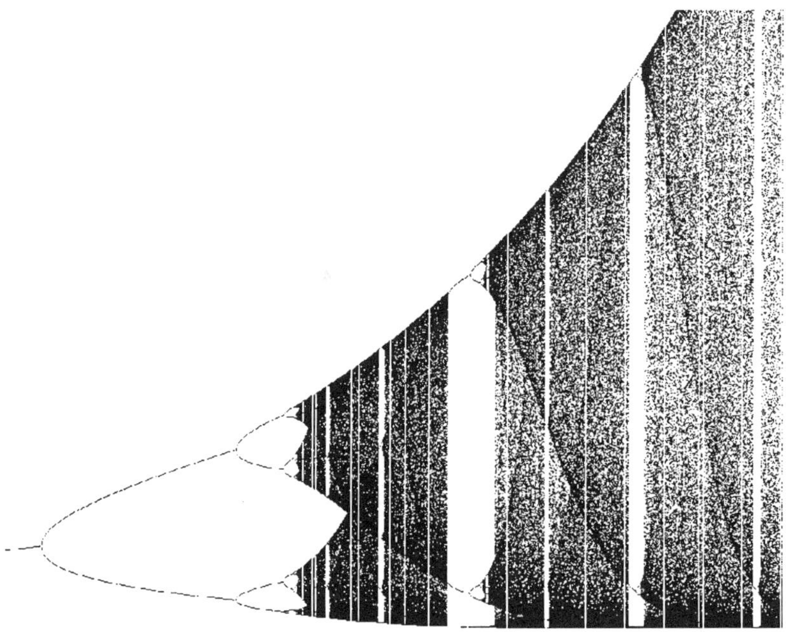

FIG. 1. *Bifurcation diagram of Ricker's model with* $k_1 = 1$. *On the horizontal axes* r_1*varies from* 1.9 *to* 4. *On the vertical axes,* x_1 *varies from* 0 *to* 15.

For Verhulst's equation (contest competition), $f_i(x_i) = r_i x_i/(x_i + k_i)$, there exists a unique positive globally stable equilibrium point, $X_i = r_i - k_i$, whenever $r_i > k_i$. The fixed point, $\{0\}$, is globally stable in $[0, \infty)$, whenever $r_i \leq k_i$. Consequently, if the local dynamics are given by Verhulst equation, $f_i(x_i) = r_i x_i/(x_i + k_i)$ with $r_i \leq k_i$, then the species goes extinct in Patch i provided there is no dispersion. Hence the species are not pioneer species.

We need the following definitions to introduce some of our results.

Definition. *(1) The local dynamics in Patch i, f_i, is a monotone concave map if $f_i'(x_i) > 0$ and $f_i''(x_i) < 0$ for each $x_i \in [0, \infty)$.*

(2) The local dynamics in Patch i, f_i, is an α-monotone concave map if $f_i'(x_i) > 0$ and $f_i''(x_i) < 0$ for each $x_i \in [0, \alpha]$.

Verhulst's model (contest competition), $f_i(x_i) = r_i x_i/(x_i + k_i)$, is a concave, monotone map on $[0, \infty)$, and, Ricker's model (scramble competition), $f_i(x_i) = x_i \exp(r_i - k_i x_i)$, is not only a $\frac{1}{k_i}$-*monotone concave map* but all positive initial populations with densities in $[0, \frac{1}{k_i}]$ approach the unique positive equilibrium point monotonically whenever $0 < r_i < 1$. In other words, in this region it behaves as a contest-competition model.

In System (2), we show that the occurrence of monotone concave local dynamics in each patch generates monotone concave dynamics in patchy environments with dispersion. This results in the full system behaving qualitatively as a single patch system.

Additional notation is needed to state our results. If $x = (x_1, x_2, ..., x_N)$ and $y = (y_1, y_2, ..., y_N) \in \mathbb{R}_+^N$ we write $x < y$ and $x \leq y$ in case the specified inequality holds componentwise. The notation $x \lneqq y$ denotes $x \leq y$ and $x \neq y$. If $x \leq y$, $[x, y] = \{z \in \mathbb{R}_+^N \mid x \leq z \leq y\}$ and $(x, y) = \{z \in \mathbb{R}_+^N \mid x < z < y\}$.

Lemma 1. *If for each Patch $i \in \{1, 2, ..., N\}$, the local dynamics f_i are modeled by a monotone concave map in $[0, \infty)$ in System (2), then*

$$\text{(i)} \qquad DF(x) > 0 \; if \; x > 0,$$

and

$$\text{(ii)} \qquad DF(y) \lneqq DF(x) \; if \; 0 < x < y.$$

The proof of Lemma 1 is in the Appendix. Ricker's model is not a monotone concave map on $[0, \infty)$. However, if the local dynamics are governed by the Ricker's equation with $k_i = 1$ and $0 < r_i < 1$ then the local dynamics, $f_i(x_i) = x_i \exp(r_i - k_i x_i)$, are modeled by 1-monotone concave maps on the closed interval $[0, 1]$ with $f_i(1) < 1$ and $X_i \in [0, 1]$. Lemma 2 below captures this last result.

Lemma 2. *If for each Patch $i \in \{1, 2, ..., N\}$, the local dynamics f_i are modeled by* α-monotone concave maps *in* $[0, \alpha] \subset \mathbb{R}_+$, *then*

$$\text{(i)} \qquad DF(x) > 0 \; if \; 0 < x < p,$$

and

$$\text{(ii)} \qquad DF(y) \lneqq DF(x) \; if \; 0 < x < y < p,$$

where $p = (\alpha, \alpha, ..., \alpha) \in int(\mathbb{R}_+^N)$.

The proof of Lemma 2 is similar to that of Lemma 1 and is omitted.

Corollary 1. *In System (2),* $\lim_{x\to 0,\ x>0} DF(x) = DF(0)$.

The proof of Corollary 1 is in the Appendix.

In System(2) the origin is an unstable fixed point $[g_i(x_i) > 1$ for each $i \in \{1,2,...,N\}]$, and therefore by standard linearization techniques the following result is immediate:

Corollary 2. *In System (2),* $\lambda = \rho(DF(0)) > 1$ *where* $\rho(DF(0))$ *denotes the spectral radius of the Jacobian matrix,* $DF(0)$.

It is also easy to show that all solutions of System (2) are bounded (Lemma 3 and Corollary 3).

Lemma 3. *In System (2), no point has an unbounded orbit.*

The proof of Lemma 3 is in the Appendix. From the proof of Lemma 3, the following result is immediate:

Corollary 3. *In System (2), the* $\omega-$*limit set of every point in* $\mathbb{R}_+^N$ *is a nonempty subset of the compact invariant set* $S \equiv \{x = (x_1, x_2, ..., x_N) \in \mathbb{R}_+^N \mid$ *for each* $i \in \{1,2,...,N\}$, $x_i \leq \max I\}$, where $\max I = \max_{i\in\{1,2,...,N\}} \{\max I_i\}$.

Lemma 3 and Corollary 3 show that there is no population explosion in System (2).

4. Identical local dynamics. In the situation where in-phase initial conditions are assumed, the population sizes in the different N patches are always the same [that is, $x = (x_1, x_2, ..., x_N) \in \mathbb{R}_+^N$ with $x_1 = x_2 = ... = x_N$] whenever there is identical local patch dynamics. However, in the situation where out-of-phase initial conditions are assumed, the population sizes in the different N patches are not always the same. In the case of identical local patch dynamics, the general $N-$ patches model with dispersion between patches, System (2), behaves qualitatively like a single patch model for the in-phase initial conditions. For out-of-phase initial population densities, we use Ricker's model to illustrate that, it is possible for System (2) with identical local patch dynamics, to exhibit dynamics that are completely different from single-patch dynamics.

Lemma 4. *In System (2), if* $g_1 = g_2 = ... = g_N$ *then the "diagonal" set of in-phase initial conditions,*

$$D \equiv \{x = (x_1, x_2, ..., x_N) \in \mathbb{R}_+^N \mid x_1 = x_2 = ... = x_N\}$$

is $F-$ *invariant with* $F_i(x) = f_i(x_i)$ *for each* $i \in \{1,2,...,N\}$.

The proof of Lemma 4 is in the Appendix. The logistic map in the chaotic regime is negative for some initial population densities. Consequently, if all the conditions of Lemma 4 are satisfied, the diagonal set D is not invariant in the positive cone whenever the local dynamics are driven by the logistic map [16]. For in-phase initial population sizes, Lemma 4 implies that the full system behaves as a single patch system whenever the underlying local dynamics are identical. Example 1 is used to illustrate that for out-of-phase initial conditions, a multiple patch system with identical underlying local dynamics can exhibit complex dynamics with fractal basins of attraction.

Example 1. Consider System (2) with $N = 2$ and with $\widetilde{x}_i(t) = x_i(t)\exp(r_i - k_i x_i(t))$ for each $i \in \{1, 2\}$. Set the following parameter values: $d_{12} = d_{21} = 0.15$, $r_1 = r_2 = 3.5$ and $k_1 = k_2 = 1$.

The local population dynamics are identical in both patches and are modeled by scramble competition maps capable of generating complex including chaotic dynamics. Lemma 4 and the fact that $r_1 = r_2 = 3.5$ imply that the dynamics for each in-phase initial population density are chaotic (see Figure 1, [20–22]). The Ricker's model has negative Schwarzian derivative and only one critical point. Therefore, Singer's theorem and the fact that $I_i \equiv f_i([0, X_i])$ is a global attractor under f_i iterations imply that the local dynamics in Example 1 have only one attractor (see Figure 1). However, the full two-patch system exhibits, numerically, the existence of a stable and positive out-of-phase period 2 orbit coexisting with the chaotic diagonal set. The points in the period 2 orbit are $(9.0228, 1.6219) \to (1.6219, 9.0228)$.

Figure 2 shows that, some out-of-phase initial population densities are attracted to the chaotic diagonal set, D, and others are attracted to the out-of-phase stable period 2 orbit. The boundary of the basins of attraction of the two coexisting attractors is complex (see Figure 2, [13]). Example 1, illustrates sensitive dependence of the long-term behavior on initial conditions. Additional numerical simulations have shown that the shape and size of the basins of attraction change with the dispersion rate [9, 26]. Hastings, in [16], used System (2) with two patches and local dynamics modeled by the logistic model to illustrate similar sensitive dependence to initial conditions. However, the qualitative features of the basins of attraction as well as the nature of the attractors in Example 1 differ from those found by Hastings (see Figure 1, [16]).

If the local dynamics are modeled by monotone concave maps then the full N-patch system behaves qualitatively like a single patch system, independent of initial population sizes and dispersion rates. Whenever monotone concave maps model the local patch dynamics in System(2) and there is no dispersion, then the dynamics of each patch are qualitatively the same as the global dynamics of the full system (proof in the Appendix). In other words, the local dynamic properties generated by contest competition transfers to the full system, System (2) and consequently, System (2) has a unique stable, positive equilibrium [Theorem 3].

Theorem 3. *Let the local dynamics f_i be a monotone concave map in $[0, \infty)$ for each Patch $i \in \{1, 2, ..., N\}$. Then System (2) has a unique positive fixed point, $q = (q_1, q_2, ..., q_N) \in \mathbb{R}_+^N$ such that $F^n(x) \to q$ as $n \to \infty$ for every point $x = (x_1, x_2, ..., x_N) > 0$.*

Proof. From Theorem 3, we notice using Lemma 1, Lemma 3, Corollary 1 and Corollary 2 that all the hypotheses of Theorem 1 are satisfied. Hence, Theorem 1 guarantees the existence of a unique positive fixed

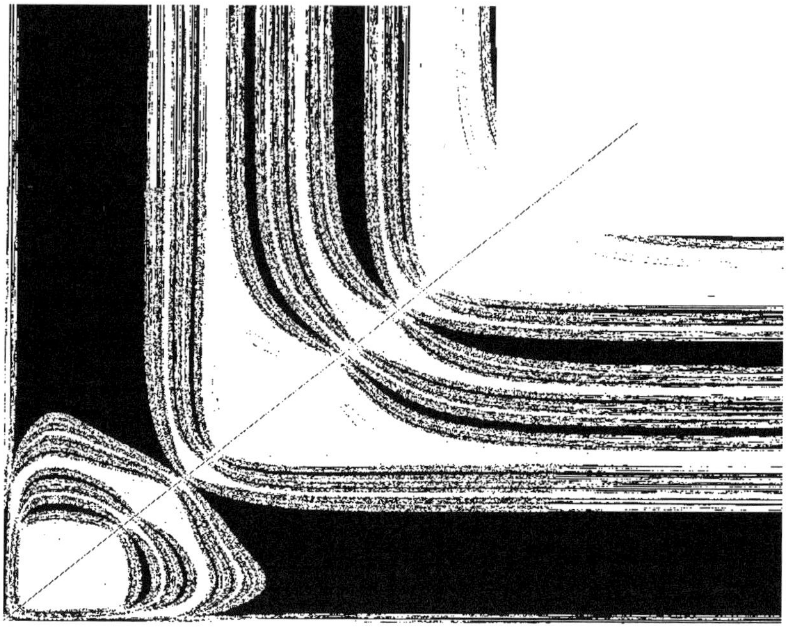

FIG. 2. *Basins of attraction of the in phase chaotic attractor (black region) and the out of phase period 2 orbit (white region).*

point $q = (q_1, q_2, ..., q_N) \in \mathbb{R}^N_+$ satisfying $\lim_{n\to\infty} F^n(x) = q$ for all points $x = (x_1, x_2, ..., x_N)$ in the interior of $\mathbb{R}^N_+$. □

In contrast to the Verhulst model [contest competition], complex dynamics can occur in single patch systems without dispersion if the equation for the local dynamics models scramble competition. Using the discrete logistic model [scramble competition] for the local dynamics in a two patch system with dispersion, Hastings illustrated the occurrence of oscillations and chaotic solutions [16]. Theorem 4 states that, if the equations for the local dynamics are monotone concave maps on a compact set (for example, Ricker's model [scramble competition] with no oscillation), then oscillations and chaotic solutions do not occur in System (2). In fact, as with the single Verhulst equation [contest competition], we obtain that the N-patch system behaves like a single patch [Theorem 4].

Theorem 4. *Let the local dynamics be modelled by* f_i, an α-monotone concave map with $f_i(\alpha) < \alpha$ and $X_i \in [0, \alpha]$, *for each Patch* $i \in \{1, 2, ..., N\}$. *Then in System (2), there exists a unique positive fixed point,* $q = (q_1, q_2, ..., q_N) \in \mathbb{R}^N_+$ *such that* $F^n(x) \to q$ *as* $n \to \infty$ *for every point* $x \in [0, p] - \{0\}$, where $p = (\alpha, \alpha, ..., \alpha) \in int(\mathbb{R}^N_+)$.

Proof. All the hypotheses in Theorem 2 are satisfied. Let $p = (\alpha, \alpha, ..., \alpha) \in int(\mathbb{R}^N_+)$, and note that $F_i(p) \leq \max\{f_i(\alpha) = \alpha g_i(\alpha),\ f_j(\alpha) = \alpha g_j(\alpha)\} < \alpha$. Hence, $F : [0,p] \to [0,p]$. It is clear using Lemma 2, Lemma 3, Corollary 1 and Corollary 2 that all the hypotheses of Theorem 2 are satisfied. Hence, Theorem 1 guarantees the existence of a unique positive fixed point $q = (q_1, q_2, ..., q_N) \in \mathbb{R}^N_+$ satisfying $\lim_{n\to\infty} F^n(x) = q$ for all points $x = (x_1, x_2, ..., x_N)$ in the interior of $\mathbb{R}^N_+$. □

For an application of Theorem 3 [or Theorem 4], consider System (2) with the local dynamics in each Patch $i \in \{1, 2\}$ being given by the Verhulst equation, $f_i(x_i) = r_i x_i/(x_i + k_i)$ with $r_i > k_i$. Then $\lambda = \rho(DF(0)) > 1$ and $X_i = r_i - k_i$. Theorem 3 implies that System (2) has a globally stable positive equilibrium population, that is, the full system behaves as a single patch system. Also, if each $r_i \leq k_i$ then the species is not a pioneer species. In fact, the species goes extinct in each patch. With dispersion, $\lambda = \rho(DF(0)) \leq 1$ and Theorem 1 implies that the origin is globally stable, that is, the full system behaves as a single patch system.

5. Scramble versus contest competition. So far, we have seen that multi-patch systems with contest competition local dynamics behave qualitatively like a single-patch model under a contest competition regime. However, multi-patch systems under local scramble competition regimes exhibit, in general, complex dynamics. Example 2 looks at a two-patch model under mixed (scramble versus contest) competitive local regimes.

Example 2. Consider System (2) with $N = 2$ and with $\widetilde{x}_1(t) = x_1(t)\exp(r_1 - k_1 x_1(t))$ and $\widetilde{x}_2(t) = r_2 x_2(t)/(x_2(t) + k_2)$. Set the following parameter values: $d_{12} = d_{21} = 0.15$, $r_1 = 2.1$, $r_2 = 2$ *and* $k_1 = k_2 = 1$.

In Example 2, Patch 1 has a stable period 2 point as the local dynamics are not given by a monotone map (Figure 1, [20–22]). Patch 2 has a globally stable equilibrium point as the local dynamics are given by a monotone map. With our choice of constants, the full system has an out-of-phase stable equilibrium population density at (2.0244, 1.2828) (Figure 3).

In this situation, the full system behaves as Patch 2, the patch with contest competition. In fact, if $0 < r_1 < 1$, $k_1 = 1$, and $r_2 > k_2$, Theorem 4 implies that the full mixed system in Example 2 behaves as Patch 2, the patch with contest competition. As we increase the parameter r_1 past 2.1745, the out-of-phase, positive fixed point for the full system undergoes period doubling bifurcation resulting in the full system behaving like the local dynamics in Patch 1, the patch with scramble competition (Figure 3). In particular, at $r_1 = 2.2$, Patch 1 has a stable period 2 point and the full system also has an out-of-phase period 2 orbit at $(2.5353, 1.3633) \to (1.7142, 1.2526)$. As r_1 is increased past 2.9, the period 2 orbit undergoes a similar period doubling bifurcation and a new stable period 4 orbit emerges (Figure 3). A dramatic period doubling reversal occurs as the parameter r_1 is increased past 3.95. The stable out-of-phase period 4 orbit "vanishes" with the emergence of an out-of-phase stable period 2 orbit (Figure 3).

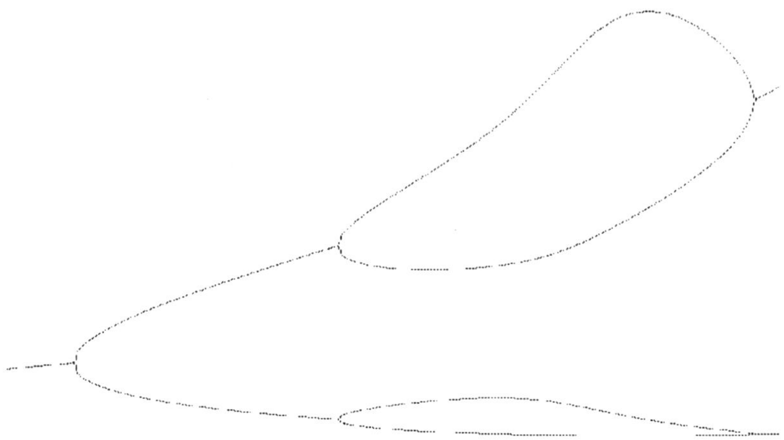

FIG. 3. *Period doubling bifurcations as r_1 increases.*

Models with mixed competitive local regimes appear to be as rich dynamically as those with only scramble competitive local regimes. However, mixed competitive local regimes are capable of, for example, stabilizing or shifting (from period four to period two or to a fixed point) the local dynamics.

6. Persistence versus extinction. In this section, we show that the possibility of altering local dynamics via dispersal is also possible in a multi-patch system with a local contest competition regime.

If all the local dynamics in the multi-patch system are given by Verhulst equation, $f_i(x_i) = r_i x_i/(x_i + k_i)$, where $r_1 > k_1$ and $r_i \leq k_i$ for each $i \neq 1 \in \{1, 2, ..., n\}$, then local persistence of the species occurs in Patch 1 [$X_1 = r_1 - k_1$is globally stable under f_1 iterations] while there is local extinction in each of the other patches[$\{0\}$ is globally stable under f_i iterations]. Without dispersion, that is, $d_{ij} = d_{ji} = 0$, the full system has an unstable fixed point at the origin [$\lambda = \rho(DF(0)) > 1$] and a stable fixed point $(X_1, 0, ..., 0)$ on the 1-axis [$\lambda = \rho(DF((X_1, 0, ...0)) < 1$]. Example 3 illustrates the persistence of species with dispersion under local contest competition regimes where there is local extinction without dispersion.

Example 3. Consider System (2) with $N = 2$ and with $\widetilde{x}_1(t) = r_1 x_1(t)/(x_1(t) + k_1)$ and $\widetilde{x}_2(t) = r_2 x_2(t)/(x_2(t) + k_2)$. Set the following parameter values: $d_{12} = d_{21} = 0$, $r_1 = 2.1$, $r_2 = 1.9$, $k_1 = 1$ and $k_2 = 2$.

Without dispersion, Example 3 has local persistence of the species in Patch 1 as $X_1 = 1.1$ is a globally stable positive equilibrium and local extinction in Patch 2 as $\{0\}$ is globally stable. With dispersion between the two patches [for example $d_{12} = d_{21} = 0.1$], Example 3 has a positive stable equilibrium population density at $(0.3682, 0.9506)$ that attracts positive initial populations. The stable positive equilibrium exists for "sufficiently" large values of the dispersion coefficients $d_{ij} = d_{ji} \in (0, 1)$.

Multi-patch systems with a local contest competition regime have the possibility of extinction of populations on some local patches, in the absence of dispersal. Example 3 exhibits the possibility of the persistence of the species in the full system with dispersion where there is local extinction without dispersion. In System (2), dispersion between patches saves endangered species from extinction. In other words, fragmented landscape with dispersal corridors are less likely to lead to extinction.

7. Connections to epidemics. Discrete-time models that incorporate complex population and disease dynamics with dispersal have rarely been studied (see [2–8]). Here, we introduce a discrete-time, susceptible-infected-susceptible (*S-I-S*) model with dispersion between two patches. In each patch, local disease dynamics occurs first followed by a dispersion phase.

In Patch $i \in \{1, 2\}$, at generation t, $S_i(t)$ denotes the population of susceptible individuals; $I_i(t)$ denotes the population of infecteds, assumed infectious; $T_i(t) \equiv S_i(t) + I_i(t)$ denotes the total population size; $T_{i\infty} \equiv \lim_{n \to \infty} T_i(t)$ denotes the demographic steady state for the total population whenever it exists (no dispersion); and, f_i denotes the recruitment function. In Patch i, individuals survive with probability γ_i (die with probability $1 - \gamma_i$) while infected individuals recover with probability $1 - \sigma_i$ (do not recover with probability σ_i) in each generation. In each generation, susceptible individuals, in Patch i, become infected with probability $1 - G_i$ (remain susceptible with probability G_i), where α_i weighs the impact of the prevalence $(\frac{I_i(t)}{T_i(t)})$ on this probability. $G_i : [0, \infty) \to [0, 1]$ is a monotone concave function with $G_i(0) = 1; G_i^{'}(x) < 0$ and $G_i^{''}(x) \geq 0$ for all $x \in [0, \infty)$.

Furthermore, it is assumed that the disease is not fatal. In other words, the nonlinear population dynamics are fixed. This assumption does not imply a constant population size as it is customarily in deterministic models. In fact, there is density-dependent mortality and complex dynamics but no disease-induced mortality. We also assume that all recruits are susceptible; the recruitment function depends on total population size; time is measured in generations; and, recovery from the disease does not give permanent or temporary immunity. The model assumes (implicitly) a sequential process. In each Patch i, at the end of each generation, a fraction $(1 - \gamma_i)$ of each class is removed (death) and surviving susceptibles become infected with probability $(1 - G_i)$ and, independently, surviving infectives recover with probability $(1 - \sigma_i)$. It is in this setting that we hope to explore disease dynamics.

Our assumptions lead to the following single-patch discrete-time *S-I-S* model:

$$\left.\begin{aligned} S_i(t+1) &= f_i(T_i(t)) + \gamma_i S_i(t) G_i(\tfrac{\alpha_i I_i(t)}{T_i(t)}) + \gamma_i I_i(t)(1-\sigma_i), \\ I_i(t+1) &= \gamma_i(1 - G_i(\tfrac{\alpha_i I_i(t)}{T_i(t)}))S_i(t) + \gamma_i \sigma_i I_i(t), \end{aligned}\right\} \tag{3}$$

where $0 < \gamma_i, \sigma_i < 1$ and $T_i(t) > 0$. System (3) is an extension of a model of Barrera *et al.* [6]. Castillo-Chavez and Yakubu have obtained thresholds for disease persistence in the single patch model, System (3) [7, 8].

As in System (2), we couple Patch 1 and Patch 2 with a simple exchange of a fixed fraction of the population per generation. Let D_S and D_I be the fraction of the susceptible and infective population that are exchanged, respectively. This leads to the following system of equations that describe the dispersal phase:

$$\left.\begin{aligned} S_1(t+1) &= (1-D_S)\widetilde{S}_1(t) + D_S\widetilde{S}_2(t) \\ I_1(t+1) &= (1-D_I)\widetilde{I}_1(t) + D_I\widetilde{I}_2(t) \\ S_2(t+1) &= D_S\widetilde{S}_1(t) + (1-D_S)\widetilde{S}_2(t) \\ I_2(t+1) &= D_I\widetilde{I}_1(t) + (1-D_I)\widetilde{I}_2(t) \end{aligned}\right\} \tag{4}$$

where $\widetilde{S}_i(t) = f_i(T_i(t)) + \gamma_i S_i(t) G_i(\frac{\alpha_i I_i(t)}{T_i(t)}) + \gamma_i I_i(t)(1-\sigma_i)$, $\widetilde{I}_i(t) = \gamma_i(1 - G_i(\frac{\alpha_i I_i(t)}{T_i(t)}))S_i(t) + \gamma_i\sigma_i I_i(t)$ and $0 < D_S, D_I < 1$. The dispersion coefficients, D_S and D_I, measure the probability of dispersion by the susceptible and infective individuals, respectively.

If there is no dispersion and Patch 2 is empty ($D_S = D_I = \widetilde{S}_2(t) = \widetilde{I}_2(t) = 0$), then System (4) reduces to the single patch model of Castillo-Chavez and Yakubu, System (3) [7, 8]. In System (4), if $D_S = 0$ and $D_I \neq 0$ [respectively, $D_I = 0$ and $D_S \neq 0$], then the susceptible [respectively, infective] individuals are confined to a patch while the infectives [respectively, susceptibles] disperse between the two patches. In the absence of dispersal we have two patches with fixed nonlinear dynamics experiencing an epidemic.

As we have seen before, it may be possible for a disease that would go extinct in Patch i with basic reproductive number $R_{0i} < 1$ to persist in the full system via dispersion (as long as one patch, Patch j, has a basic reproductive number $R_{0j} > 1$). Hence, corridors (migration, complex-life cycles, transportation and so on) may promote disease persistence or re-emergence. In this short note, we have illustrated how host persistence may be enhanced by dispersal in models without disease. Preliminary simulations suggest that disease re-emergence and eventual persistence in patches without disease is likely in the presence of dispersal.

8. Conclusions. The determination of the type of local intra-specific competition is important in understanding the aggregate dynamics in patchy environments. Local dynamics are qualitatively the same as the aggregate dynamics whenever the local dynamics are under contest or pseudo-contest competitions. However, if the local dynamics are driven by oscillatory scramble or mixed competitions with oscillations, then the aggregate dynamics are the result of delicate trade-offs between dispersal and local dynamics. Hence, the fragmentation of the landscape (increasing the number of patches) gives rise to drastically different aggregate dynamics, and these results may have serious implications in the fields of conservation and evolutionary biology. Furthermore, changes in dispersal patterns may lead to local population extinctions with serious ecological consequences or it may lead to novel (re-establishment of corridors) conservation policies.

However, re-establishing mechanisms that promote host-survival in multi-patch systems may also promote disease re-emergence or disease growth in populations where it was absent. What would be the evolutionary consequences of increasing the connectivity between populations? The possibilities are endless as the recent article by Kolata [17] on the role of air-transportation on the potential spread of tuberculosis has shown (see Aparicio *et al.* [4] in this volume, for example).

In continuous-time deterministic models it is customary to look at disease dynamics in populations that have reached a demographic equilibrium. Hence, a huge literature of the study of disease dynamics on populations with no demography (constant population size) has emerged. In the last two decades, the study of the role of disease in regulating population growth has been studied. The focus has been on the study of the effects of disease on populations that would otherwise grow exponentially. It is possible to fix complex (local) population dynamics and then build epidemics on them. In fact, the local population dynamics can match those given by any nonlinear function, that is, they can be fixed to be of the form $T(t+1) = f(T(t))$. Hence, with an interesting f, for example, Ricker's equation, the local dynamics can be as complicated as we wish. In other words (at some price) we can now look at disease dynamics on populations with arbitrarily complex dynamics. In the past, it has been customary to look at the impact of externally driven factors on the spread of disease with seasonality on the transmission parameters the most explored possibility. Here, we focus on internally driven complex dynamics.

Several questions of interest emerge including whether or not complex internally driven population dynamics "drive" disease dynamics. It has been shown that this is not always the case (see [6, 7]). In other words, we have built examples where the local population dynamics and the local disease dynamics differ. Under our framework, it is possible to explore systematically the role of dispersal and disease on local (complex) population dynamics. Questions that we hope to address is under what circumstances dispersal by susceptibles (or infectives) increases (or decreases) the likelihood of disease persistence in multi-patch systems. On the other hand, there may be systems in which disease may increase the ability to disperse (behavioral changes in the host). Whether or not disease-induced dispersal actually plays a significant role on disease persistence and on the qualitative nature of the local dynamics and under what conditions are some of the questions that we hope to address in the future.

APPENDIX

Proof of Lemma 1. $DF(x) = \begin{bmatrix} \frac{\partial F_1(x)}{\partial x_1} & \frac{\partial F_1(x)}{\partial x_2} & \cdots & \frac{\partial F_1(x)}{\partial x_n} \\ \frac{\partial F_2(x)}{\partial x_1} & \frac{\partial F_2(x)}{\partial x_2} & \cdots & \frac{\partial F_2(x)}{\partial x_n} \\ \vdots & \vdots & \vdots & \vdots \\ \frac{\partial F_n(x)}{\partial x_1} & \frac{\partial F_n(x)}{\partial x_2} & \cdots & \frac{\partial F_n(x)}{\partial x_n} \end{bmatrix} =$

$$\begin{bmatrix} (1-\sum_{\substack{j=1\\j\neq 1}}^N d_{1j})f_1'(x_1) & d_{21}f_2'(x_2) & \dots & d_{n1}f_n'(x_n) \\ d_{12}f_1'(x_1) & (1-\sum_{\substack{j=1\\j\neq 2}}^N d_{2j})f_2'(x_2) & \dots & d_{n2}f_n'(x_n) \\ \vdots & \vdots & \vdots & \vdots \\ d_{1n}f_1'(x_1) & d_{2n}f_2'(x_2) & \dots & (1-\sum_{\substack{j=1\\j\neq n}}^N d_{nj})f_n'(x_n) \end{bmatrix}.$$

Recall that $0 < d_{ij} < 1$, $0 < \sum_{\substack{j=1\\j\neq i}}^N d_{ij} < 1$. Hence, $f_i'(x_i) > 0$ for each $x_i \in [0, \infty)$ imply that $DF(x) > 0$ *if* $x > 0$. In addition, $f_i''(x_i) < 0$ for each $x_i \in [0, \infty)$ imply that $DF(y) \lneqq DF(x)$ *if* $0 < x < y$. This establishes Lemma 1.

Proof of Corollary 1. From the proof of Lemma 1 and the fact that $f_i'(x_i) = g_i(x_i) + x_i g_i'(x_i)$ we have that $DF(x) =$

$$\begin{bmatrix} (1-\sum_{\substack{j=1\\j\neq 1}}^N d_{1j})\cdot (g_1(x_1)+x_1g_1'(x_1)) & d_{21}(g_2(x_2)+x_2g_2'(x_2)) & \dots & d_{n1}(g_n(x_n)+x_ng_n'(x_n)) \\ d_{12}(g_1(x_1)+x_1g_1'(x_1)) & (1-\sum_{\substack{j=1\\j\neq 2}}^N d_{2j})\cdot (g_2(x_2)+x_2g_2'(x_2)) & \dots & d_{n2}(g_n(x_n)+x_ng_n'(x_n)) \\ \vdots & \vdots & \vdots & \vdots \\ d_{1n}(g_1(x_1)+x_1g_1'(x_1)) & d_{2n}(g_2(x_2)+x_2g_2'(x_2)) & \dots & (1-\sum_{\substack{j=1\\j\neq n}}^N d_{nj})\cdot (g_n(x_n)+x_ng_n'(x_n)) \end{bmatrix}$$

Hence, $DF(0) =$

$$\begin{bmatrix} (1-\sum_{\substack{j=1\\j\neq 1}}^N d_{1j})g_1(0) & d_{21}g_2(0) & \dots & d_{n1}g_n(0) \\ d_{12}g_1(0) & (1-\sum_{\substack{j=1\\j\neq 2}}^N d_{2j})g_2(0) & \dots & d_{n2}g_n(0) \\ \vdots & \vdots & \vdots & \vdots \\ d_{1n}g_1(0) & d_{2n}g_2(0) & \dots & (1-\sum_{\substack{j=1\\j\neq n}}^N d_{nj})g_n(0) \end{bmatrix}$$

and $\lim_{x\to 0,\ x>0} DF(x) = DF(0)$.

Proof of Lemma 3. We need to show that for each $i \in \{1, 2, ..., N\}$, the sequence $\{F_i^n(x)\}_{n\geq 0}$ is bounded, where $x = (x_1, x_2, ..., x_N) \in \mathbb{R}_+^N$ is an arbitrary point.

For each $i, j \in \{1, 2, ..., N\}$, $F_i(x) = (1 - \sum_{\substack{j=1 \\ j \neq i}}^{N} d_{ij}) x_i g_i(x_i) + \sum_{\substack{j=1 \\ j \neq i}}^{N} d_{ji} x_j g_j(x_j)$ and $d_{ij} = d_{ji}$. Thus, if $x_i g_i(x_i) \geq x_j g_j(x_j)$ then $F_i(x) \leq x_i g_i(x_i)$. However, if $x_i g_i(x_i) < x_j g_j(x_j)$ then $F_i(x) < x_j g_j(x_j)$. Hence, for each $i \in \{1, 2, ..., N\}$, $F_i(x) \leq \max\{f_i(x_i) = x_i g_i(x_i),\ f_j(x_j) = x_j g_j(x_j)\}$.

If $x_i \leq \max I_i$, then $f_i(x_i) = x_i g_i(x_i) \leq \max I_i$ but if $x_i > \max I_i$ then $f_i(x_i) = x_i g_i(x_i) < x_i$. Therefore, for each $i \in \{1, 2, ..., N\}$ and each point $x = (x_1, x_2, ..., x_N) \in \mathbb{R}_+^N$ we have
$F_i(x) \leq \max_{i \in \{1,2,...,N\}}\{x_i, \max I_i\}$. Hence, each sequence $\{F_i^n(x)\}_{n \geq 0}$ is bounded and, consequently, no point in System (2) has an unbounded orbit.

Proof of Lemma 4. Let the point $(x_1, x_2, ..., x_N) \in \mathbb{R}_+^N$. Since $g_1(x_1) = g_2(x_2) = ... = g_N(x_N)$ and $d_{ij} = d_{ji}$ we have that $F_1(x) = f_1(x_1) = F_2(x) = f_2(x_2) = ... = F_N(x) = f_N(x_N)$ and, consequently, the set D is $F-$*invariant* with $F_i(x) = f_i(x_i)$ for each $i \in \{1, 2, ..., N\}$.

The following results of Hal Smith [27] for monotone systems will be useful in the proof of global stability results for System (2), under a contest competition regime.

Theorem 1 [27]. *Let $T : \mathbb{R}_+^N \to \mathbb{R}_+^N$ be continuous, C^1 in $int(\mathbb{R}_+^N)$ and suppose $DT(0)$ exists with $\lim_{x \to 0,\ x > 0} DT(x) = DT(0)$. In addition, assume*

$$(i) \qquad DT(x) > 0 \; if \; x > 0$$

and

$$(ii) \qquad DT(y) \leq DT(x) \; if \; 0 < x < y.$$

If $T(0) = 0$, let $\lambda = \rho(DT(0))$. If $\lambda \leq 1$, then for every $x \geq 0$, $T^n(x) \to 0$ as $n \to \infty$. If $\lambda > 1$, then either $T^n(x) \to \infty$ as $n \to \infty$ for every $x \gneqq 0$ or there exists a unique nonzero fixed point q of T. In the later case, $q > 0$ and for every $x \gneqq 0$, $T^n(x) \to q$ as $n \to \infty$.

If $T(0) \neq 0$, then either $T^n(x) \to \infty$ as $n \to \infty$ for every $x \geq 0$ or there exists a unique fixed point q of T. In the later case, $q > 0$ and for every $x \geq 0$, $T^n(x) \to q$ as $n \to \infty$.

For Ricker's model (scramble competition), the monotonicity condition (condition (i), of Theorem 1) and the concavity condition (condition (ii), of Theorem 1) are not satisfied on all of $\mathbb{R}_+^N$. The following second result of Hal Smith [27], Theorem 2, is helpful in the analysis of models for scramble competition.

Theorem 2 [27]. *Let $p \in int(\mathbb{R}_+^N)$ and $T : [0, p] \to [0, p]$ be continuous, C^1 in $(0, p)$ and suppose $DT(0)$ exists with $\lim_{x \to 0,\ x > 0} DT(x) = DT(0)$. In addition, assume conditions (i) and (ii) of Theorem 1 hold for $0 < x < y < p$ and that $Tp < p$.*

If $T(0) = 0$, let $\lambda = \rho(DT(0))$. If $\lambda \leq 1$, then for every $x \in [0, p]$, $T^n(x) \to 0$ as $n \to \infty$. If $\lambda > 1$, then T has a unique nonzero fixed point q. Moreover, $q \in (0, p)$ and $T^n(x) \to q$ as $n \to \infty$ for every $x \in [0, p] - \{0\}$.

If $T(0) \gneqq 0$, *then* T *has a unique fixed point* $q \in [0,p]$. *Moreover,* $q \in (0,p)$ *and* $T^n(x) \to q$ *as* $n \to \infty$ *for every* $x \in [0,p]$.

Acknowledgments. This study was partially supported by grants from National Science Foundation (NSF Grant DMS 9977919); National Security Agency (NSA Grant MDA 9149710074); Presidential Mentoring Award (NSF Grant HRD 9724850) to Carlos Castillo-Chavez. We also thank the office of the provost of Cornell University for its support. We also thank the Intel Technology for Education 200 Equipment Grant. The examples that lead to this research were part of a summer research experience supported by the above grants. The related work of Ms. Beatriz Salguero-Rivera and Eratό stenes Flores (under our supervision) has been published as Biometrics Department Technical Reports (see references). Simulations were carried out using Dynamics: Numerical Explorations by Helena E. Nusse and James A. Yorke.

REFERENCES

[1] L.J. Allen, Persistence, extinction, and critical patch number for island populations, *J. Math. Biol.* **24**, 617–625 (1987).

[2] L.J. Allen, Some discrete-time SI, SIR and SIS epidemic models. *Math. Biosci.* **124**: 83–105 (1994).

[3] R.M. Anderson and R.M. May, Infectious diseases of humans: Dynamics and control. Oxford University Press, Oxford (1992).

[4] J.P. Aparicio, A.F. Capurro, and C. Castillo-Chavez, Contact networks and the spread of infectious diseases, IMA volume.

[5] N.T.J. Bailey, The simple stochastic epidemic: a complete solution in terms of known functions. *Biometrika* **50**, 235–240 (1963).

[6] J.H. Barrera, A. Cintron-Arias, N. Davidenko, L.R. Denogean, and S.R. Franco-Gonzalez, Dynamics of a two-dimensional discrete-time SIS model, *MTBI Cornell University Technical Report* (1999).

[7] C. Castillo-Chavez and A.A. Yakubu, "Discrete-time *S-I-S* models with complex dynamics", Nonlinear Anal. TMA (Accepted).

[8] C. Castillo-Chavez and A.A. Yakubu, "Discrete-time *S-I-S* models with simple and complex population dynamics", Mathematical Approaches for Emerging and Reemerging Infectious Diseases: Models, Methods and Theory, edited by Carlos Castillo-Chavez with Pauline van den Driessche, Denise Kirschner and Abdul-Aziz Yakubu, Vol. **1**.

[9] Erastóthenes Flores Torres, "Interaction between dispersal and dynamics: Coupled Ricker's Equation", *MTBI Cornell University Technical Report* (1999).

[10] J.E. Franke and A.-A. Yakubu, "Extinction and persistence of species in discrete competitive systems with a safe refuge", *J. Math. Anal. Appl.* **23**: 746–761 (1996).

[11] J.E. Franke and A.-A. Yakubu, "Geometry of exclusion principles in discrete systems", *J. Math. Anal. Appl.* **168**: 385–400 (1992).

[12] J.E. Franke and A.-A. Yakubu, "Mutual exclusion versus coexistence for discrete competitive systems", *J. Math. Biol.* **30**: 161–168 (1991).

[13] C. Grebogi, E. Ott, and J.A. Yorke, "Chaos, strange attractors, and fractal basin boundaries in nonlinear dynamics", *Science.* **228**: 632–638 (1987).

[14] M.P. Hassell, "The dynamics of competition and predation", *Studies in Biol.* **72**, The Camelot Press Ltd. (1976).

[15] M.P. Hassell, J.H. Lawton, and R.M. May, "Patterns of dynamical behavior in single species populations", *J. Anim. Ecol.* **45**: 471–486 (1976).

[16] A. Hastings, "Complex interactions between dispersal and dynamics: Lessons from coupled logistic equations", *Ecology.* **75**: 1362–1372 (1993).

[17] G. Kolata, "First documented case of TB passed on airliner is reported by the U.S., *New York Times* (March 3, 1995).

[18] S.A. Levin: "Dispersion and population interactions", *Amer. Naturalist* **108**: 207–228 (1974).

[19] S.A. Levin, "The problem of pattern and scale in ecology", *Ecology.* **73**: 1943–1967 (1992).

[20] R.M. May and G.F. Oster, "Bifurcations and dynamic complexity in simple ecological models", *Amer. Naturalist* **110**: 573–579 (1976).

[21] R.M. May, "Simple mathematical models with very complicated dynamics", *Nature* **261**: 459–469 (1977).

[22] R.M. May, "Stability and complexity in model ecosystems", *Princeton University Press* (1974).

[23] A.J. Nicholson, "Compensatory reactions of populations to stresses, and their evolutionary significance", *Aust. J. Zool.* **2**: 1–65 (1954).

[24] W.E. Ricker, "Stock and recruitment", *Journal of Fisheries Research Board of Canada* **II(5)**: 559–623 (1954).

[25] T. Royama, "Analytical population dynamics", *Pop & Comm. Biol. Series.* **10**, Chapman & Hall (1992).

[26] B. Salguero-Rivera, " Scramble versus contest competition in a two patch system", *MTBI Cornell University Technical Report* (1999).

[27] H.L. Smith, "Cooperative systems of differential equations with concave nonlinearities", *Nonlinear Anal. Theor. Methods & Appl.* **10**: 1037–1052 (1986).

THE IMPACT OF LONG-RANGE DISPERSAL ON THE RATE OF SPREAD IN POPULATION AND EPIDEMIC MODELS

LINDA J.S. ALLEN* AND RALYNN K. ERNEST*

Abstract. The growth and dispersal of a population are modeled using an integrodifference equation. The model assumes that growth and dispersal occur in separate stages and that spread is over a continuous spatial region R. The model takes the following form:

$$P_{t+1}(x) = \int_R f(P_t(y))k(x,y)dy,$$

where $P_t(x)$ represents the population density at time t and position $x \in R$. The function k is the dispersal kernel and the function f determines the rate of population growth. The model is applied to an SIS epidemic with general force of infection, where P represents infected individuals.

Integrodifference equations have been used extensively to investigate the rate of spread of populations. However, they have not been applied to epidemics. Kot, Lewis and van den Driessche [11] investigated the rate of spread for various types of dispersal kernels and showed for kernels with leptokurtic distributions that the asymptotic rate of spread may increase over time. We exploit this relation between leptokurtic distributions and the asymptotic rate of spread by investigating the moments of the kernel and the corresponding asymptotic rate of spread of the model. It is shown that the moments of the kernel and the asymptotic rate of spread of the model increase significantly when long range dispersal is added to the model. The small amount of long-range dispersal may be overlooked in estimates of the variability of spread and hence, asymptotic rate of spread can be seriously underestimated.

1. Introduction. Biological invasions have been documented for many types of species including mammals, birds, insects, and plants (e.g., [8, 14, 17]). Shigesada and Kawasaki [14] discuss three different phases during an invasion of an alien species, establishment phase, expansion phase, and saturation phase. Endemic infections follow these three phases of invasion also. After disease becomes established within a plant or animal community, if left unchecked, the disease spreads throughout the community until it reaches an endemic level of infection.

The rate of spread during the expansion phase varies greatly between species and locality. It is the asymptotic rate of spread during the expansion phase that concerns this investigation. In particular, the effect of short and long range dispersal capabilities on the asymptotic rate of spread is investigated. It is assumed that the greatest proportion of the population is spread locally with small variation in the distance spread from the point of origin. However, a small proportion of the population has a wide variability in its dispersal capabilities. A few individuals have the capability of

*Department of Mathematics and Statistics, Texas Tech University, Lubbock, Texas 79409-1042.

spreading distances which may be many orders of magnitude larger than those individuals whose spread is confined to a local area.

The growth and dispersal of a population are modeled using an integrodifference equation. The model assumes that growth and dispersal occur in separate stages and that spread is over a continuous spatial region R. The model takes the following form:

$$P_{t+1}(x) = \int_R f(P_t(y))k(x,y)dy, \tag{1}$$

where $P_t(x)$ is the population density at time t and position $x \in R$. The function f determines the rate of growth of the population and k is the dispersal kernel; $k(x,y)$ is the probability that individuals move from position y to position x. Such types of models have been used extensively to investigate rate of spread of populations [1, 3, 4, 10–13, 16]. Kot et al. [11] investigated the rate of spread for various types of dispersal kernels and showed for some kernels with leptokurtic distributions that the asymptotic rate of spread may increase over time.

In our investigation, the population model is extended to epidemic models and the single dispersal kernel is separated into two kernels, a composite kernel of the form:

$$k(x,y) = (1-p)k_1(x,y) + pk_2(x,y). \tag{2}$$

It is assumed that a proportion $1-p$ of the population disperses according to probability distribution k_1 (short-range) and the remaining proportion p disperses according to the probability distribution k_2 (long-range). Kernels which yield a constant rate of asymptotic spread and kernels with a linear increasing rate of spread are considered. The kurtosis is investigated for the composite kernel k as a function of p. It is shown that the kurtosis and some normalized higher order moments are inversely proportional to p^{m-1} for some parameter values and $m > 1$. For example, large values of the kurtosis (leptokurtic) are associated with small values of p. The leptokurtosis of the kernel may account for the large increase in the asymptotic rate of spread associated with small values of p.

In the next section, the model components are described, the time-dependent epidemic model and the spatially-dependent dispersal kernel. The kurtosis and higher order moments of the dispersal kernels are defined and their relation to p discussed. In Section 3, the asymptotic rate of spread is discussed. Numerical examples are presented and discussed in Section 4. Extensions and conclusions are presented in the final section.

2. Mathematical model. The mathematical model is an integrodifference equation of the form (1), where the difference equation, $P_{t+1} = f(P_t)$, represents the change in population density over time, in the absence of spatial spread. Kot et al. [11] used models with Ricker and Beverton-Holt dynamics. The Beverton-Holt growth function f is represented by

$$f(P_t) = \frac{rKP_t}{K + (r-1)P_t}, \quad r > 1$$

and the Ricker form is

$$f(P_t) = P_t \exp\left[r\left(1 - \frac{P_t}{K}\right)\right], \quad 0 < r < 2.$$

Integrodifference equations have not been applied to epidemic models.

A simple epidemic model is considered here, an SIS epidemic. Individuals become infected, recover, and immediately become susceptible again. The epidemic dynamics can be described by a single difference equation. The two model components of (1), SIS epidemic and dispersal kernel, are discussed separately below.

2.1. SIS Epidemic. The full system of difference equations for an SIS epidemic includes equations for susceptibles and infectives:

$$\begin{aligned} S_{t+1} &= S_t(1 - \lambda(I_t)) + (\mu + \gamma)I_t \\ I_{t+1} &= I_t(1 - \mu - \gamma) + \lambda(I_t)S_t, \end{aligned} \tag{3}$$

where it is assumed that the parameters and initial conditions are positive:

$$\alpha > 0, \quad 0 < \mu + \gamma \leq 1, \quad S_0 > 0, \quad I_0 > 0, \quad \text{and} \quad S_0 + I_0 = N. \tag{4}$$

For this model, it follows that the total population size $S_t + I_t$ remains constant for all time, $S_t + I_t = N$. Thus, system (3) can be simplified to a single difference equation in I:

$$I_{t+1} = I_t(1 - \mu - \gamma) + \lambda(I_t)(N - I_t) \equiv f(I_t) \tag{5}$$

System (3) has a general force of infection given by $\lambda(I_t)$. Some well-known forms for the force of infection are

$$\text{(a)} \quad \frac{\alpha}{N}I_t \quad \text{and} \quad \text{(b)} \quad \beta I_t,$$

where the expression $\lambda(I_t)S_t$ in (a) is referred to as standard incidence and in (b) as mass action incidence, $\alpha > 0$ and $\beta > 0$ [9]. Since N is constant, forms (a) and (b) are equal if $\beta = \alpha/N$. Another form for the force of infection that has been studied is

$$\text{(c)} \quad 1 - \exp\left(-\frac{\alpha}{N}I_t\right),$$

where $\alpha > 0$ [7, 15].

With certain restrictions on the force of infection, λ, it can be shown that the asymptotic behavior of the model is determined by the basic reproductive number [5]. The basic reproductive number for model (3) is given by the expression,

$$\mathcal{R}_0 = \frac{\alpha}{\mu + \gamma},$$

which is the number of secondary infections caused by one infective in an entirely susceptible population [6]. These restrictions on λ also ensure that solutions to (3) are positive and that a unique endemic equilibrium I^* exists [5],

(i) $0 < \lambda(I) \le \alpha I/N$ for $I \in (0, N]$.
(ii) $\lambda(I) \in C^2[0, N]$, $d\lambda(I)/dI > 0$, and $d\lambda^2(I)/dI^2 \le 0$ for $I \in [0, N]$.
(iii) $\lambda(I)|_{I=0} = 0$ and $d\lambda(I)/dI|_{I=0} = \alpha/N$ and
(iv) $0 < \alpha \le 1$.

If λ satisfies the conditions (i)–(iv), the following asymptotic results hold [5]:

If $\mathcal{R}_0 \le 1$, then $\lim_{t\to\infty} I_t = 0$ and if $\mathcal{R}_0 > 1$, then $\lim_{t\to\infty} I_t = I^*$, where I^* is the unique positive solution of

$$(\mu + \gamma)I^* = \lambda(I^*)(N - I^*),$$

on $(0, N)$.

In the case of the force of infection (c), I^* is the unique positive solution of

$$\exp\left(-\frac{\alpha}{N}I^*\right) = 1 - \frac{(\beta + \gamma)I^*}{N - I^*}.$$

The conditions (i)–(iv) are sufficient but not necessary. In the case of the force of infection (c), there are no additional conditions required, other than the conditions in (4), for the asymptotic results to hold [7, 15]. In addition, in the case of force of infection (a), a less restrictive condition than (iv) is needed [2]:

$$0 < \alpha < \min\left\{\, (2 + \mu + \gamma),\ (1 + \sqrt{\mu + \gamma}\,)^2 \right\}.$$

In the epidemic-dispersal model (1), the population variable P will be denoted as I, for the infected population. In addition, for this model, it is assumed that the population is located throughout the region R, so that the infection can spread anywhere in R, i.e., for $x \in R$, $S_t(x) + I_t(x) = N$. The function f in (1) is given by (5):

$$f(I) = I(1 - \mu - \gamma) + \lambda(I)(N - I), \tag{6}$$

where $I \equiv I_t(y) = P_t(y)$.

2.2. Dispersal kernels. The dispersal kernels k_i in (2) are assumed to be of convolution type,

$$k_i(x, y) = k_i(|x - y|), \quad i = 1, 2,$$

where the dispersal depends on the distance from the source. In particular, $k_i(x, y) \equiv k_i(u)$, where $u = |x - y|$, $\int_R k_i(u)du = 1$ and the mean $\int_R k_i(u)du = 0$, $i = 1, 2$. In addition, the variances satisfy

$$\sigma_1^2 = \int_R u^2 k_1(u)du \ll \int_R u^2 k_2(u)du = \sigma_2^2.$$

The variance of kernel k_1 is much less than that of k_2. In addition, it is assumed that the variance of k_1, representing short-range dispersal, is normalized to one, $1 \ll \sigma_2^2$. Long-range dispersal, k_2, has a large variance.

With these assumptions on k_i, the kernel functions depend on a single variable u which is the distance from the source. For convenience, the variable for distance is denoted as x, so that the kernel functions are denoted $k_i(x)$. The kernels also depend on a parameter D which is related to the variance. The dependence of the individual kernels k_i or the composite kernel k on the parameters will be explicitly noted at times by denoting them as $k_i(x; D)$ or $k(x; p, D)$. For example, the composite kernel,

$$k(x; p, D) = (1 - p)k_1(x) + pk_2(x; D) \tag{7}$$

depends on parameters p and D, where the dependence on D is via long-range dispersal; variance σ_2^2 is directly related to D^2.

Three types of kernels k_i are considered in the numerical examples:

$$k_n(x; D) = \frac{1}{\sqrt{2D^2\pi}} \exp\left(-\frac{x^2}{2D^2}\right) \tag{8}$$

$$k_{be}(x; D) = \frac{1}{2D} \exp\left(-\frac{|x|}{D}\right) \tag{9}$$

$$k_{es}(x; D) = \frac{1}{D} \exp\left(-2\sqrt{\frac{|x|}{D}}\right). \tag{10}$$

The subscript notation refers to the type of kernel, normal density (n), bilateral exponential density (be) and exponential square root density (es). Note that the mean for each of these kernels is zero. Their variances and higher order moments are given in Table 1.

A graph of each of the kernels is given in Figure 1, where in each case the variance is normalized to one. Note that $\sigma^2 = 1$ implies the value of D^2 for each of the kernels in (8), (9), and (10) equals 1, 1/2, or 2/15, respectively.

TABLE 1
Values for the variance, σ^2, kurtosis, κ, and higher order moments for the normal, bilateral exponential and exponential square root kernels.

	Kernels		
Statistics	Normal	Bilateral Exponential	Exponential Square Root
σ^2	D^2	$2D^2$	$(15/2)D^2$
$E(X^4)$	$3D^4$	$24D^4$	$(2835/2)D^4$
$E(X^6)$	$15D^6$	$720D^6$	$(6081075/4)D^6$
κ	3	6	126/5
M^6	15	90	18018/5

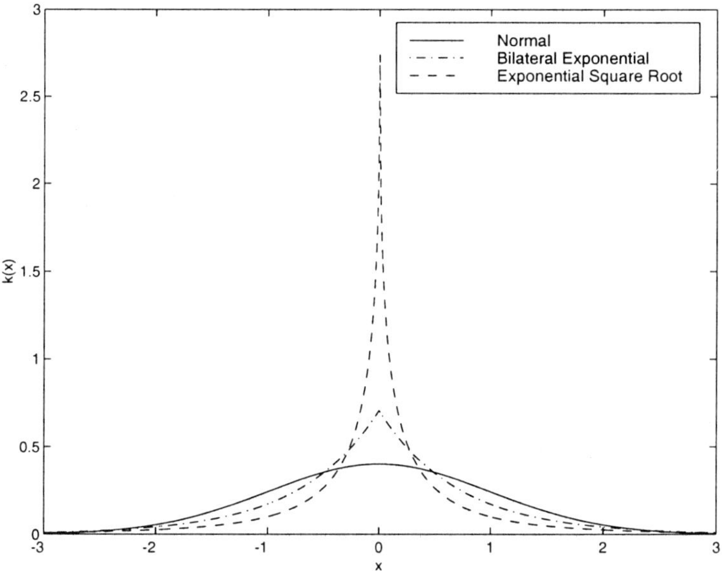

FIG. 1. *Graphs of the dispersal kernels $k_n(x)$, $k_{be}(x)$, and $k_{es}(x)$, where each kernel has a mean of zero and a variance of one.*

2.3. Kurtosis and higher order moments of the kernels. The kurtosis is a measure related to the peakedness and the size of the tail of the distribution. The kurtosis is defined as follows for a density function $f(x)$ of the random variable X, with mean and variance given by μ and σ^2:

$$Kur(f(x)) = \frac{E(X-\mu)^4}{[E(X-\mu)^2]^2} = \frac{E(X-\mu)^4}{\sigma^4} = \kappa.$$

Normalized higher order moments are also related to the thickness of the tail of the distribution. The $2m$th normalized moment is defined by

$$M^{2m}(f(x)) = \frac{E(X-\mu)^{2m}}{[E(X-\mu)^2]^m}, \quad m = 1, 2, 3, \dots .$$

Note that $M^2 = 1$ and $M^4 = \kappa$.

The kurtosis for the normal density function $k_n(x)$ is $\kappa = 3$. This value often serves as a reference for other density functions. Large values of the kurtosis or higher order moments indicate longer and fatter tailed distributions. For example, density functions with $\kappa \gg 3$ are known as leptokurtic distributions. The kurtosis and the higher order moment M^6 are given in Table 1 for each of the kernels (8), (9), and (10). Note that the kurtosis and M^6 are independent of D. This is not the case for the composite kernel (7).

The kurtosis and higher order moments of the composite kernel can be calculated in terms of the moments of each of the kernels k_i. Let κ_i, σ_i^2, and $E(X_i)^{2m}$ represent the kurtosis, variance and $2m$th moment of the kernel k_i, $i = 1, 2$, and $\sigma_1^2 = 1$. Then, the kurtosis of the composite kernel (7) is

$$Kur(k(x;p,D)) = \frac{(1-p)\kappa_1 + pE(X_2)^4}{[1-p+p\sigma_2^2]^2} = \kappa_{1,2}(p,D),$$

where the subscript 1, 2 refers to the two kernels in the composite kernel (2). For the composite normal kernel,

$$\kappa_{n,n}(p,D) = 3\frac{1-p+pD^4}{[1-p+pD^2]^2}. \tag{11}$$

The $2m$th normalized moment for the composite kernel is defined by

$$M_{1,2}^{2m}(p,D) = \frac{(1-p)E(X_1)^{2m} + pE(X_2)^{2m}}{[1-p+p\sigma_2^2]^m}. \tag{12}$$

Figure 2 illustrates the kurtosis, $\kappa_{n,n}(p,D)$, as a function of p for different values of D^2.

Some properties of the moments for the composite kernel can easily be verified. Note that $\kappa_{1,2}(0,D) = \kappa_1 = \kappa_{1,2}(p,0)$, $\kappa_{1,2}(1,D) = \kappa_2$, $M_{1,2}^{2m}(0,D) = M_1^{2m}$ and $M_{1,2}^{2m}(1,D) = M_2^{2m}$. Also, composite kernels with k_i one of the following forms, (8), (9), or (10), satisfy

$$\lim_{\sigma_2^2\to\infty} \kappa_{1,2}(p,D) = \lim_{D\to\infty} \kappa_{1,2}(p,D) = \frac{\kappa_2}{p}, \quad 0 < p \le 1.$$

This follows because the variance of k_2 is proportional to D^2 and the fourth moment is proportional to D^4 (Table 1). In general, higher order moments of composite kernels with k_i one of the forms (8), (9), or (10) satisfy

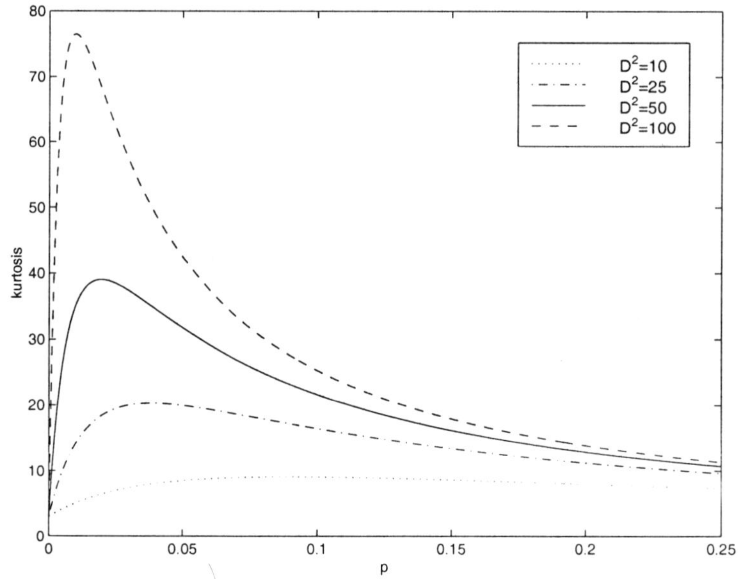

FIG. 2. *The kurtosis for the dispersal kernel,* $k(x;p,D) = (1-p)k_n(x)+pk_n(x,D)$, *as a function of* p *for various values of* D^2 $(=\sigma_2^2)$.

$$\lim_{D\to\infty} M_{1,2}^{2m}(p,D) = \frac{C}{p^{m-1}}, \quad 0 < p \leq 1,$$

where C is a constant. This latter identity follows because in (12), $E(X_1)^{2m}$ is constant, $E(X_2)^{2m}$ is proportional to D^{2m} and σ_2^2 is proportional to D^2. The composite kernel becomes extremely leptokurtic for small values of p as the variance increases (Figure 2). In addition, for kernels k_i of the form (8), (9) or (10), as $D \to \infty$, the value of p at which the maximum value of the kurtosis occurs approaches zero and the maximum value of the kurtosis increases at a rate proportional to D^2 when $D \gg 1$.

3. Rate of spread. It has been shown by Weinberger [16] that models of the form (1) with kernels having exponentially bounded tails, such as (8) and (9), have traveling wave solutions with a constant wave speed. This asymptotic wave speed is given by the formula:

$$c = \min_{\mu>0}\left(\frac{1}{\mu}\ln[f'(0)\int_{\mathbf{R}} \exp(\mu z)k(z)dz]\right), \quad f'(0) > 1. \tag{13}$$

For kernels of the form (8) and (9), the asymptotic wave speed c simplifies to

$$c = \sqrt{2D^2\ln[f'(0)]} \tag{14}$$

and

$$c = \min_{0<\mu D<1} \frac{1}{\mu} \ln \left[\frac{f'(0)}{1-\mu^2 D^2} \right], \tag{15}$$

respectively. For the epidemic-dispersal model (1) with f given by (6) satisfying assumptions (i)–(iv), $\mathcal{R}_0 > 1$ is equivalent to $f'(0) > 1$ since $f'(0) = 1 + \alpha - \mu - \gamma = 1 + [\mathcal{R}_0 - 1](\mu + \gamma)$. If $\mathcal{R}_0 > 1$ and the kernel is of the type (8) or (9), then the epidemic will eventually spread at the rate given by (14) or (15) until it reaches an endemic level I^* across the entire domain.

For kernels of the form (10), Kot et al. [11] showed that the asymptotic wave speed c is not constant but is approximately linear in t. It satisfies

$$c(t) \approx \frac{D}{4}[\ln f'(0)]^2 t + O(\sqrt{t}).$$

The formula for the asymptotic wave speed given in (14) and (15) are for single kernels, not for composite kernels. For composite kernels of the form (7), where k_1 or k_2 are given by (8) or (9), the model has a constant asymptotic wave speed which can be calculated numerically using formula (13). For composite kernels with k_i given by (10), the asymptotic speed $c(t)$ must also be calculated numerically.

Several examples are given in the next section to illustrate the impact of a small proportion, $p \ll 1$, of long-range dispersal, $\sigma_2^2 \gg 1$, on the asymptotic wave speed.

4. Numerical examples. It is assumed that the dominant method of spread for a population or an infectious disease is via short-range dispersal, e.g., local contacts. However, a small proportion, $p \ll 1$, of the population or disease is spread via long-range dispersal. Long-range dispersal is characterized by having a much greater variance than short-range dispersal. In particular, it is assumed that the composite kernel is of the form (7), where the variance for short-range dispersal is normalized to one and the variance for long-range dispersal is proportional to D^2.

Consider a model of the form (1), where f is given by (6) and the force of infection λ satisfies

$$\lambda(I) = 1 - \exp\left(-\frac{\alpha}{N} I\right).$$

In the numerical examples, it is assumed that $\alpha = 1.5$, $\gamma + \mu = 0.5$, so that $\mathcal{R}_0 = 3$ and $f'(0) = 2$. Then, the endemic equilibrium is $I^* \approx 51.995$.

Solutions to model (1) are calculated for an initial density of infectives given by

$$I_0(x) > 0, \quad x \in [-\epsilon, \epsilon] \text{ and } I_0(x) = 0, \quad x \notin [-\epsilon, \epsilon],$$

for ϵ small. Graphs of the solutions to (1) for $t = 0, 1, \ldots, 25$ are given in Figure 3 for dispersal governed by a composite kernel (7) with a (a) normal density, (b) bilateral exponential density, and (c) exponential square root density, i.e.,

$$k(x;p,D) = (1-p)k_i(x) + pk_i(x;D), \quad i = n, be, es. \tag{16}$$

It can be seen for cases (a) and (b) that there exists a traveling wave solution with a constant wave speed. However, for case (c), the wave speed is increasing.

The asymptotic wave speed for a normal composite kernel as in case (a), equation (16) with $i = n$, is calculated and graphed in Figure 4. The wave speed is graphed for $0 \le p \le 1$ and for different values of the variance for long-range dispersal, $\sigma_2^2 = D^2$. For small values of p and large values of D, the kurtosis of the kernel is large and the asymptotic wave speed is much greater than the speed when $p = 0$, where the kurtosis of the kernel is $\kappa_n = 3$ and there is no long-range dispersal. For example, when $D^2 = 100$ and $p = 0$, the asymptotic wave speed is $c = 1.177$; for $p = 0.1$, $c = 5.785$ and for $p = 1$, $c = 11.77$. The rate of increase in the speed is extremely large as p increases above zero, as can be seen from the slope of the wave speed curves at $p = 0$ (Figure 4). Table 2 gives the wave speeds for model (1) with composite normal and composite bilateral exponential kernels for different values of p.

TABLE 2

Asymptotic wave speed for model (1) with the composite normal and composite bilateral exponential kernels of the form (16) when the variance of long-range dispersal is 100.

	Wave Speed, c	
p	Normal	Bilateral Exponential
0.000	1.177	1.343
0.001	2.732	5.233
0.010	3.637	5.800
0.100	5.785	7.616
1.000	11.770	13.430

The asymptotic wave speed for model (1) with the composite normal and composite bilateral exponential kernels are compared in Figure 5. It is assumed that long-range dispersal has a variance of 100. The rate of increase of the speed is greatest at $p = 0$.

In the final example, the asymptotic wave speed, $c(t)$, is calculated numerically for $p = 0$, 0.005, and 0.01 when the composite kernel has an exponential square root form,

$$k(x;p,D) = (1-p)k_{es}(x) + pk_{es}(x;D).$$

A graph of the wave speed as a function of t is given in Figure 6. It can be seen that $c(t)$ increases at an approximately linear rate for $t > 15$, as

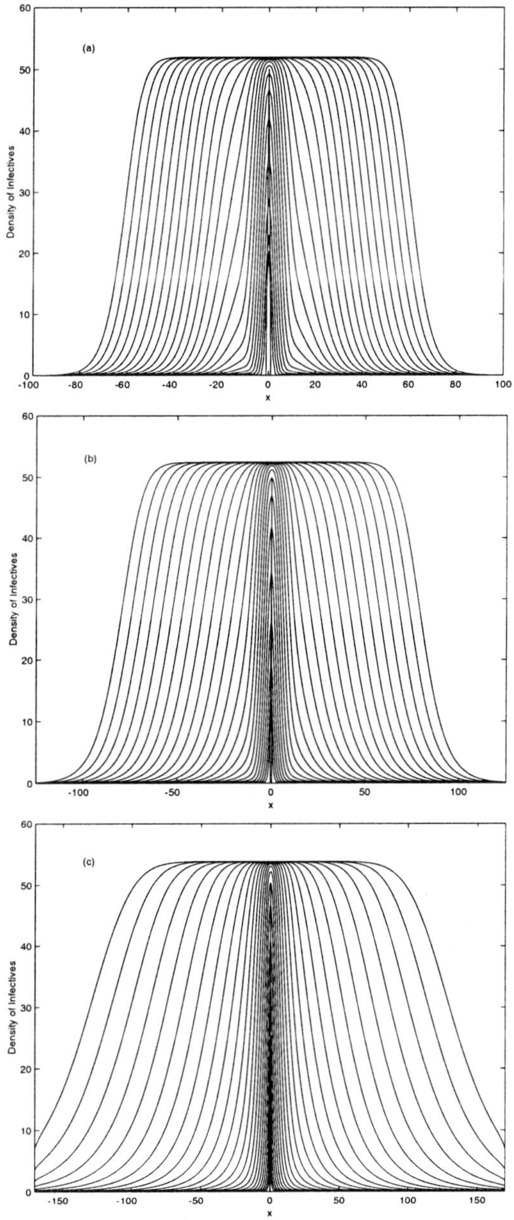

FIG. 3. *Traveling wave for the density of infectives for model (1) with (a) the normal dispersal kernel,* $k(x;D) = 0.99k_n(x) + 0.01k_n(x;D)$ *(b) the bilateral exponential kernel,* $k(x;D) = 0.99k_{be}(x) + 0.01k_{be}(x;D)$ *and (c) the exponential square root kernel,* $k(x;D) = 0.99k_{es}(x) + 0.01k_{es}(x;D)$, *where the variance for long-range dispersal is 100,* $f'(0) = 2$.

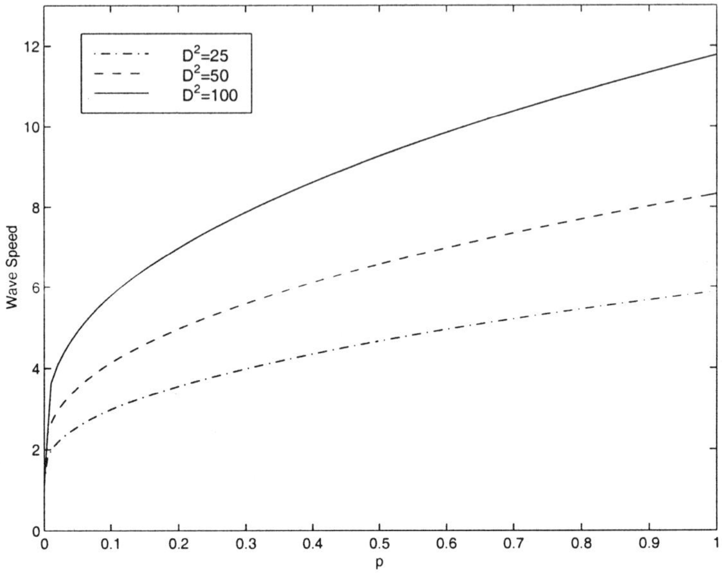

FIG. 4. *The asymptotic wave speed as a function of p for various values of D^2 for model (1) with the composite normal kernel, $k(x; p, D) = (1-p)k_n(x) + pk_n(x; D)$. The variance for long-range dispersal is D^2, $f'(0) = 2$.*

predicted by Kot et al. [11]. This linear rate is much greater when p is slightly greater than zero than when $p = 0$.

5. Summary and extensions. An integrodifference equation model for the spatial spread of a population is extended to an SIS epidemic model with general force of infection. Two methods of dispersal are incorporated into the model by assuming that the composite kernel is a linear combination of two kernels, one representing short-range dispersal and the other long-range dispersal. Local contacts are frequently the primary method of spread in infectious diseases. However, long-range movements of infectious individuals may result in establishment and spread of the disease far from the source. In the model, the two dispersal methods are differentiated by assuming the variance for long-range dispersal is much greater than for short range, $\sigma_2^2 \gg 1$.

It was shown for some composite kernels that the kurtosis and higher order moments are inversely proportional to p^{m-1} for large values of σ_2^2. In addition, it was shown numerically that small values of p and large values of σ_2^2 lead to large increases in the wave speed. This relation between the moments or shape of the kernel and the asymptotic wave speed was noted by Kot et al. [11]; in their formulation, models with single kernels having "fat-tails" (leptokurtic) had greater wave speeds than those having exponentially bounded tails.

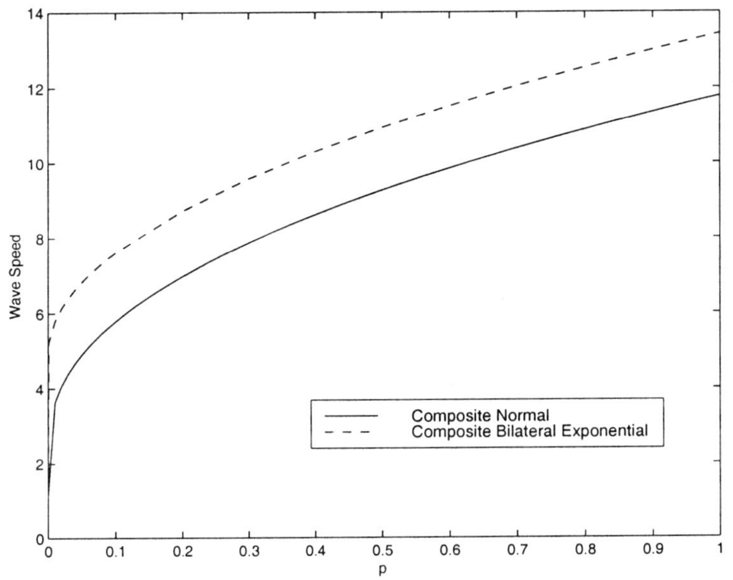

FIG. 5. *The asymptotic wave speed as a function of p for model (1) with the composite normal and composite bilateral kernels,* $k(x;p,D) = (1-p)k_n(x) + pk_n(x;D)$ *and* $k(x;p,D) = (1-p)k_{be}(x) + pk_{be}(x;D)$. *The variance for long-range dispersal is 100,* $f'(0) = 2$.

In applications, where the proportion p of spread due to long-range dispersal is significant but very small, it will be difficult to estimate p from data. If the spread due to long-range dispersal is neglected, the models indicate that the rate of spread will be seriously underestimated. Therefore, it is important to obtain data on long-range dispersal.

The model developed here for two methods of dispersal can be easily extended to more than two methods. For example, a model with n methods of dispersal would have a kernel of the form:

$$k(x;p_1,\dots,p_{n-1}) = \sum_{i=1}^{n} p_i k_i(x),$$

where $\sum_{i=1}^{n} p_i = 1$ and $p_i > 0$. In addition, each dispersal kernel k_i may have different means and variances. In this case, the moments of the composite kernel k and the wave speed will depend on the proportions p_i and the moments for each of the kernels k_i.

Acknowledgments. L.J.S. Allen and R.K. Ernest gratefully acknowledge the support of NSF grant DMS-9626417 (Allen) and the support of the Ronald E. McNair Scholars program at Texas Tech University (Ernest).

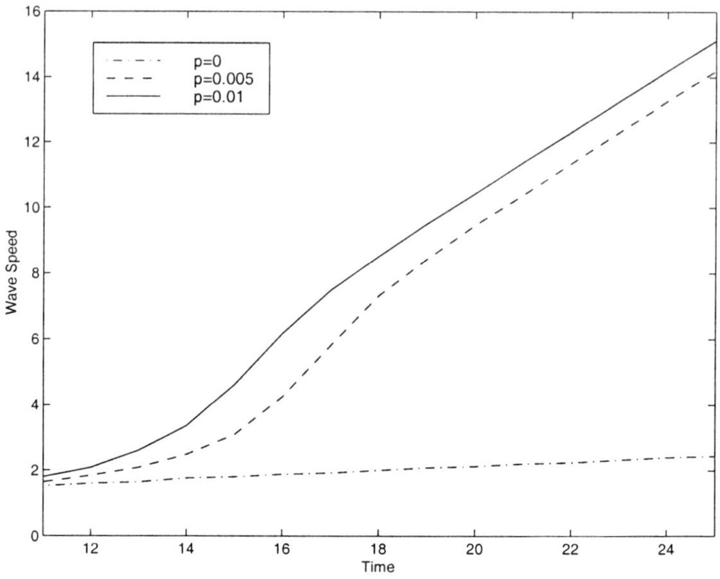

FIG. 6. *Wave speed* $c(t)$ *for model (1) with the composite exponential square root kernel,* $k(x;p,D) = (1-p)k_{es}(x) + pk_{es}(x,D)$*, as a function of* t*, when* $p = 0$*, 0.005, and 0.01,* $f'(0) = 2$*. The variance for long-range dispersal is 100,* $D^2 = 200/15$.

REFERENCES

[1] Allen, E.J., L.J.S. Allen, and X. Gilliam. 1996. Dispersal and competition models for plants. *J. Math. Biol.* 34:455–481.

[2] Allen, L.J.S. 1994. Some discrete-time SI, SIR, and SIS epidemic models. *Math. Biosci.* 124:83–105.

[3] Allen, L.J.S., E.J. Allen, and D.N. Atkinson. 1999. Integrodifference equations applied to plant dispersal, competition, and control. *Fields Inst. Comm.* 21:15–30.

[4] Allen, L.J.S., E.J. Allen, and X. Ponweera. 1996. A mathematical model for weed dispersal and control. *Bull. Math. Biol.* 58:815–834.

[5] Allen, L.J.S. and A.M. Burgin. 2000. Comparison of deterministic and stochastic SIS and SIR models. *Math. Biosci.* 163:1–33.

[6] Anderson, R.M. and R.M. May. 1991. *Infectious Diseases of Humans, Dynamics and Control.* Oxford University Press, Oxford.

[7] Cooke, K.L., D.F. Calef, and E.V. Level. 1977. Stability or chaos in discrete epidemic models. In *Nonlinear Systems and Applications.* V. Lakshmikantham (Ed.) pp. 73–93, Academic Press, New York.

[8] Hengeveld, R. 1989. *Dynamics of Biological Invasions.* Chapman & Hall, London.

[9] Hethcote, H.W. 1994. A thousand and one epidemic models. In: *Frontiers in Mathematical Biology*, Lecture Notes in Biomathematics, 100, (Edited by S.A. Levin), pp. 504–515. Springer-Verlag, Berlin-Heidelberg, New York.

[10] Kot, M. 1992. Discrete-time travelling waves: ecological examples. *J. Math. Biol.* 30:413–436.

[11] Kot, M., M.A. Lewis, and P. van den Driessche. 1996. Dispersal data and the spread of invading organisms. *Ecology.* 77:2027–2042.

[12] Kot, M. and W.M. Schaffer. 1986. Discrete-time growth-dispersal models. *Math. Biosci.* 80:109–136.

[13] Lewis, M. 1997. Variability, patchiness, and jump dispersal in the spread of an invading population. In: *Spatial Ecology The Role of Space in Population Dynamics and Interspecific Interactions.* D. Tilman and P. Kareiva (Eds.) pp. 46–69, Princeton University Press.

[14] Shigesada, N. and K. Kawasaki. 1997. *Biological Invasions: Theory and Practice.* Oxford Series in Ecology and Evolution. Oxford University Press, Oxford, New York and Tokyo.

[15] Sumpter, K.J. 1995. The dynamics of some epidemic models. Master's Thesis, Texas Tech University, Lubbock, TX, USA.

[16] Weinberger, H.F. 1982. Long-time behavior of a class of biological models. *SIAM J. Math. Anal.* 13:353–396.

[17] Williamson, M. 1996. *Biological Invasions.* Chapman & Hall, London.

ENDEMICITY, PERSISTENCE, AND QUASI-STATIONARITY*

INGEMAR NÅSELL†

Abstract. The concept of quasi-stationarity is basic for the study of stochastic models for endemic infections. Information about both the endemicity and the persistence of an endemic infection is contained in the quasi-stationary distribution. We describe and summarize the contents of several recent papers, dealing with both the univariate SIS model and the bivariate endemic SIR model. Qualitative results generalizing the threshold behaviour of the corresponding deterministic models are emphasized. The deterministic SIS model serves well as an approximation of the stochastic SIS model, while the deterministic endemic SIR model is unacceptable as an approximation of the corresponding stochastic model. Unsolved problems for the stochastic endemic SIR model are discussed.

Key words. Endemic infections, persistence, time to extinction, quasi-stationarity, demographic stochasticity, persistence threshold.

AMS(MOS) subject classifications. 60J27, 92D40.

1. Introduction. Epidemic infections are characterized by short outbreaks as contrasted to endemic infections that are present in a population for a long time period. Mathematically one deals with transients for epidemic infections, while one studies stationary (or almost stationary) behaviour for endemic infections.

We discuss two different types of mathematical models, denoted by SIS and SIR, respectively. The letters S, I, and R refer to Susceptible, Infected, and Recovered individuals. The letters in the type designation refer to the consecutive possible states of an individual. Thus, susceptible individuals can become infected in both SIS and SIR models. On the other hand, infected individuals are immediately susceptible again after recovery in the SIS model, but not in the SIR model. SIR models are used for infections that confer immunity, and SIS models for infections that give no immunity.

Models for the spread of infections are based on hypotheses about such mechanisms as infection and recovery. Additional hypotheses about demographic mechanisms are important when one wishes to study the spread of the infection over longer time periods, where demographic changes in the population are important. It turns out that SIR models without demography lead to epidemic infections, while both SIR models with demography

*This paper is based on two talks that were presented at the IMA tutorial "Introduction to Epidemiology and Immunology" at the University of Minnesota in Minneapolis in May 1999. I thank Carlos Castillo-Chavez and the IMA for inviting me to attend the tutorial and the IMA for providing excellent facilities during my stay in Minneapolis.

†Department of Mathematics, The Royal Institute of Technology, S-100 44 Stockholm, Sweden. Email: ingemar@math.kth.se.

and SIS models, without or with demography, are associated with endemic infections.

Both stochastic and deterministic models have been used to study both epidemic and endemic infections. Among these, stochastic models have played a major role in the work on epidemic infections, while deterministic models have dominated in the work on endemic infections.

An important message of the present paper is that one needs to resort to stochastic models in the study of those endemic infections that confer immunity, namely the endemic SIR models. The reason is that the alternative mode of modelling, via deterministic models, leads to qualitatively incorrect conclusions. On the other hand, deterministic models appear to give good approximations for SIS models.

The importance of stochastic modelling for endemic SIR models was emphasized already by Bartlett (1956-1960), and is described by Bailey (1975). It is remarkable that many papers dealing with deterministic endemic SIR models have appeared after Bartlett published his important work more than 40 years ago, but that only few papers have been published that deal with stochastic models. The reason is that Bartlett's ideas were ahead of their time. Bartlett had a remarkable intuition that gave him an insight into the intricate behaviour of his stochastic model. His insight was, however, not matched by available theory. Developments of stochastic theory since then have changed the scenario. Some of the model behaviour can now be analyzed in a mathematically satisfactory way. This does not mean that we understand all aspects of the behaviour of the model. Open problems remain that continue to pose a challenge for mathematicians that are eager to analyze the intricacies of the stochastic setup. The time has come to follow up on Bartlett's ideas.

We analyze only the simple model formulations for which the deterministic versions lead to one or several ordinary differential equations, while the stochastic versions take the form of a Markov chain with discrete state space and continuous time. More realistic models with additional assumptions concerning heterogeneity, age dependence, spatial distribution, isolation, and duration of infection have been studied by a number of authors. We refrain from a discussion of such models. Our modest goal is to understand the qualitative properties of the simple models.

The deterministic models allow us, at least in principle, to predict the values of the state variables at any time $t > 0$ from specified initial values at time $t = 0$. The emphasis is on the long-term behaviour as $t \to \infty$. The common approach is to use methods and results from the qualitative theory of ordinary differential equations. The most powerful mathematical result is a bifurcation phenomenon. It says that there are two regions in parameter space with qualitatively different solution behaviours. In one of the regions most solutions approach a critical point that corresponds to an endemic infection level, while the infection ultimately disappears in the complementary region. The boundary between these two regions is called a threshold. It is customary to define a function on parameter space that is denoted by R_0 and referred to as the basic reproduction ratio. In many situations, and certainly for the simple models considered here, R_0 takes the value 1 on the threshold.

Each deterministic model has a natural stochastic counterpart. The state variables, which take values on the nonnegative real axis in the deterministic model, are stochastic variables that are restricted to take nonnegative integer values. In this sense, the stochastic model is the more realistic one, since populations always come in units of one. The deterministic model predicts exact future values of the state variables, while the stochastic model predicts future probability distributions. The counterpart to the initial-value problem for the deterministic model is the so-called Markov property, which says that the probability distribution at some future date, given the present state, is independent of the past. The stochastic process that forms the model is a Markov chain. Indeed, it is a special case of a Markov chain called a birth-death process. This means that the possible transitions are to one of the nearest neighbor states (only one birth, or one death, or one infection, etc.).

The term transition rate is used to describe the hypotheses in both deterministic and stochastic models. This usage is convenient in the comparison between the two model types, and it makes it obvious how to formulate the stochastic counterpart of a deterministic model or vice versa. Note however that the mathematical meanings of the coinciding terms are different in the two settings. Thus, a transition rate in the deterministic model is a rate of change of a state variable, while it is a rate of change of a corresponding transition probability in the stochastic model.

The deterministic and stochastic models are counterparts to each other, with both of them based on the same transition rates. However, the two models do not carry the same power. The stochastic model is the basic one. Indeed, the deterministic model can be derived from the stochastic one by first introducing scaled state variables that are equal to the original state variables divided by the population size N, and thereafter taking the limit as $N \to \infty$.

This means that among the two types of model, only the stochastic one is able to deal with a finite population size N. Since every population that we encounter is finite, we can also conclude that the deterministic model is an approximation of the stochastic one, and that this approximation is acceptable if N is large enough. It is an important mathematical problem to establish how large N must be in order for the approximation to be acceptable. This question can only be answered by a careful analysis of the stochastic model.

The stochastic features that we are concerned with are related to the fact that the state variables are all discrete. These features are referred as "demographic stochasticity".

The population size N is an essential parameter for the stochastic model, but if it appears at all in the deterministic model, then it serves only as an innocent parameter. Indeed, it can be removed completely from the deterministic model equations by simply rescaling the state variables. Conceptually, the deterministic model can not deal with actual population sizes, but only with proportions. This will be apparent in the model results, where we expect N to play an important role for the stochastic model, but only to appear in an innocent role for the deterministic model.

The counterpart to a stationary solution in the deterministic model is a stationary distribution for the stochastic model. It turns out, however, that the stochastic models we consider have absorbing states where the number of infected individuals is equal to zero. This has the consequence that the stationary distributions are degenerate and uninformative. Indeed, the stationary distribution describes the state after absorption has occurred. The absorption phenomenon constitutes a qualitative difference between deterministic and stochastic models, since absorption will occur in finite time in the stochastic models we consider, but never in the deterministic ones.

The time to extinction can in some cases be very long. It is then of interest to find the distribution of the state variable(s) under the condition that absorption has not yet occurred. This distribution is approximated by the so-called quasi-stationary distribution, and it is actually equal to this distribution when the initial distribution is. It is not possible to solve for the quasi-stationary distribution in explicit form.

The time to extinction depends on the state that the process is in initially. If it is only known that the process is non-extinct initially, then our lack of precise knowledge is reflected by the assumption that the initial distribution equals the quasi-stationary distribution. The time to extinction from the quasi-stationary distribution is therefore a measure of the persistence of the infection. One of the results of the mathematical analysis is that the distribution of the time to extinction from quasi-stationarity can be determined if the quasi-stationary distribution is known.

We study two models for endemic infections in this paper, namely the SIS model (without demography), and the endemic SIR model (with demography). Results from four recent papers (Nåsell (1996, 1999a, 1999b, 2001)) and one unpublished manuscript (Nåsell (2000)) are summarized and described, while we refer to the original papers for mathematical details and derivations. The SIS model takes the form of a univariate birth-death process, while the endemic SIR model is a bivariate birth-death process. A rather satisfactory mathematical analysis can be carried through for the former of these models, while the latter still presents substantial mathematical difficulties. A description of the SIS model and its properties is given in Section 3, while what is known for the endemic SIR model is treated in Section 4. The results for the SIS model in Section 3 make heavy use of the powerful mathematical method of asymptotic approximations. The

SIS model results allow us to indicate the open problems for the endemic SIR model in Section 4. Section 2 is devoted to the analysis of a general univariate birth-death process, of which the SIS model is a special case.

2. A birth-death process with finite state space and with absorbing state at the origin. In Subsection 2.1 we formulate a univariate birth-death process with finite state space, and for which the origin is an absorbing state. Two auxiliary processes without absorbing states are then formulated in Subsection 2.2, and their stationary distributions are determined. The quasi-stationary distribution of the original process is studied in Subsection 2.3. It is shown to satisfy a recursion relation where the coefficients can be interpreted in terms of the stationary distributions of the two auxiliary processes. The time to extinction is studied in Subsection 2.4, both when the initial distribution equals the quasi-stationary distribution, and when the initial state is fixed. We show that the time to extinction from the quasi-stationary distribution has an exponential distribution. This distribution is completely determined by its expectation, which in turn is simply related to the probability of taking the value 1 (the state from which transitions to the absorbing state 0 can take place) in quasi-stationarity. The expected time to extinction from a fixed state is determined by an explicit expression whose coefficients can be interpreted in terms of the stationary distributions of the two auxiliary processes. A diffusion approximation is treated in Subsection 2.5.

Our presentation follows Nåsell (2000) closely. Another discussion of these issues is given by Nisbet and Gurney (1982). Our results prepare for the treatment of the SIS model via asymptotic approximations in Section 3.

2.1. Formulation of the birth-death process. We study a birth-death process $\{X(t), t \geq 0\}$ with finite state space $\{0, 1, \ldots, N\}$ and where the origin is an absorbing state. Transitions in the process are only allowed to neighboring states. The rate of transition from state n to state $n+1$ (the population birth rate) is denoted λ_n, and the rate of transition from the state n to the state $n-1$ (the population death rate) is denoted by μ_n. It is convenient to also have notation for the sum of λ_n and μ_n: we put $\kappa_n = \lambda_n + \mu_n$. We assume that μ_0 and λ_N are equal to zero, to be consistent with the assumption that the state space is limited to $\{0, 1, \ldots, N\}$. Furthermore, we assume that λ_0 also equals zero, to be consistent with the assumption that the origin is an absorbing state. All other transition rates are assumed to be strictly positive.

The Kolmogorov forward equations for the state probabilities $p_n(t) = P\{X(t) = n\}$ can be written

$$p_n'(t) = \mu_{n+1} p_{n+1}(t) - \kappa_n p_n(t) + \lambda_{n-1} p_{n-1}(t), \quad n = 0, 1, \ldots, N. \tag{2.1}$$

(Put $\mu_{N+1} = \lambda_{-1} = p_{N+1}(t) = p_{-1}(t) = 0$, so that (2.1) makes sense formally for all n-values indicated.) The state probabilities depend on the initial distribution $p_n(0)$.

An alternative way of writing this system of equations is in the form

$$p' = pA, \tag{2.2}$$

where $p(t) = (p_0(t), p_1(t), \ldots, p_N(t))$ is the row vector of state probabilities and A is a square matrix with $N + 1$ rows and $N + 1$ columns. The elements of the matrix A (the infinitesimal generator) are determined from the transition rates λ_n and μ_n as follows: Let the rows and columns of A be numbered from 0 to N. Each nondiagonal element a_{mn} then equals the rate of transition from state m to state n. Hence $a_{mn} = 0$ if $|m - n| > 1$, while $a_{m,m+1} = \lambda_m$ and $a_{m,m-1} = \mu_m$. Furthermore, the diagonal element a_{nn} equals the sum of the rates of transition from the state n, multiplied by -1. Hence $a_{nn} = -\kappa_n$. It follows that the matrix A can be written as follows:

$$A = \begin{pmatrix} -\kappa_0 & \lambda_0 & 0 & \ldots & 0 \\ \mu_1 & -\kappa_1 & \lambda_1 & \ldots & 0 \\ 0 & \mu_2 & -\kappa_2 & \ldots & 0 \\ \ldots & \ldots & \ldots & \ldots & \ldots \\ 0 & 0 & 0 & \ldots & -\kappa_N \end{pmatrix}. \tag{2.3}$$

Note that A is a tridiagonal matrix with all row sums equal to 0. Thus the determinant of A equals zero, so A is noninvertible. Note also that $\lambda_0 = \kappa_0 = 0$, so the first row of A is a row of zeros.

A stationary distribution is found by putting the time derivative equal to zero, i.e. by solving $pA = 0$. It is readily shown that the process $\{X(t)\}$ has a degenerate stationary distribution $p = (1, 0, \ldots, 0)$. The distribution of $\{X(t)\}$ approaches the stationary distribution as time t approaches infinity. This says that ultimate absorption is certain. In many cases, the time to absorption is long. It is therefore of interest to study the distribution of $\{X(t)\}$ before absorption has taken place. This is done via the concept of quasi-stationarity, which is introduced in Subsection 2.3.

2.2. Two auxiliary processes. In this subsection we study two birth-death processes $\{X^{(0)}(t)\}$ and $\{X^{(1)}(t)\}$ that both are close to the original process $\{X(t)\}$, but lack absorbing states. The state space of each of the two auxiliary processes coincides with the set of transient states $\{1, 2, \ldots, N\}$ for the original process. We determine the stationary distribution of each of the two auxiliary processes. The importance of these stationary distributions was pointed out in the context of the SIS model by Kryscio and Lefèvre (1989).

The process $\{X^{(0)}(t)\}$ can be described as the original process with the origin removed. Its rate of transition from the state 1 to the state 0, namely the death rate $\mu_1^{(0)}$, is equal to 0, while all other transition rates are equal to the corresponding rates for the original process.

The process $\{X^{(1)}(t)\}$ is found from the original process by allowing for one immortal individual. Here, each death rate μ_n is replaced by $\mu_n^{(1)} =$

μ_{n-1}, while each of the birth rates $\lambda_n^{(1)}$ equals the corresponding birth rate for the original process.

The state probabilities for the two processes are denoted by $p^{(0)}(t) = (p_1^{(0)}(t), p_2^{(0)}(t), \ldots, p_N^{(0)}(t))$ and $p^{(1)}(t) = (p_1^{(1)}(t), p_2^{(1)}(t), \ldots, p_N^{(1)}(t))$, respectively.

Stationary distributions are easy to determine explicitly for both of the auxiliary processes. In order to describe them we introduce two sequencies of parameters ρ_n and π_n as follows:

$$\rho_1 = 1, \quad \rho_n = \frac{\lambda_1 \lambda_2 \cdots \lambda_{n-1}}{\mu_1 \mu_2 \cdots \mu_{n-1}}, \qquad n = 2, 3, \ldots, N, \tag{2.4}$$

$$\pi_n = \frac{\mu_1}{\mu_n} \rho_n, \quad n = 1, 2, \ldots, N. \tag{2.5}$$

The two stationary distribution can be simply expressed in terms of these parameter sequencies. The stationary distribution of the process $\{X^{(0)}(t)\}$ equals

$$p_n^{(0)} = \pi_n p_1^{(0)}, \quad n = 1, 2, \ldots, N, \quad \text{where} \quad p_1^{(0)} = \frac{1}{\sum_{n=1}^N \pi_n}, \tag{2.6}$$

while the stationary distribution of the process $\{X^{(1)}(t)\}$ equals

$$p_n^{(1)} = \rho_n p_1^{(1)}, \quad n = 1, 2, \ldots, N, \quad \text{where} \quad p_1^{(1)} = \frac{1}{\sum_{n=1}^N \rho_n}. \tag{2.7}$$

Both of these stationary distributions will serve as approximations of the quasi-stationary distribution defined in the next section. Furthermore, the related parameter sequencies ρ_n and π_n play important roles in a recursion relation for the quasi-stationary distribution, and in an explicit expression for the expected time to extinction from a fixed state n.

2.3. The quasi-stationary distribution q. We define and study the quasi-stationary distribution q for the process $\{X(t)\}$. The concept of quasi-stationarity for finite Markov chains in continuous time goes back to the paper by Darroch and Seneta (1967).

We partition the state space into two subsets, one contaning the absorbing state 0, and the other equal to the set of transient states $\{1, 2, \ldots, N\}$. Corresponding to this partition, we write the equation (2.2) in block form. The vector $p(t)$ is expressed as $p(t) = (p_0(t), p_Q(t))$, where $p_Q(t) = (p_1(t), \ldots, p_N(t))$ is the row vector of state probabilities in the set of transient states. The corresponding block form of the matrix A contains four blocks. The first row of A gives rise to two blocks of row vectors of zeroes. The remaining two blocks contain a column vector a of length N and a square matrix A_Q of order N. The first entry of a equals μ_1, while all other entries are equal to 0. Thus, a contains the rate of transition from the transient state 1 to the absorbing state 0. The matrix A_Q is formed be deleting the first row and the first column from A. It contains (on the diagonal above and below the main diagonal) the rates of transition between transient states. With this notation one can rewrite (2.2) in the form

$$(p_0', p_Q') = (p_0, p_Q) \begin{pmatrix} 0 & 0 \\ a & A_Q \end{pmatrix}. \tag{2.8}$$

By carrying out the product on the right-hand side and equating the block components of the two sides of the equation, we are led to the following two differential equations:

$$p_0' = p_Q a = p_1 \mu_1 \tag{2.9}$$

and

$$p_Q' = p_Q A_Q. \tag{2.10}$$

Before absorption, the process takes values in the set of transient states. The state of the process at time t is restricted to this set if the initial distribution is supported on this set, i.e. if $P\{X(0) > 0\} = 1$, and if absorption at the origin has not yet occurred at time t, i.e. if $X(t) > 0$. The corresponding conditional state probabilities are denoted $q_n(t)$. We introduce $q(t) = (q_1(t), \dots, q_N(t))$ to denote the row vector of conditional state probabilities. We note that $q(t)$ depends on the initial distribution $q(0)$. The conditioning on non-absorption at time t leads to the relation

$$q_n(t) = P\{X(t) = n | X(t) > 0\} = \frac{p_n(t)}{1 - p_0(t)}. \tag{2.11}$$

Hence the vector of conditional state probabilities $q(t)$ can be determined from the vector $p_Q(t)$ of state probabilities on the set of transient states via the relation

$$q(t) = \frac{p_Q(t)}{1 - p_0(t)}. \tag{2.12}$$

By differentiating this relation and using expression (2.9) for p_0' we get

$$q' = \frac{p_Q'}{1 - p_0} + \mu_1 q_1 \frac{p_Q}{1 - p_0}. \tag{2.13}$$

By using (2.10) and (2.12) we get the following equation for the vector of conditional state probabilities q:

$$q' = q A_Q + \mu_1 q_1 q. \tag{2.14}$$

The quasi-stationary distribution q can now be defined. It is the stationary solution of this equation. Thus, it satisfies the equation

$$q A_Q = -\mu_1 q_1 q. \tag{2.15}$$

This shows that the quasi-stationary distribution q is a left eigenvector of the matrix A_Q corresponding to the eigenvalue $-\mu_1 q_1$. This result is useful for numerical evaluations. The eigenvalue $-\mu_1 q_1$ is the maximum eigenvalue of the matrix A_Q.

It is not possible to determine the quasi-stationary distribution explicitly in the general situation that we consider here. The best we can do is to derive a recursion relation for the probabilities q_n that involves the parameters ρ_n and π_n that are used to describe the stationary distributions of the two auxiliary processes $X^{(0)}(t)$ and $X^{(1)}(t)$. This recursion relation takes the following form:

$$q_n = \pi_n \sum_{k=1}^{n} \frac{1 - \sum_{j=1}^{k-1} q_j}{\rho_k} q_1, \quad n = 1, 2 \ldots, N, \quad \sum_{n=1}^{N} q_n = 1. \tag{2.16}$$

A derivation of this result is given by Nåsell (2000). Note that the sequencies π_n and ρ_n are known explicitly in terms of the transition rates λ_n and μ_n. This recursion relation is used to derive an explicit approximation for the quasi-stationary distribution for the SIS model that is given in the next section.

We emphasize that the relation in (2.16) is not an explicit solution. It can be used to successively determine the values of q_2, q_3 etc. if q_1 is known. But the crux is that q_1 can only be determined from the relation $\sum_{n=1}^{N} q_n = 1$, which requires knowledge of all the q_n.

Two iteration methods for numerically determining the quasi-stationary distribution can be based on (2.16). One of these methods uses iteration for determining q_1. It starts with an initial guess for q_1, determines successively all the q_n from (2.16), computes the sum of the q_n, and determines the result of the first iteration as the initial guess divided by this sum. The process is repeated until successive iterates are sufficiently close. Nisbet and Gurney (1982) describe essentially the same iteration method.

The second method uses iteration on the whole distribution. It starts with an initial guess for the whole quasi-stationary distribution ($p^{(0)}$ and $p^{(1)}$ discussed in the previous subsection are candidates), uses this distribution as input in the numerators of the terms that are summed over k, and solves (2.16) for the q_n. The process is repeated until successive iterates are sufficiently close. The iteration of the second numerical method can be formally described as follows:

$$q_n^{(i+1)} = \pi_n \sum_{k=1}^{n} \frac{1 - \sum_{j=1}^{k-1} q_j^{(i)}}{\rho_k} q_1^{(i+1)}, \tag{2.17}$$

where the quasi-stationary distribution of iteration number i is denoted $q^{(i)}$. Numerical evaluations and explicit approximations of the quasi-stationary distribution for the SIS model in Section 3 are based on this method.

2.4. The time to extinction. The time to extinction τ is a random variable that clearly depends on the initial distribution. We denote this random variable by τ_Q when the initial distribution $p(0)$ equals the quasi-stationary distribution q, and by τ_n when $X(0) = n$.

We study first τ_Q. As mentioned above, this random variable is an important measure of the persistence of the infection. It turns out to be possible to get a simple form for the state probabilities p in this case, i. e. when the initial distribution equals q. To derive this we note from (2.13) that

$$p'_Q = -\mu_1 q_1 p_Q, \quad p_Q(0) = q. \tag{2.18}$$

This says essentially that probability is leaking from each transient state with the same rate. This equation has the solution

$$p_Q(t) = q \exp(-\mu_1 q_1 t). \tag{2.19}$$

From this solution one can also determine $p_0(t)$, since (2.9) gives a differential equation for p_0 in terms of p_1, and the initial value is $p_0(0) = 0$. Thus p_0 satisfies the initial value problem

$$p'_0 = \mu_1 p_1, \quad p_0(0) = 0. \tag{2.20}$$

The solution of this problem is

$$p_0(t) = 1 - \exp(-\mu_1 q_1 t). \tag{2.21}$$

The expressions in (2.19) and (2.21) combine to give the solution of the Kolmogorov forward equations in this case. It is noteworthy that it is possible to get such a simple expression for this solution. The solution is, however, not explicit, since we have no explicit expression for q_1.

If absorption has occurred at time t, then clearly the waiting time to extinction τ_Q is less than or equal to t, and the state of the process $X(t)$ is equal to 0. By computing the probabilities of these events we get $P\{\tau_Q \le t\} = P\{X(t) = 0\} = p_0(t)$. We conclude that the time to extinction from the quasi-stationary distribution, τ_Q, has an exponential distribution with the expectation

$$\mathbf{E}\tau_Q = \frac{1}{\mu_1 q_1}. \tag{2.22}$$

The distribution of τ_Q is thus completely determined from the probability q_1.

The distribution of the time to extinction τ_n from the fixed initial state n is more complicated. Some insight into its behaviour may be gained by considering its expectation. It is a standard result for birth-death processes that this expectation can be determined explicitly. The result is given e.g.

by Karlin and Taylor (1975), Nisbet and Gurney (1982), and Renshaw (1991). We rewrite this result using our notation:

$$\mathbf{E}\tau_n = \frac{1}{\mu_1} \sum_{k=1}^{n} \frac{\sum_{j=k}^{N} \pi_j}{\rho_k}. \tag{2.23}$$

Note that the two parameter sequencies ρ_n and π_n both appear here. Since these parameter sequencies are related to the two stationary distributions $p^{(1)}$ and $p^{(0)}$ we can interpret both numerator and denominator of each term in the sum with the aid of these distributions.

By putting $n = 1$ in the above formula we find that the expected time to extinction from the state 1 can be written as follows:

$$\mathbf{E}\tau_1 = \frac{1}{\mu_1} \sum_{j=1}^{N} \pi_j = \frac{1}{\mu_1 p_1^{(0)}}. \tag{2.24}$$

The expected time to extinction from state n can hence be written

$$\mathbf{E}\tau_n = \mathbf{E}\tau_1 \sum_{k=1}^{n} \frac{1 - \sum_{j=1}^{k-1} p_j^{(0)}}{\rho_k}. \tag{2.25}$$

Both Nisbet and Gurney (1982) and Renshaw (1991) describe the exact analytic expression that they give for $\mathbf{E}\tau_n$ as cumbersome and claim that it does not allow an intuitive understanding. Our different notation and our interpretation of ρ_n and π_n in terms of the stationary distributions $p^{(1)}$ and $p^{(0)}$ improves this situation. Additional improvement is reached for particular models where the functional dependencies of λ_n and μ_n on n are known. Insight into the functional dependencies of ρ_n and π_n on n can then be reached by derivation of asymptotic approximations.

It is useful to note that our expressions for expected times to extinction are dimensionally correct. Each expectation is proportional to $1/\mu_1$, the rate μ_1 has the dimension inverse time, and $1/\mu_1$ is a natural time constant for the process.

2.5. Diffusion approximation. The powerful method of approximating the discrete-state process with a continuous-state diffusion process can be used to derive an approximation of the quasi-stationary distribution. Such an approximation is derived by Nisbet and Gurney (1982). They show that the quasi-stationary distribution is approximated by a normal distribution if N is sufficiently large. We denote the mean and the variance of the approximating distribution by $\bar{Y}$ and σ_D^2, respectively. Both of them can be determined from the transition rates λ_Y and μ_Y. Indeed, the mean is equal to the positive stationary solution of the corresponding deterministic model. This model leads to a differential equation for the state variable $Y(t)$. This equation takes the form

$$Y' = \lambda_Y - \mu_Y. \tag{2.26}$$

Thus $\bar{Y}$ is found as a solution of the equation $\lambda_Y = \mu_Y$. The variance σ_D^2 of the same distribution is found by evaluating the functions λ_Y and μ_Y, and their derivatives with respect to Y, at the particular value $Y = \bar{Y}$. The expression for the variance can be written

$$\sigma_D^2 = \frac{1}{2}\frac{\lambda_{\bar{Y}} + \mu_{\bar{Y}}}{\mu'_{\bar{Y}} - \lambda'_{\bar{Y}}}. \tag{2.27}$$

One condition for the validity of this approximation is that the model shows density dependence, as described by Kurtz (1970), or the more general concept of asymptotic density dependence as introduced by Pollett (1990).

3. The SIS model. The SIS model that we consider in this section is concerned with an infection with no immunity. Recovered individuals are immediately susceptible to reinfection. No demographic forces are assumed; all individuals in the population are assumed to live forever. The model is therefore clearly unrealistic, especially since we are concerned with its behaviour over long time intervals. However, the model is important from a methodological standpoint, since it allows a mathematically satisfactory analysis. In this way, it points the way to follow in the analysis of the more complicated endemic SIR model of the next section. In particular, our analysis brings out qualitative properties that can be expected to have counterparts in more realistic settings.

Mathematically, we are concerned with analysis of the stochastic version of the model. It can be formulated as a univariate birth-death process on a finite state space, and with the origin as an absorbing state. It is thus a special case of the birth-death process considered in the previous section. We confine ourselves to a discussion of the results and to an indication of the methods that are used to derive them. The results are not new; most of them are contained in Nåsell (1996) and Nåsell (1999a). The derivations are based on the results of the preceding section. They are similar to the derivations used in the study of the Verhulst model in Nåsell (2000). The SIS model is a special case of the Verhulst logistic model.

The model is formulated in Subsection 3.1. Its deterministic version is briefly analysed in Subsection 3.2. Its threshold at $R_0 = 1$ partitions the one-dimensional parameter space into the two intervals $R_0 > 1$ and $0 < R_0 < 1$.

The parameter space for the stochastic model is two-dimensional, containing both R_0 and the population size N. We identify three regions of this parameter space in which both the quasi-stationary distribution and the time to extinction show qualitatively different behaviours. The new one, compared to the deterministic case, is a transition region near $R_0 = 1$. The remaining two are described by saying that R_0 is distinctly larger than 1 and distinctly smaller than 1, respectively.

The analysis of the stochastic version of the model proceeds by applying the results of the previous section for a finite-state birth-death process with an absorbing state at the origin. We derive asymptotic approximations wherever possible. This applies also for the stationary distributions of the two auxiliary processes, even though explicit expressions are available for them. Approximations of the quasi-stationary distribution and of the time to extinction are given in Subsections 3.3 and 3.4 for the two cases when R_0 is distinctly larger than 1 and distinctly smaller than 1, respectively. The rescaling of R_0 needed to identify the transition region is discussed in Subsection 3.5, and approximations of the quasi-stationary distribution and of the time to extinction in the transition region are given in Subsection 3.6. The transition region is mathematically the most difficult one to treat. The approximations given for this region in Nåsell (1996) are rather crude. Considerable improvement of these crude results are contained in Nåsell (1999a), and also in Subsection 3.6 below. Some comments on the persistence threshold for the SIS model are made in Subsection 3.7, while Subsection 3.8 deals with the diffusion approximation.

3.1. Formulation of the stochastic SIS model. We formulate a stochastic SIS model in the form of a finite-state birth-death process with an absorbing state at the origin. The main step is to define the transition rates λ_n and μ_n as functions of n. We consider a constant population with N individuals, and use $S(t)$ and $I(t)$ to denote the number of susceptible and infected individuals at time t, respectively. The infection rate, which is the rate of transition from the state (S, I) to the state $(S-1, I+1)$, is equal to $\beta SI/N$, where β is the contact rate. Furthermore, the recovery rate, which is the rate of transition from the state (S, I) to the state $(S+1, I-1)$, equals γI, where γ is the rate of recovery per infected individual. Since $S(t) = N - I(t)$ we find that the number of infected individuals $I(t)$ is described by a birth-death process with state space $\{0, 1, 2, \ldots, N\}$, and with transition rates

$$\lambda_n = \beta \left(1 - \frac{n}{N}\right) n, \quad \text{and} \quad \mu_n = \gamma n. \tag{3.1}$$

Our expressions for λ_n and μ_n define implicitly the three parameters N, β, and γ. Among these, the maximum population size N is a large positive integer, and the rates β and γ are strictly positive real numbers.

3.2. The deterministic model and reparametrization. It is always useful to formulate and analyze the deterministic counterpart of any stochastic model. One advantage with this is that the deterministic formulation leads in a simple and natural way to a reparametrization that is important also for the stochastic version of the model. Let $Y(t)$ denote the number of infected individuals at time t in the deterministic model. It follows then that Y satisfies the following differential equation:

$$Y' = \lambda_Y - \mu_Y = \beta \left(1 - \frac{Y}{N}\right) Y - \gamma Y. \tag{3.2}$$

This nonlinear differential equation has a bifurcation behaviour when $\beta = \gamma$. The ratio β/γ is therefore important. We denote it by

$$R_0 = \frac{\beta}{\gamma} \tag{3.3}$$

and refer to it as the basic reproduction ratio.

The differential equation for Y can then be rewritten in the form

$$Y' = \gamma \left(R_0 - 1 - R_0 \frac{Y}{N} \right) Y. \tag{3.4}$$

For $R_0 = 1$ this equation can be written

$$Y' = -\frac{\gamma Y^2}{N}, \quad R_0 = 1, \tag{3.5}$$

while it takes the form of the logistic equation

$$Y' = \gamma(R_0 - 1) \left(1 - \frac{Y}{\bar{Y}} \right) Y, \quad R_0 \neq 1, \tag{3.6}$$

where

$$\bar{Y} = \frac{R_0 - 1}{R_0} N, \tag{3.7}$$

for R_0 different from 1.

The importance of the parameter R_0 is shown by its role in describing a threshold result for the deterministic model. To describe it we study the asymptotic behaviour of the solution $Y(t)$ of the differential equation for Y as $t \to \infty$ with the initial value $Y(0) \geq 0$. It is straightforward to show that $Y(t)$ approaches the positive value $\bar{Y}$ as $t \to \infty$ if $Y(0) > 0$ and $R_0 > 1$, while $Y(t)$ approaches 0 as $t \to \infty$ for all nonnegative initial values if $R_0 \leq 1$. Thus, the infection is predicted to approach a constant and positive level for $R_0 > 1$ if $Y(0) > 0$, while it approaches 0 for large t if $R_0 \leq 1$.

In what follows we use the three parameters N, R_0, and γ for both the stochastic and the deterministic versions of the model. Parameters can be classified as either essential or innocent. We use the term innocent to refer to a parameter that can be eliminated from the model by a rescaling of either the state variable or the time, while all other parameters are essential. It is easy to see that the parameter R_0 is essential for both versions of the model, and that the parameter γ is innocent for both. The third parameter, N, is special, since it is essential for the stochastic model and innocent for the deterministic one. One explanation for this special behaviour of N is that the deterministic model can be derived from the stochastic one by introducing scaled (nondimensional) state variables and taking the limit as $N \to \infty$. In this way, N disappears from the scene as we go from the stochastic to the deterministic setting. The conclusion that there are two essential parameters for the stochastic model, but only one for the deterministic model, is of importance for the further analysis.

The threshold result for the deterministic model shows that the solution behaves in qualitatively different ways in two different regions of the one-dimensional parameter space where the only essential parameter R_0 takes its values. The boundary between the two regions is given by the threshold where $R_0 = 1$. We shall establish a certain counterpart to this result for the stochastic model. It takes the form of a partition of the two-dimensional parameter space where the two essential parameters R_0 and N for the stochastic model take their values. Three parameter regions are identified where asymptotic approximations of both the quasi-stationary distribution and of the time to extinction show qualitatively different behaviours. The transition region, where R_0 is close to 1, becomes empty in the limit as $N \to \infty$, while the remaining two coincide with the two parameter regions that describe the threshold behaviour for the deterministic model. This establishes a certain consistency between the qualitative results for the stochastic and the deterministic model.

It should be noted that neither of the two boundaries between the three regions in $N - R_0$-space is equal to the threshold for the stochastic model.

3.3. Approximations when R_0 is distinctly above the deterministic threshold value 1. Two approximations are given for the quasi-stationary distribution q when $R_0 > 1$ is fixed as $N \to \infty$. The first approximation is valid in the body of the distribution, and the second one in the left tail. The approximation in the body of the distribution takes the following form:

$$(3.8) \quad q_n \approx \frac{1}{\bar{\sigma}_1}\varphi(y_1(n)), \quad R_0 > 1, \quad R_0 \text{ fixed}, \quad y_1(n) = \mathrm{O}(1), \quad N \to \infty,$$

while the approximation in the left tail can be written

$$(3.9) \quad \begin{aligned} q_n &\approx \frac{R_0 - 1}{R_0}\sqrt{N}\frac{R_0^n - 1}{n}\varphi(\beta_1), \\ &\qquad R_0 > 1, \quad R_0 \text{ fixed}, \quad n = \mathrm{o}(\sqrt{N}), \quad N \to \infty. \end{aligned}$$

Here we use the following notation:

$$\bar{Y} = \frac{R_0 - 1}{R_0} N, \tag{3.10}$$

$$\bar{\sigma}_1 = \sqrt{\frac{N}{R_0}}, \tag{3.11}$$

$$y_1(n) = \frac{n - \bar{Y}}{\bar{\sigma}_1}, \tag{3.12}$$

$$\beta_1 = \operatorname{sign}(R_0 - 1)\sqrt{2N\left(\log R_0 - \frac{R_0 - 1}{R_0}\right)}. \tag{3.13}$$

Furthermore, $\varphi(x) = \exp(-x^2/2)/\sqrt{2\pi}$ denotes the normal density function.

The first of these expressions shows that the quasi-stationary distribution is approximately normal in its body, and that the mean of this normal distribution equals the stationary value $\bar{Y}$ of the deterministic model. The second of the expressions shows that this normality does not extend to the important left tail of the distribution.

In the parameter region that we are concerned with here we find that $\bar{Y}$ is of the order $O(N)$ and that $\bar{\sigma}_1$ is of the order $O(\sqrt{N})$. The coefficient of variation of the quasi-stationary distribution is therefore of the order $O(1/\sqrt{N})$. Hence it becomes negligibly small if N is sufficiently large. This supports the arguments May (1974) uses to justify the use of deterministic modelling for large populations. Our results have the additional power of allowing us to evaluate quantitatively what is meant by the term "N is sufficiently large". Indeed, this requirement is met exactly when R_0 is distinctly larger than 1. The boundary for this parameter region is discussed in Subsection 3.5.

A plot of the body of the quasi-stationary distribution is shown in Figure 1, together with its normal distribution approximation (3.8). The left tail of the quasi-stationary distribution is shown together with two approximations in Figure 2. Approximation 1 is given in (3.9) above, and Approximation 2 is that given via the diffusion approximation in Subsection 3.7. It is actually the left tail of the normal distribution whose body is illustrated in Figure 1. The second approximation is seen to be much less satisfactory than the first one.

We noted in Subsection 2.4 that the time to extinction τ_Q from quasi-stationarity for a birth-death process with finite state space and with absorbing state at the origin has an exponential distribution with expectation equal to $\mathbf{E}\tau_Q = 1/(\mu_1 q_1)$. Our approximation for this expectation takes the following form:

$$\mathbf{E}\tau_Q \approx \frac{1}{\gamma}\frac{R_0}{(R_0 - 1)^2}\frac{1}{\sqrt{N}\,\varphi(\beta_1)}, \qquad R_0 > 1, \quad R_0 \text{ fixed}, \quad N \to \infty. \tag{3.14}$$

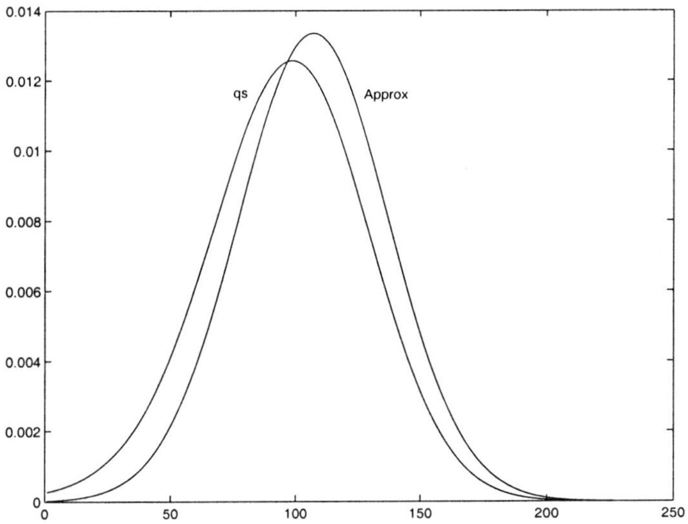

FIG. 1. *The quasi-stationary distribution of the SIS model is shown together with its normal approximation for* R_0 *distinctly larger than 1. The parameters are* $N = 1000$ *and* $R_0 = 1.12$. *The approximation improves as* N *is increased.*

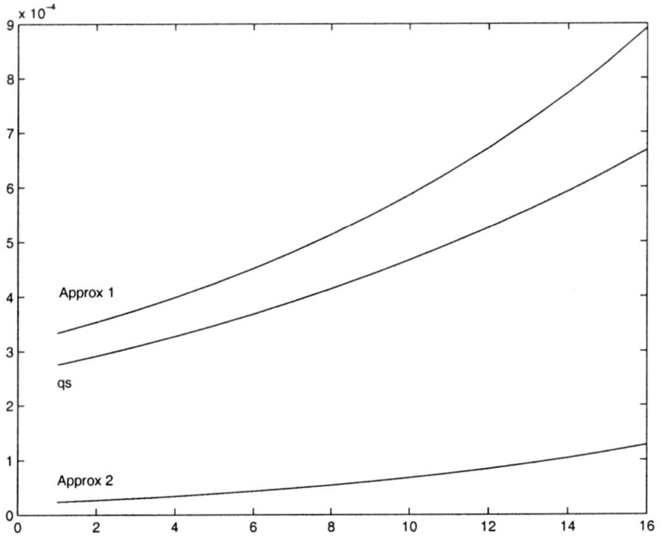

FIG. 2. *The left tail of the quasi-stationary distribution for the SIS model is shown together with two approximations for* R_0 *distinctly larger than 1. The parameters are* $N = 1000$ *and* $R_0 = 1.12$ *(same as in Figure 1). The first approximation is given by* (3.9), *while the second one is the normal distribution* (3.8) *derived via diffusion approximation.*

This result shows that $\mathbf{E}\tau_Q$ grows exponentially with N as $N \to \infty$ because of the factor $\varphi(\beta_1)$ in the denominator.

Our approximation of the expected time to extinction from the state n can be written

$$\mathbf{E}\tau_n \approx \frac{1}{\gamma} \frac{R_0}{(R_0 - 1)^2} \frac{1}{\sqrt{N}\,\varphi(\beta_1)} \left(1 - \frac{1}{R_0^n}\right), \tag{3.15}$$
$$R_0 > 1, \quad R_0 \text{ fixed}, \quad N \to \infty.$$

Note that this approximation of the expected time to extinction from the state n increases monotonically with n from the approximation of $\mathbf{E}\tau_1$ toward the approximation of $\mathbf{E}\tau_Q$. Note also that the approximation of the ratio $\mathbf{E}\tau_Q/\mathbf{E}\tau_1 \approx R_0/(R_0 - 1)$ for $R_0 > 1$ is bounded as $N \to \infty$.

It should be noted that the time to extinction from state n, τ_n, is a random variable whose location is poorly measured by its expectation $\mathbf{E}\tau_n$ for small values of n. The reason for this is that its distribution is bimodal. In fact, τ_n can be seen as a mixture of two random variables with widely different expectations. After starting in the state n, the process will either reach the absorbing state 0 very quickly, with probability $1/R_0^n$, or it will with the complementary probability reach the set of states where the quasi-stationary distribution describes its behaviour, and where the time to extinction is close to τ_Q.

3.4. Approximations when R_0 is distinctly below the deterministic threshold value 1. The time to extinction decreases drastically for large N if R_0 is lowered from a fixed value larger than 1 to a fixed value smaller than 1. We give approximations of the quasi-stationary distribution and of the time to extinction in the latter case.

The quasi-stationary distribution q is approximated by the geometric distribution

$$q_n \sim (1-R_0)R_0^{n-1}, \quad R_0<1, \quad R_0 \text{ fixed}, \quad n=\mathrm{o}(\sqrt{N}), \quad N\to\infty. \tag{3.16}$$

The time to extinction from quasi-stationarity has an exponential distribution whose expectation is asymptotically approximated as follows:

$$\mathbf{E}\tau_Q = \frac{1}{\mu_1 q_1} \sim \frac{1}{\gamma}\frac{1}{1 - R_0}, \quad R_0 < 1, \quad R_0 \text{ fixed}, \quad N \to \infty. \tag{3.17}$$

Similarly, the expected time to extinction from the state 1 is asymptotically approximated by

$$\mathbf{E}\tau_1 = \frac{1}{\mu_1 p_1^{(0)}} \sim \frac{1}{\gamma}\frac{\log(1/(1-R_0))}{R_0}, \quad R_0<1, \quad R_0 \text{ fixed}, \quad N\to\infty. \tag{3.18}$$

We note that these approximations of expectations of time to extinction are independent of N, while the results in Subsection 3.3 show that the corresponding approximations grow exponentially with N when R_0 is distinctly larger than 1.

3.5. Scaling of R_0 in the transition region. We recall that the quasi-stationary distribution q is for $R_0 > 1$ and N sufficiently large approximated in its body by a normal distribution with mean $\bar{Y}$ and standard deviation $\bar{\sigma}_1$. The random variable having q as its distribution takes only positive values. The normal approximation can therefore be expected to be acceptable only if the ratio of $\bar{Y}$ to $\bar{\sigma}_1$ is large. We find from (3.10) and (3.11) that this ratio equals

$$\frac{\bar{Y}}{\bar{\sigma}_1} = \frac{(R_0 - 1)\sqrt{N}}{\sqrt{R_0}}. \tag{3.19}$$

The normal distribution is a good approximation if the ratio approaches infinity as $N \to \infty$, as it does in the parameter region defined by $R_0 > 1$ being constant as $N \to \infty$, but a poor approximation if the ratio is small. Smallness in an asymptotic analysis context is interpreted as not approaching infinity as $N \to \infty$, or, equivalently, as the condition $\bar{Y}/\bar{\sigma}_1 = \mathrm{O}(1)$. The expression for the ratio $\bar{Y}/\bar{\sigma}_1$ above shows that this ratio remains bounded if the quantity ρ defined by

$$\rho = (R_0 - 1)\sqrt{N} \tag{3.20}$$

remains bounded. The introduction of ρ represents a rescaling of R_0 that makes R_0 a function of N. If ρ remains bounded as $N \to \infty$ then R_0 approaches 1. The parameter region described by the condition $\rho = \mathrm{O}(1)$ defines the transition region that will be studied in the following subsection. A natural condition that guarantees boundedness of ρ is that ρ is fixed. We note the rule of thumb that the transition region is for practical purposes described by the inequality $|\rho| < r$, where r equals 3 or 4. This choice of r is related to the fact that a normally distributed random variable takes values within 3 or 4 standard deviations of its mean with high probability.

3.6. Approximations in the transition region. The quasi-stationary distribution q is approximated as follows in the transition region:

$$q_n \approx \frac{1}{\varphi(\rho)(1+\rho H(\rho))} \frac{1}{n} \left(1 - \frac{1}{R_1^n(\rho, N)}\right) \varphi(y_3(n)), \qquad \rho \text{ fixed}, \quad n = \mathrm{O}(\sqrt{N}), \quad N \to \infty. \tag{3.21}$$

Here, we use the notation

$$y_3(n) = \frac{n - \bar{\mu}_3}{\bar{\sigma}_3}, \tag{3.22}$$

where

$$\bar{\mu}_3 = \rho\sqrt{N} \quad \text{and} \quad \bar{\sigma}_3 = \sqrt{N}. \tag{3.23}$$

Furthermore, the function H is defined implicitly by the relation

$$H(\rho) = \frac{1}{\rho + 1/H(\rho)} \int_{-1/H(\rho)}^{\rho} \frac{\Phi(y)}{\varphi(y)}\, dy, \tag{3.24}$$

while the function R_1 is defined by

$$R_1(\rho, N) = 1 + \frac{\rho + 1/H(\rho)}{\sqrt{N}}, \tag{3.25}$$

and Φ denotes the normal distribution.

The definition of the function H shows that $H(\rho)$ is equal to the average of the function H_1 defined by $H_1(y) = \Phi(y)/\varphi(y)$ over the interval $(-1/H(\rho), \rho)$, whose left end-point depends on $H(\rho)$. The dependence of H on ρ is illustrated in Figures 3 and 4.

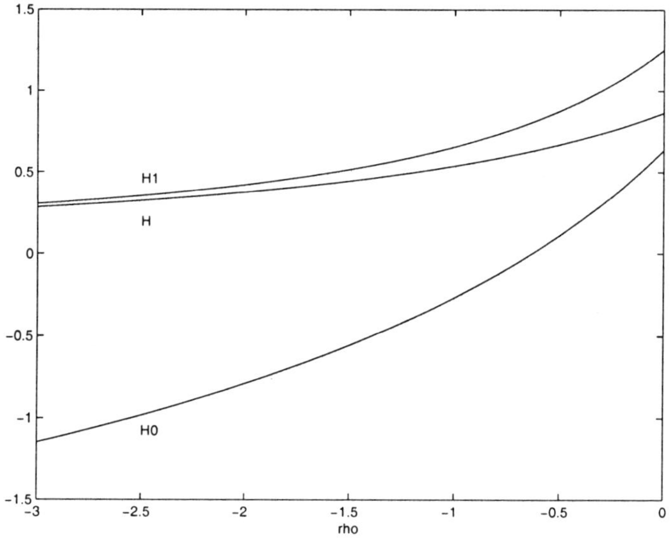

FIG. 3. *The functions H, H_0 and $H_1 = \Phi/\varphi$ are shown as functions of ρ for negative values of ρ. Note that the vertical scale is linear.*

Note that the approximation of q_n above covers the body of the distribution, where $y_3(n) = O(1)$. Note also that in this case the important n-value $n = 1$ belongs to the body of the distribution and is covered by the same approximation. The important probability q_1 is approximated by

$$q_1 \approx \frac{1}{\sqrt{N} H(\rho)}, \quad \rho \text{ fixed}, \quad N \to \infty. \tag{3.26}$$

The quasi-stationary distribution q is shown in the transition region in Figure 5 together with two approximations. As in Figure 2, the first

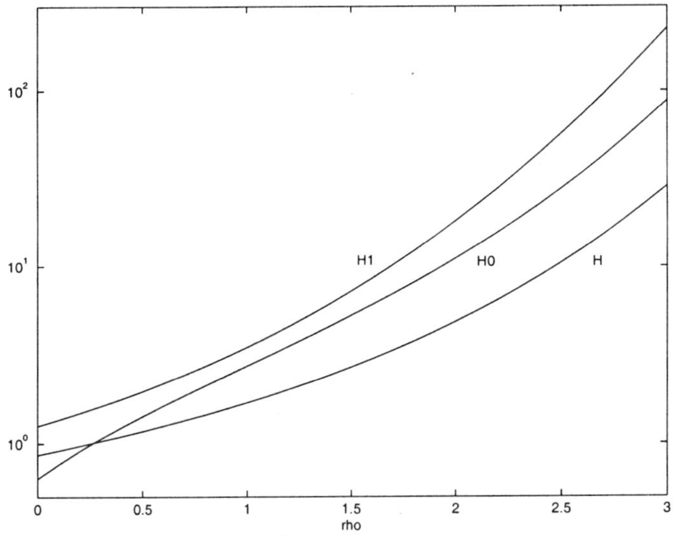

FIG. 4. *The functions H, H_0 and $H_1 = \Phi/\varphi$ are shown as functions of ρ for positive values of ρ. Note that the vertical scale is logarithmic.*

approximation is that derived by use of asymptotic approximation in the discrete-state process, while the second one is derived by diffusion approximation. The latter is formally equal to the normal distribution in (3.8), modified by truncation at 0.5. The first of the two approximations is clearly superior to the second one.

The expected time to extinction from quasi-stationarity is approximated by

$$\text{(3.27)} \qquad \mathbf{E}\tau_Q = \frac{1}{\mu_1 q_1} \approx \frac{\sqrt{N} H(\rho)}{\gamma}, \quad \rho \text{ fixed}, \quad N \to \infty.$$

Furthermore, the expected time to extinction from the state 1 is approximated by

$$\text{(3.28)} \qquad \mathbf{E}\tau_1 = \frac{1}{\mu_1 p_1^{(0)}} \approx \frac{1}{\gamma}\left(\frac{1}{2}\log N + H_0(\rho)\right), \quad \rho \text{ fixed}, \quad N \to \infty.$$

The function H_0 that appears here is defined in Nåsell (1999a). It is shown in Figures 3 and 4 as a function of ρ.

These two results show that the expected time to extinction from the state n, $\mathbf{E}\tau_n$, grows quite strongly with n in the transition region. The reason is that $\mathbf{E}\tau_Q$ is of the order $\sqrt{N}$, while $\mathbf{E}\tau_1$ is of the order $\log N$. Hence the relation $\mathbf{E}\tau_Q = \sum_{n=1}^{N} q_n \mathbf{E}\tau_n$ implies that there are n-values for which $\mathbf{E}\tau_n$ is at least of the order $\sqrt{N}$. This is turn implies that the

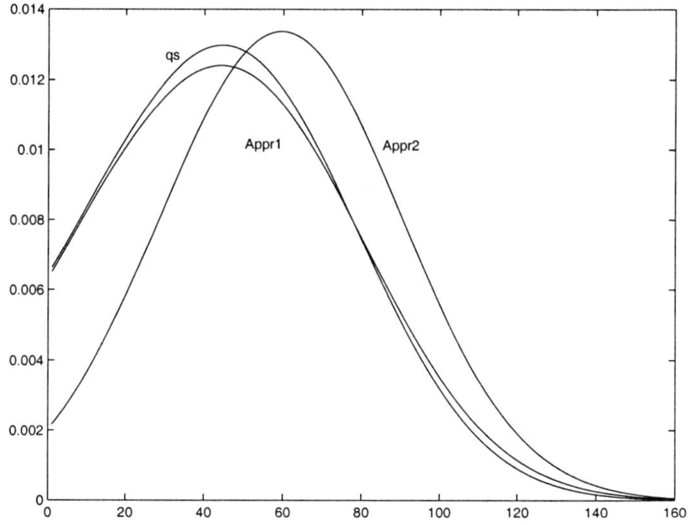

FIG. 5. *The quasi-stationary distribution for the SIS model is shown together with two approximations for R_0 in the transition region. The parameters are $N = 1000$ and $\rho = 2$. The first approximation is given by* (3.21), *while the second one is the normal distribution* (3.8) *derived via diffusion approximation, modified with truncation at 0.5.*

ratio $\mathbf{E}\tau_n/\mathbf{E}\tau_1$ is at least of the order $\sqrt{N}/\log N$ for these values of n. This behaviour is clearly different from the case when R_0 is distinctly larger than 1. For that case we showed above that the ratio $\mathbf{E}\tau_n/\mathbf{E}\tau_1 \approx R_0/(R_0 - 1)$ is bounded and independent of N.

The parameter region where R_0 is distinctly larger than 1 is the most important one for the SIS model. It is in this parameter region that the deterministic model gives an acceptable approximation of the stochastic model. The transition region for the SIS model is very narrow. As an example, we note that if $N = 10\,000$, then the transition region is confined to the interval $R_0 = 1 \pm r/\sqrt{N} = 1 \pm 0.03$ if we choose $r = 3$. The third parameter region, where R_0 is distinctly smaller than 1, turns out to be important for the persistence threshold.

3.7. The persistence threshold. The persistence threshold R_{0P} is defined by Nåsell (1995) as that value of R_0 for which the expected time to extinction $\mathbf{E}\tau_Q$ from quasi-stationarity equals an acceptable waiting time. As can be expected, the persistence threshold depends on the population size N. By specifying the waiting time to be equal to K/γ one finds that the function $R_{0P}(N)$ is determined implicitly by the relation $\mathbf{E}\tau_Q = K/\gamma$, where $\mathbf{E}\tau_Q$ depends on R_0 and N. A numerical evaluation in Nåsell (1996) indicates that the dependence of the persistence threshold on the population size takes the form $R_{0P} \approx 1 - 1/K + C/N$, where C is a constant independent of N. As argued by Nåsell (1999b), there is a close relation between the concept of persistence threshold and the concept of critical community size introduced by Bartlett. Indeed, the critical community size N_C is a function of R_0, and for each fixed value of K it is the inverse of the function R_{0P}. For reasonably large values of K and N we conclude that the persistence threshold for the stochastic version of the SIS model is quite close to the threshold $R_0 = 1$ for the deterministic model. As already noted, the persistence threshold appears in the parameter region where R_0 is distinctly smaller than 1.

3.8. Diffusion approximation. The diffusion approximation method of Subsection 2.5 does not give as sharp results as the method of asymptotic approximations that lies behind the results of the preceding subsections. It is straightforward to show that the diffusion approximation of the quasi-stationary distribution coincides with the normal distribution in (3.8). It is natural to modify this distribution by truncation at 0.5. This choice of truncation point accounts for the continuity correction in using the continuous normal distribution as an approximation of the discrete quasi-stationary distribution. A weakness with the diffusion method is that information is missing concerning the left tail of the quasi-stationary distribution when R_0 is distinctly larger than 1, and about the deviation from normality in the body of the distribution in the transition region.

4. The endemic SIR model. Infections that give permanent immunity to recovered individuals have intriguing properties. With measles as an outstanding example, it is known that recurrence of the infection can occur, and also that extinction of the infection is possible. Both of these phenomena can be explained by stochastic models. The basic idea goes back to Bartlett (1956-1960). The deterministic version of the endemic SIR model is treated in Subsection 4.1, and the stochastic version in Subsection 4.2. We show that the deterministic model is unable to capture the main qualitative features of the infection.

4.1. The deterministic model and reparametrization. We formulate the deterministic version of the endemic SIR model, and use the results to introduce a reparametrization that is important also for the stochastic version of the model.

The deterministic endemic SIR model leads to the following pair of differential equations:

$$S' = \mu N - \frac{\beta}{N} SI - \mu S, \tag{4.1}$$

$$I' = \frac{\beta}{N} SI - (\gamma + \mu) I. \tag{4.2}$$

Here, the state variables S and I stand for the number of susceptible and infective individuals, respectively. There are four parameters, namely the population size N, the death-rate per individual μ, the contact rate β, and the recovery rate per infected individual γ.

We reparametrize by introducing R_0 to denote the basic reproduction ratio, defined as the ratio of the contact rate β to the sum of the recovery rate γ and the death rate μ. Furthermore, we use α to denote the ratio of the sum of the recovery rate γ and the death rate μ to the death rate μ. Thus,

$$R_0 = \frac{\beta}{\gamma+\mu}, \tag{4.3}$$

$$\alpha = \frac{\gamma+\mu}{\mu}. \tag{4.4}$$

This means that α is the ratio of the average life length to the average duration of infection. Thus, α is large for the common childhood infections. After the reparametrization we still have four parameters, namely N, R_0, α, and μ. Among these, R_0 and α are essential parameters for both stochastic and deterministic versions of the model, μ is innocent for both, while N is innocent for the deterministic model and essential for the stochastic one.

The system of differential equations for S and I can be written as follows after the reparametrization:

$$S' = \mu\left(N - \frac{\alpha R_0}{N} SI - S\right), \tag{4.5}$$

$$I' = \mu\alpha\left(\frac{R_0}{N} S - 1\right) I. \tag{4.6}$$

This model has its threshold at $R_0 = 1$. If any amount of infection is introduced into the community, then it will ultimately disappear if $R_0 < 1$, while it will establish itself at an endemic level if $R_0 > 1$. The corresponding critical point $(\bar{S}, \bar{I})$ of the above system of differential equations is determined as

$$\bar{S} = \frac{N}{R_0}, \tag{4.7}$$

$$\bar{I} = \frac{R_0 - 1}{\alpha R_0} N. \tag{4.8}$$

The solution of this model shows damped oscillations for realistic values of α and $R_0 > 1$. The angular frequency of the damped oscillations can be approximated by the standard method of linearization of the right-hand side of the system of differential equations about the critical point $(\bar{S}, \bar{I})$. The Jacobian matrix J, evaluated at the critical point $(\bar{S}, \bar{I})$, equals

$$J = \mu \begin{pmatrix} -R_0 & -\alpha \\ R_0 - 1 & 0 \end{pmatrix}. \tag{4.9}$$

Damped oscillations are associated with complex conjugate eigenvalues of this matrix. The condition for this is that $R_0^2 < 4\alpha(R_0 - 1)$. This inequality is easily satisfied by the parameters for the common childhood infections. The eigenvalues can be written $a_0 \pm i\omega_0$, where

$$a_0 = -\mu\frac{R_0}{2}, \tag{4.10}$$

$$\omega_0 = \mu\sqrt{\alpha(R_0 - 1) - R_0^2/4}. \tag{4.11}$$

For large values of α we find that the frequency ω_0 can be approximated by

$$\omega_0 \sim \mu\sqrt{\alpha(R_0 - 1)}, \quad \alpha \to \infty. \tag{4.12}$$

The main properties of this model are concerned with recurrence, extinction, and threshold behaviour. Recurrence is studied in a rather similar model, an endemic SEIR model, in Nåsell (2001). Here, the letter E stands for the state of being "exposed", which accounts for the state of being infected but not yet infective. The deterministic versions of the endemic SIR and SEIR models differ in the sense that chaos is possible in the latter but not in the former, but there does not appear to be any qualitative differences between the stochastic versions of the two models.

Concerning recurrence, the deterministic endemic SIR model predicts damped oscillations, with quasi-frequency given by ω_0 above. The damping is not realistic and is essentially absent in the stochastic model. It is caused by the fact that the solution of the deterministic model is an approximation over all realizations of the stochastic model. This expectation is a poor approximation of any individual realization. The damping in the deterministic model is a measure of the stochastic variability in the lengths of the time intervals between the essentially undamped successive outbreaks in the stochastic model. The value of ω_0 derived from the deterministic model is the one result from the deterministic model that is useful. It appears to give a good approximation of the quasi-period of both the deterministic and the stochastic model.

Extinction is a purely stochastic phenomenon. It cannot be studied at all with the deterministic model. This phenomenon is of basic importance for the stochastic model, since the stochastic model persistence threshold is defined with the help of the time to extinction. It turns out to lead to very different threshold value for R_0 than the deterministic threshold value $R_0 = 1$, as evident from a comparison with the numerical evaluations of the persistence threshold in the next subsection.

4.2. The stochastic model. The stochastic process corresponding to the above deterministic model for the endemic SIR model takes the form of a bivariate process for the two state variables $S(t)$ and $I(t)$. The state space is the set of all nonnegative values (m, n) of S and I. Among these states, the states $(m, 0)$ where the infection is absent are absorbing, while the states (m, n) with $n \geq 1$ where the infection is present are transient.

The quasi-stationary distribution q_{mn} is supported on the set of transient states. It serves to describe the state of the process before absorption. The time to extinction τ_Q from the quasi-stationary distribution has an exponential distribution. Its expected value is equal to

$$\mathbf{E}\tau_Q = \frac{1}{\mu\alpha q_{\cdot 1}}. \tag{4.13}$$

Here, $q_{\cdot n}$ denotes the marginal distribution of the number of infected individuals in quasi-stationarity. It is therefore an important goal of the analysis to derive good approximations of this distribution, and more generally of the bivariate quasi-stationary distribution q_{mn}. It turns out to be appreciably more difficult to derive an approximation of this bivariate distribution, or of the corresponding marginal distributions, than it is to derive an approximation of the quasi-stationary distribution for the univariate birth-death process used for the SIS model in Section 3. The only method available today appears to be the method of diffusion approximation. An application of this method to the endemic SIR model in Nåsell (1999b) leads to the result that the marginal distribution of the number of infected individuals in quasi-stationarity is approximated by a normal distribution whose mean μ_I and standard deviation σ_I are as follows:

$$\mu_I = \frac{R_0 - 1}{\alpha R_0} N, \tag{4.14}$$

$$\sigma_I = \frac{\sqrt{R_0 - 1}}{R_0} \sqrt{N}. \tag{4.15}$$

These expressions are derived under the assumptions that both the population size N and the parameter α are large, and that $R_0 > 1$. This restriction of R_0 has the consequence that no conclusions can be drawn about the parameter regions where R_0 is distinctly smaller than 1, or where R_0 is in the transition region.

We determine the condition under which the normal distribution with the above mean and standard deviation gives an acceptable approximation of the marginal distribution $q_{\cdot n}$. This condition will at the same time identify the parameter region where R_0 is distinctly large. The condition is that the inverse of the approximation of the coefficient of variation μ_I/σ_I is reasonably large, say larger than 3. We reparametrize by introducing $\rho = \mu_I/\sigma_I$. This leads to the following expression:

$$R_0 = 1 + \frac{\alpha^2 \rho^2}{N}. \tag{4.16}$$

The region where R_0 is distinctly large is thus given by $R_0 > 1 + 9\alpha^2/N$. Thus we get $R_0 > 1 + 81 \cdot 10^6/N$ with $\alpha = 3000$. This value of α is appropriate for an infection that lasts about 1 week in a population whose average life length is 60 years. Thus we conclude that R_0 must exceed the value 82 (811) in a population of 1 million (100 000) in order to allow the conclusion that R_0 is distinctly large, and that lower R_0-values put us in the transition region. We conclude that the transition region is very wide indeed for infections with such large α-values. Since estimated values of R_0 for childhood infections are of the order of 10, we draw the important conclusion that the transition region is the most important one for such infections.

The marginal distribution of infected individuals $q_{\cdot n}$ is definitely non-normal in the transition region. Since the number of infected individuals I in quasi-stationarity takes only positive values, we modify the result from the diffusion approximation in an ad hoc fashion by truncation at 0.5. The result is that the marginal distribution of the number of infected individuals in quasi-stationarity is approximated by the following expression in the transition region:

$$q_{\cdot n} \approx \frac{1}{\sigma_I} \frac{\varphi((n - \mu_I)/\sigma_I)}{\Phi((\mu_I - 0.5)/\sigma_I)}. \tag{4.17}$$

This approximation holds also when R_0 is distinctly large, since the truncation point then lies in the left tail of the distribution, and the probability of lying to the left of the truncation point is asymptotically small.

By putting $n = 1$ in the above approximation for $q_{\cdot n}$ we get an approximation for $q_{\cdot 1}$ which can be used to approximate $\mathbf{E}\tau_Q$. The result is

$$\mathbf{E}\tau_Q \approx \frac{\rho}{\mu(1 + \rho^2/M)} \frac{\Phi(\rho)}{\varphi(\rho)}, \tag{4.18}$$

where $M = N/\alpha^2$. This approximation is not at all as good as the approximation of the corresponding quantity for the SIS model, but numerical evaluations by Nåsell (1999b) show that it gives the correct order of magnitude. Observe that although the stochastic model has three essential parameters, namely R_0, α, and N, the above approximation of $\mathbf{E}\tau_Q$ depends on only two essential parameters, namely ρ and M. The approximation can easily be evaluated numerically.

The persistence threshold R_{0P} for the endemic SIR model is determined as that value of R_0 for which the expected time to extinction from quasi-stationarity, $\mathbf{E}\tau_Q$, is equal to an acceptable waiting time. It is natural to express it as a function of N. We choose the acceptable waiting time equal to K/μ for some K. The persistence threshold $R_{0P}(N)$ can then be interpreted as that value of R_0 for which the expected time to extinction from quasi-stationarity is equal to K times the average life length of each individual.

The persistence threshold R_{0P} is shown as a function of the population size N for three different values of α in Figure 6 with $K = 1$. For all three α-values we plot the approximation based on the above approximation of

$\mathbf{E}\tau_Q$. For the two smaller α-values 250 and 500 we show also the results of Monte Carlo simulation. The simulation requires longer time for larger α-values, and would be very time-consuming for the value $\alpha=$ 3000. The simulation results for the two smaller α-values are the ones that are slightly larger for N=10 000. The figure shows that the deterministic threshold value $R_0 = 1$ is utterly unrealistic for the larger α-value unless N is very much larger than 100 000.

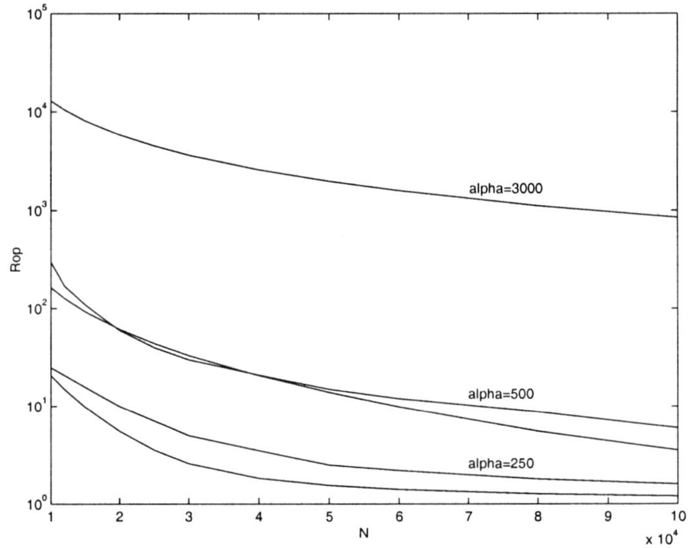

FIG. 6. *Approximations of the persistence threshold R_{0P} for the endemic SIR model are shown as a function of the population size N for three values of α. The approximations are based on the approximation* (4.18) *of the expected time to extinction $\mathbf{E}\tau_Q$. The approximations for the two lower values of α are compared with numerical evaluations based on Monte Carlo simulation.*

We noted above for the SIS model that the diffusion approximation results are considerably weaker than the results based on asymptotic approximation of the discrete state space model. In the case of the endemic SIR model all our approximation results are based on diffusion approximation. As can be expected, these results are rather weak. The SIS model results give us reason to expect that the normality of the body of the quasi-stationary distribution when R_0 is distinctly large does not extend to the important left tail. The diffusion approximation gives no information about this deviation from normality in the left tail. Furthermore, the SIS model results cause us to expect that the deviation from normality in the transition region is not as simple as the truncation that we have assumed above. These two weaknesses with the diffusion approximation indicate two important open problems to be solved for quasi-stationary distributions of bivariate or multivariate birth-death processes that are used as models of endemic infections.

REFERENCES

[1] N.T.J. Bailey, The Mathematical Theory of Infectious Diseases and Its Applications (1975), London: Griffin.

[2] M.S. Bartlett, *Deterministic and stochastic models for recurrent epidemics*, In Proc. 3rd Berkeley Symp. Math. Stat. and Prob., **4** (1956) 81–109, Berkeley: University of California Press.

[3] M.S. Bartlett, *Measles periodicity and community size (with discussion)*, J. Roy. Stat. Soc. A, **120** (1957), 48–70.

[4] M.S. Bartlett, *Stochastic Population Models in Ecology and Epidemiology* (1960a), London: Methuen.

[5] M.S. Bartlett, *Some stochastic models in ecology and epidemiology*, In Contributions to Probability and Statistics: Essays in Honor of Harold Hotelling (eds I. Olkin, S.G. Ghurye, W. Hoeffding, W.G. Madow and H.B. Mann) (1960b), 89–96, Stanford: Stanford University Press.

[6] M.S. Bartlett, *The critical community size for measles in the United States*, J. Roy. Stat. Soc. A, **123** (1960c), 37–44.

[7] J.N. Darroch and E. Seneta, *On quasi-stationary distributions in absorbing continuous-time finite Markov chains*, J. Appl. Prob., **4** (1967), 192–196.

[8] S. Karlin and H.M. Taylor, *A First Course in Stochastic Processes*, Academic Press, New York, 1975.

[9] R.J. Kryscio and C. Lefèvre, *On the extinction of the S-I-S stochastic logistic epidemic*, J. Appl. Prob., **27** (1989), 685–694.

[10] T.G. Kurtz, *Limit theorems for sequencies of jump Markov processes approximating ordinary differential processes*, J. Appl. Prob., **8** (1971), 344–356.

[11] R.M. May, *Stability and Complexity in Model Ecosystems*, Princeton University Press, Princeton, N.J. (1974).

[12] I. Nåsell, *The threshold concept in stochastic epidemic and endemic models*, In Epidemic Models: Their Structure and Relation to Data (ed. D. Mollison), Publications of the Newton Institute, Cambridge University Press, Cambridge, 1995.

[13] I. Nåsell, *The quasi-stationary distribution of the closed endemic SIS model*, Adv. Appl. Prob., **28** (1996), 895–932.

[14] I. Nåsell, *On the quasi-stationary distribution of the stochastic logistic epidemic*, Math. Biosci., **156** (1999a), 21–40.

[15] I. Nåsell, *On the time to extinction in recurrent epidemics*, J. Roy. Statist. Soc., Series B, **61**, Part 2 (1999b), 309–330.

[16] I. Nåsell, *Extinction and quasi-stationarity in the Verhulst logistic model* (2000) unpublished manuscript.

[17] I. Nåsell, *Measles outbreaks are not chaotic* (2001), this issue.

[18] R.M. Nisbet and W.S.C. Gurney, *Modelling Fluctuating Populations*, Wiley, New York, 1982.

[19] P.K. Pollett, *On a model for interference between searching insect parasites*, J. Austr. Math. Soc. Series B32 (1990), 133–150.

[20] E. Renshaw, *Modelling Biological Populations in Space and Time*, Cambridge University Press, Cambridge, 1991.

ON THE COMPUTATION OF $\mathcal{R}_0$ AND ITS ROLE ON GLOBAL STABILITY

CARLOS CASTILLO-CHAVEZ*, ZHILAN FENG†, AND WENZHANG HUANG‡

Abstract. In this paper we outline the second generation operator approach developed by Diekmann and collaborators for the computation of the basic reproductive number, $\mathcal{R}_0$. The use of this method is illustrated on epidemic models, mostly developed by the authors, that incorporate various degree of host and pathogen heterogeneity. Finally, conditions that clarify the connections between $\mathcal{R}_0$ and its relationship to the global asymptotic stability of the disease-free equilibrium are discussed.

Introduction. Threshold phenomena is prevalent in the study of scientific phenomena. The computation of nondimensional quantities that determine the nature of dynamic transitions, "tipping" or bifurcation points, have a long tradition in epidemiology. Sir Ronald Ross, who received the Nobel Prize for his work on malaria (1902), founded the field of mathematical epidemiology with his quest for establishing (within the epidemiology community) what must have appeared obvious to him, that is, that *it is not necessary to drive a vector (mosquito) population to extinction to eliminate malaria.* He made his point effectively only after he introduced a mathematical model for malaria in 1911. He used his model to show that bringing a mosquito population below a certain threshold was sufficient to eliminate malaria. This threshold naturally depended on biological factors such as the biting rate and vectorial capacity (ratio of the vector to host population). His mathematical work has been used extensively not only in the study malaria (MacDonald 1957) but also in the study of other diseases (see Anderson and May 1982; Busenberg and Cooke 1993).

The importance of contact processes (well recognized by Ross on his work on malaria) is at the center of the study of threshold phenomena (see Busenberg and Castillo-Chavez 1991; Castillo et al. 1994). In their recent book Diekmann and Heesterbeek (2000) present an extensive and systematic study of threshold phenomena. The following tutorial notes also used the next generation approach for the systematic computation of the basic reproductive number. The examples used come mostly from our own work. Connections between threshold phenomena and stability are also explored.

The basic reproductive number $\mathcal{R}_0$ is *typically* defined (see Diekmann and Heestterbeek, 2000) as: *the average number of secondary cases produced by a "typical" infected (assumed infectious) individual during his/her*

*Biometrics, Statistics and Theoretical and Applied Mechanics Departments, Cornell University, Ithaca, NY 14853, USA; Email: cc32@cornell.edu.

†Department of Mathematics, Purdue University, West Lafayette, IN 47907-1395, USA; Email: zfeng@math.purdue.edu.

‡Department of Mathematics, University of Alabama, Huntsville, AL 35899, USA; Email: huang@math.uah.edu.

entire life as infectious (infectious period) when introduced in a population of susceptibles. This nondimensional quantity cannot be computed explicitly in most cases because the mathematical description of what is a "typical" infectious individual is difficult to quantify in populations with high degree of heterogeneity.

Regardless of whether or not $\mathcal{R}_0$ can be computed explicitly, its role on the study of the stability of equilibria can still be determined. Most reasonable epidemic models support at least two type of equilibria: a disease-free equilibria and a positive (endemic) equilibria. "Typically" one can show that the disease-free equilibrium is locally asymptotically stable (l.a.s.) if $\mathcal{R}_0 < 1$ and unstable whenever $\mathcal{R}_0 > 1$. Furthermore, in many examples, it has been shown that $\mathcal{R}_0 > 1$ implies the existence of a unique (l.a.s.) endemic equilibrium. Many models found in the literature have been used to show that when $\mathcal{R}_0$ crosses the threshold, $\mathcal{R}_0 = 1$, a transcritical bifurcation takes place. That is, asymptotic local stability is transferred from the infectious-free state to the new (emerging) endemic (positive) equilibria. In some situations, it can be shown that the transfer of asymptotic stability is indepenedent of initial conditions, that is, it is global (Feng et al., 2000; Zhou et al. 2001; Song et al. 2001).

In this article, we revisit several models of infectious diseases involving a discrete and continuous stratification of host and pathogen. We compute $\mathcal{R}_0$ for each model using the approach developed by Diekmann and his collaborators. Finally, we look at the role of $\mathcal{R}_0$ on the global stability of the disease-free equilibrium.

This paper is organized as follows: Section 1 outlines the next generation operator approach for the computation of $\mathcal{R}_0$. Section 2 gives a series of examples with various degrees of host and pathogen heterogeneity. The models used come from the study of communicable, vector and sexually-transmitted diseases. Examples are drawn from our published work, work in progress, or the work of others. These models have been used in the study of questions associated with the dynamics of Tuberculosis, HIV, Dengue, Gonorrhea and childhood diseases. Our examples include group, gender, host-structure, and pathogen heterogeneity. Section 3 states and proves a theorem on the relationship between local and global asymptotic stability for the infection free state. The tutorial ends with an example where the conditions of the last theorem are not met: a model that is capable of supporting multiple endemic equilibria when $\mathcal{R}_0 < 1$.

1. The next generation operator approach. $\mathcal{R}_0$ is often found through the study and computation of the eigenvalues of the Jacobian at the disease- or infectious-free equilibrium. Diekmann *et al. 1990* follow a different approach: *the next generation operator approach.* They define $\mathcal{R}_0$ as the spectral radius of the "next generation operator". The details of this approach are outlined in the rest of this section. First, we consider the case where heterogeneity is discrete, that is, the case where heterogeneity is defined using groups defined by fixed characteristics, that is, for epidemiological models that can be written in the form:

$$\begin{aligned} \frac{dX}{dt} &= f(X,Y,Z), \\ \frac{dY}{dt} &= g(X,Y,Z), \\ \frac{dZ}{dt} &= h(X,Y,Z), \end{aligned} \tag{1.1}$$

where $X \in \mathbb{R}^r$, $Y \in \mathbb{R}^s$, $Z \in \mathbb{R}^n$, $r, s, n \geq 0$, and $h(X,0,0) = 0$. The components of X denote the number of susceptibles, recovered, and other classes of non-infected individuals. The components of Y represent the number of infected individuals who do not transmit the disease (various latent or non-infectious stages). The components of Z represent the number of infected individuals capable of transmitting the disease (e.g., infectious and non-quarentined individuals).

Let $\mathbf{U}_0 = (X^*, 0, 0) \in \mathbb{R}^{r+s+n}$ denote the disease-free equilibrium, that is,

$$f(X^*,0,0) = g(X^*,0,0) = h(X^*,0,0) = 0.$$

Assume that the equation $g(X^*, Y, Z) = 0$ implicitly determines a function $Y = \widetilde{g}(X^*, Z)$. Let $A = D_Z h(X^*, \widetilde{g}(X^*, 0), 0)$ and further assume that A can be written in the form $A = M - D$, with $M \geq 0$ (that is, $m_{ij} \geq 0$) and $D > 0$, a diagonal matrix.

The spectral bound of matrix B is denoted by $m(B) = \sup\{\Re\lambda : \lambda \in \sigma(B)\}$, where $\Re\lambda$ means the real part of λ, while $\rho(B) = \lim_{n\to\infty} \|B^n\|^{\frac{1}{n}}$ denotes the spectral radius of B. The proof of the following theorem involving matrix A is found in Diekmann et al., (1990):
Either

$$m(A) < 0 \Longleftrightarrow \rho(MD^{-1}) < 1$$

or

$$m(A) > 0 \Longleftrightarrow \rho(MD^{-1}) > 1.$$

The *basic reproductive number* is defined as the spectral radius (dominant eigenvalue) of the matrix MD^{-1}, that is,

$$\mathcal{R}_0 = \rho(MD^{-1}). \tag{1.2}$$

Examples using (1.1) to compute $\mathcal{R}_0$ are provided in Section 2.

An analogous formula for $\mathcal{R}_0$ when a heterogenous population is stratified by continuous characteristics (see Diekmann et al. 1990) can be similarly computed. In fact, let $S(\xi)$ denote the population density function that describes the (steady) demographic state in the absence of disease where $\xi \in \Omega_h$ (h stands for heterogeneity). Furthermore, let $A(\tau,\xi,\eta)$ denote the current (expected) infectivity of an individual who was infected τ units of time ago while at stage η, that is, $A(\tau,\xi,\eta)$ denotes the average infectivity that can be exercised on an uninfected individual at stage ξ (provided the uninfected population finds itself at the steady demographic state $S(\xi)$). The function $A(\tau,\xi,\eta)$ combines information on the probability (per unit of time) that contacts between certain stages take place and the probability that, given a contact, the disease agent is actually transmitted.

Under the special assumption of proportionate-mixing (see Busenberg and Castillo-Chavez, 1991), $A(\tau,\xi,\eta)$ can be written in the form $A(\tau,\xi,\eta) = f(\xi)g(\tau,\eta)$. $\mathcal{R}_0$, the spectral radius of the "next generation operator", can be computed under proportionate mixing. In fact, it is given by the following formula:

$$R_0 = \int_{\Omega}\int_0^{\infty} g(\tau,\eta)S(\eta)f(\eta)d\tau d\eta. \tag{1.3}$$

The key element, in the computation of $\mathcal{R}_0$ in formula (1.3), is the infectivity function $A(\tau,\xi,\eta)$.

2. Examples. Several models taken from prior work by others or us are used to illustrate the computation of $\mathcal{R}_0$ via Formulas (1.2) and (1.3).

Example 1(a). McKendrick, like Sir Ronald Ross, was a physician commissioned by the English Army to India. McKendrick became involved in the study of epidemic diseases using mathematical models through the direct encouragement of Ross. His simple epidemic model was published in a joint paper with Kermack (Kermack and McKendrick, 1927). It involved the study of the transmission dynamics of a communicable disease that provide permanent immunity after recovery. Their model was used to study single epizootic outbreaks. Their mathematical work led to the first widely recognized threshold theorem in epidemiology (the threshold theorem of Ross came from the study of vector-transmitted diseases sisxteen years earlier). Kermack and Mckendrick's model is an SIR (Susceptible-Infected-Recovered) model without vital (births and deaths) dynamics. The model equations are:

$$\begin{aligned}
\frac{dS}{dt} &= -\beta S\frac{I}{N},\\
\frac{dI}{dt} &= \beta S\frac{I}{N} - \gamma I,\\
\frac{dR}{dt} &= \gamma I,\\
N &= S + I + R.
\end{aligned}$$

S denotes the number of susceptibles, I is the number of infected (assumed infectious), and R is the number of recovered individuals (assumed to be permanently immune). β is the average number of susceptibles infected by one infectious individual per unit of time while γ is the per capita recovery rate (at which an infected individual leaves the I class). Note that $X = (S, R)$, $Z = I$, $\mathbf{U}_0 = (S^*, R^*, I^*) = (N, 0, 0)$, $A = \beta - \gamma$ (there are no latent classes, that is, $s = 0$). Hence, $M = \beta, \quad D = \gamma$ and

$$\mathcal{R}_0 = MD^{-1} = \frac{\beta}{\gamma}.$$

The threshold theorem of Kermack and McKendrick says that if $\mathcal{R}_0 > 1$ then an outbreak will take place while if $\mathcal{R}_0 < 1$ there will be no outbreaks.

Example 1(b). The addition of vital dynamics to the SIR model of Kermack and McKendrick, leads to the follwing system:

$$\begin{aligned}
\frac{dS}{dt} &= \Lambda - \beta S\frac{I}{N} - \mu S,\\
\frac{dI}{dt} &= \beta S\frac{I}{N} - (\mu + \gamma)I,\\
\frac{dR}{dt} &= \gamma I - \mu R,\\
N &= S + I + R.
\end{aligned}$$

Λ is the birth rate and μ is the per capita natural death rate both assumed constant. Note that in this case $X = (S, R)$, $Z = I$, $\mathbf{U}_0 = (\frac{\Lambda}{\mu}, 0, 0)$, and $A = \beta - (\mu + \gamma)$. Hence, $M = \beta, \quad D = \mu + \gamma$ and

$$R_0 = MD^{-1} = \frac{\beta}{\mu + \gamma}.$$

The threshold theorem of Kermack and McKendrick in this setting says that if $\mathcal{R}_0 > 1$ then an outbreak will take place and the disease will persist while if $\mathcal{R}_0 < 1$ the disease will die out.

Remark. Note that β is the average number of susceptibles infected by one infectious individual per unit of time and $\frac{1}{\mu+\gamma}$ is the (death-adjusted) mean length of infectious period (see Thieme's paper in this volume for extensions and clarifications of this interpretation). Therefore $\mathcal{R}_0 = \frac{\beta}{\mu+\gamma}$ gives the number of secondary infectious cases produced by an infectious individual who has been introduced into a population of susceptibles during the individual's period of infectiousness. The expressions for $\mathcal{R}_0$ computed here, agree with those found by Brauer in his tutorial epidemiological notes included in this volume.

Example 2. Many communicable diseases can be modeled using models that include compartments for the suceptible, exposed, infected and recovered epidemiological classes. An $SEIR$ model for a homogeneously mixing population is given by the following set of equations:

$$\begin{aligned}\frac{dS}{dt} &= \Lambda - \beta S\frac{I}{N} - \mu S,\\ \frac{dE}{dt} &= \beta S\frac{I}{N} - (\mu+k)E,\\ \frac{dI}{dt} &= kE - (\gamma+\mu)I,\\ \frac{dR}{dt} &= \gamma I - \mu R,\end{aligned}$$

where E is the number of latent individuals and k is the rate at which a latent individual becomes infectious. Letting $X = (S, R)$, $Y = E$, $Z = I$, $\mathbf{U}_0 = (\frac{\Lambda}{\mu}, 0, 0, 0)$ and $\widetilde{g}(X^*, Z) = \frac{\beta I}{\mu+k}$ gives $M = \frac{k\beta}{\mu+k}$ and $D = \gamma + \mu$. Hence

$$\mathcal{R}_0 = MD^{-1} = \frac{k\beta}{(\mu+k)(\mu+\gamma)}.$$

Example 3. The following model (see Castillo-Chavez and Feng, 1997) describes the disease transmission dynamics of both drug-sensitive and drug-resistant strains of TB. The host population is divided into the following epidemiological subgroups: Susceptibles (S); Latent with strain i ($i = 1$ represents the sensitive strain and $i = 2$ the resistant strain) of TB (E_i); Infectious with strain i (I_i); and (effectively) Treated (T) individuals. The two-strain model for the dynamics of TB is given by:

$$\begin{aligned}\frac{dS}{dt} &= \Lambda - \beta_1 S\frac{I_1}{N} - \beta_2 S\frac{I_2}{N} - \mu S,\\ \frac{dE_1}{dt} &= \beta_1 S\frac{I_1}{N} - (\mu+k_1)E_1 - rE_1 + p\tilde{r}I_1 + \sigma\beta_1 T\frac{I_1}{N} - \beta_2 E_1\frac{I_2}{N},\\ \frac{dI_1}{dt} &= k_1E_1 - (\mu+d_1+\tilde{r})I_1,\\ \frac{dT}{dt} &= rE_1 + (1-p-q)\tilde{r}I_1 - \sigma\beta_1 T\frac{I_1}{N} - \beta_2 T\frac{I_2}{N} - \mu T,\\ \frac{dE_2}{dt} &= q\tilde{r}I_1 - (\mu+k_2)E_2 + \beta_2(S+E_1+T)\frac{I_2}{N},\\ \frac{dI_2}{dt} &= k_2E_2 - (\mu+d_2)I_2,\\ N &= S + E_1 + I_1 + T + E_2 + I_2,\end{aligned}$$

where d_i ($i = 1, 2$) denotes the per capita disease induced death rate due to strain i; r, $\tilde{r}$ denote the per capita treatment rates; $p+q$ the proportion of treated individuals who did not complete the treatment; $\sigma \leq 1$ the reduction in infection rate due to the immunity obtained from treatment. The proportion p modifies the rate of departure from the latent class while $q\tilde{r}I_1$ denotes the rate at which individuals acquire resistant-TB as a result of not completing treatment for active TB.

Letting $X = (S,T)$, $Y = (E_1, E_2)$, $Z = (I_1, I_2)$, $\mathbf{U}_0 = (\Lambda/\mu, 0, 0, 0)$ and $\widetilde{g}(X^*, Z) = (\widetilde{g}_1(X^*, Z), \widetilde{g}_2(X^*, Z))$ with

$$\begin{aligned}\widetilde{g}_1(X^*, Z) &= \frac{(\beta_1 + p\tilde{r})I_1}{\mu\beta_2 I_2/\Lambda + \mu + k_1 + r},\\ \widetilde{g}_2(X^*, Z) &= \frac{q\tilde{r}I_1 + \beta_2 I_2}{\mu + k_2} + O(2),\end{aligned}$$

where $O(2)$ denotes terms of order two and higher in I_i gives

$$M = \begin{pmatrix} \frac{k_1(\beta_1+p\tilde{r})}{\mu+k_1+r} & 0 \\ c_1 & \frac{k_2\beta_2}{\mu+k_2} \end{pmatrix} \quad \textit{and} \quad D = \begin{pmatrix} -(\mu + d_1 + \tilde{r}) & 0 \\ c_2 & -(\mu + d_2) \end{pmatrix}.$$

The two eigenvalues λ_1 and λ_2 of MD^{-1} are:

$$\lambda_1 = \frac{k_1(\beta_1 + p\tilde{r})}{(\mu + k_1 + r)(\mu + d_1 + \tilde{r})} \quad \textit{and} \quad \lambda_2 = \frac{k_2\beta_2}{(\mu + k_2)(\mu + d_2)}.$$

It follows that $\mathcal{R}_0 = \max\{\lambda_1, \lambda_2\}$.

Example 4. In this example, we introduce a minimal degree of host heterogeneity by dividing the host population in two groups. Such division could be the result of differences in socio economic status or other characteristics that are likely to remain fixed in the time scale of the epidemic process. To illustrate the computation of $\mathcal{R}_0$ in this case, we use the following SIR model with two groups:

$$\begin{aligned}\frac{dS_i}{dt} &= \Lambda_i - S_i\big(\beta_{ii}\frac{I_i}{N} + \beta_{ij}\frac{I_j}{N}\big) - \mu S_i,\\ \frac{dI_i}{dt} &= S_i\big(\beta_{ii}\tfrac{I_i}{N} + \beta_{ij}\tfrac{I_j}{N}\big) - \mu I_i - k_i I_i,\\ \frac{dR_i}{dt} &= k_i I_i - \mu R_i, \qquad i = 1, 2.\end{aligned}$$

where the subscript i identifies each group (i = 1 or i = 2). In this case, $Z = (I_1, I_2)$,

$$M = \begin{pmatrix} \beta_{11}\frac{\Lambda_1}{\Lambda_1+\Lambda_2} & \beta_{12}\frac{\Lambda_1}{\Lambda_1+\Lambda_2} \\ \beta_{21}\frac{\Lambda_2}{\Lambda_1+\Lambda_2} & \beta_{22}\frac{\Lambda_2}{\Lambda_1+\Lambda_2} \end{pmatrix}, \qquad D = \begin{pmatrix} \mu + k_1 & 0 \\ 0 & \mu + k_2 \end{pmatrix},$$

and

$$MD^{-1} = \begin{pmatrix} \frac{\beta_{11}}{\mu+k_1}\frac{\Lambda_1}{\Lambda_1+\Lambda_2} & \frac{\beta_{12}}{\mu+k_2}\frac{\Lambda_1}{\Lambda_1+\Lambda_2} \\ \frac{\beta_{21}}{\mu+k_1}\frac{\Lambda_2}{\Lambda_1+\Lambda_2} & \frac{\beta_{22}}{\mu+k_2}\frac{\Lambda_2}{\Lambda_1+\Lambda_2} \end{pmatrix} =: (\alpha_{ij}).$$

Since the dominant eigenvalue of MD^{-1} is

$$\lambda = \frac{1}{2}\left(\alpha_{11} + \alpha_{22} + \sqrt{(\alpha_{11} - \alpha_{22})^2 + 4\alpha_{12}\alpha_{21}}\right)$$

then $\mathcal{R}_0 = \lambda$.

Example 5. The following model was developed to study the dynamics of multiple strains of a sexually transmitted diseases (like gonorrhea) on a population that included a high degree of host heterogeneity (see Castillo-Chavez, Huang & Li 1997). The model included populations of males and females as well as a highly active female population (core group) since one of our main goals was to study the impact of female prostitution on disease persistence. The model equations are:

$$\begin{aligned}
\frac{dS^m}{dt} &= \Lambda^m - B^m - \mu S^m + \sum_{i=1}^{2} \gamma_i^m I_i^m, \\
\frac{dI_i^m}{dt} &= B_i^m - (\mu + \gamma_i^m) I_i^m, \\
\frac{dS^f}{dt} &= \Lambda^f - B^f - \mu S^f + \sum_{i=1}^{2} \gamma_i^f I_i^f, \\
\frac{dI_i^f}{dt} &= B_i^f - (\mu + \gamma_i^m) I_i^f, \\
\frac{dS^c}{dt} &= \Lambda^c - B^c - \mu^c S^c + \sum_{i=1}^{2} \gamma_i^c I_i^c, \\
\frac{dI_i^c}{dt} &= B_i^c - (\mu + \gamma_i^c) I_i^c, \qquad i = 1, 2,
\end{aligned} \tag{2.1}$$

where

$$\begin{aligned}
B_i^m &= r^m(T^m, T^f, T^c) S^m \left(\beta_i^f \frac{I_i^f}{T^f} + \beta_i^c \frac{I_i^c}{T^c}\right), \\
B_i^f &= r^f(T^m, T^f, T^c) S^f \beta_i^m \frac{I_i^m}{T^m}, \\
B_i^c &= r^c(T^m, T^f, T^c) S^c \beta_i^m \frac{I_i^m}{T^m}, \quad i = 1, 2, \\
B^m &= \sum_{i=1}^{2} B_i^m, \;\; B^f = \sum_{i=1}^{2} B_i^f, \;\; B^c = \sum_{i=1}^{2} B_i^c,
\end{aligned}$$

with the natural constraint

$$r^m(T^m, T^f, T^c) T^m = r^f(T^m, T^f, T^c) T^f + r^c(T^m, T^f, T^c) T^c.$$

Here Λ^k ($k = m$ (male), f (female), c (core group, females)) denote the input flow or (constant) recruitment into the corresponding sexually active sub-population; $1/\mu^c$ is the average sexual life span for group c while $1/\mu$ is the average sexual life span for individuals not in group c; γ_i^k are the per capita rates of recovery; $T^k = S^k + \sum_j I_j^k$ are the total number of males or females (group f and group c), respectively; r^k, as functions of T^m, T^f, T^c, denote the numbers of partners per individual per unit of time; and, β_i^k denote the rates of infection. The constraint simply states that the total number of partners per unit of time for each gender (this is a purely heterosexual model) must match.

The dynamics of the above system are equivalent to those of limiting system (see Castillo-Chavez and Huang and Li, 1997) below:

$$
\begin{aligned}
\frac{dI_i^m}{dt} &= -(\mu+\gamma_i^m)I_i^m + b^m\Big(\frac{\Lambda^m}{\mu} - \sum_j I_j^m\Big)\Big(\beta_i^f \frac{\mu}{\Lambda^f} I_i^f + \beta_i^c \frac{\mu^c}{\Lambda^c} I_i^c\Big), \\
\frac{dI_i^f}{dt} &= -(\mu+\gamma_i^m)I_i^f + \frac{\mu b^f \beta_i^m}{\Lambda^m}\Big(\frac{\Lambda^f}{\mu} - \sum_j I_j^f\Big) I_i^m, \qquad (2.2) \\
\frac{dI_i^c}{dt} &= -(\mu^c+\gamma_i^c)I_i^c + \frac{\mu b^c \beta_i^m}{\Lambda^m}\Big(\frac{\Lambda^c}{\mu^c} - \sum_j I_j^c\Big) I_i^m, \quad i = 1,2.
\end{aligned}
$$

where

$$
\begin{aligned}
\sigma_i^c &= (\mu^c + \gamma_i^c),\ p^c = \frac{\Lambda^c}{\mu^c},\ \sigma_i^k = (\mu + \gamma_i^k),\ p^k = \frac{\Lambda^k}{\mu}, \quad k = m, f, \\
a_i^m &= \frac{b^m \beta_i^f}{p^f},\ a_i^f = \frac{b^f \beta_i^m}{p^m},\ a_i^c = \frac{b^c \beta_i^m}{p^m},\ a_i^{mc} = \frac{b^m \beta_i^c}{p^c}. \quad i = 1,2.
\end{aligned}
$$

System (2.2) can be rewritten as

$$
\begin{aligned}
\frac{dI_i^m}{dt} &= -\sigma_i^m I_i^m + (p^m - \sum_j I_j^m)(a_i^m I_i^f + a_i^{mc} I_i^c), \\
\frac{dI_i^f}{dt} &= -\sigma_i^f I_i^f + a_i^f (p^f - \sum_j I_j^f) I_i^m, \qquad (2.3) \\
\frac{dI_i^c}{dt} &= -\sigma_i^c I_i^c + a_i^c (p^c - \sum_j I_j^c) I_i^m, \quad i = 1,2.
\end{aligned}
$$

Linearizing about the infection-free equilibrium of (2.3) gives

$$
\begin{pmatrix} \frac{dI_i^m}{dt} \\ \frac{dI_i^f}{dt} \\ \frac{dI_i^c}{dt} \end{pmatrix} = \begin{pmatrix} -\sigma_i^m & p^m a_i^m & p_i^m a_i^{mc} \\ p^f a_i^f & -\sigma_i^f & 0 \\ p^c a_i^c & 0 & -\sigma_i^c \end{pmatrix} \begin{pmatrix} I_i^m \\ I_i^f \\ I_i^c \end{pmatrix}, \quad i = 1,2.
$$

In this case

$$
Z = (Z_1, Z_2), \quad M = \begin{pmatrix} M_1 & 0 \\ 0 & M_2 \end{pmatrix}, \quad D = \begin{pmatrix} D_1 & 0 \\ 0 & D_2 \end{pmatrix},
$$

where $Z_i = (I_i^m, I_i^f, I_i^c)$,

$$M_i = \begin{pmatrix} 0 & p^m a_i^m & p^m a_i^{mc} \\ p^f a_i^f & 0 & 0 \\ p^c a_i^c & 0 & 0 \end{pmatrix} \quad and \quad D_i = \begin{pmatrix} \sigma_i^m & 0 & 0 \\ 0 & \sigma_i^f & 0 \\ 0 & 0 & \sigma_i^c \end{pmatrix}.$$

$\mathcal{R}_0 = \max\{\mathcal{R}_1, \mathcal{R}_2\}$ where $\mathcal{R}_i$ is the dominant eigenvalue of $M_i D_i^{-1}$. Since the characteristic equation of $M_i D_i^{-1}$ is

$$\lambda(\lambda^2 - \frac{a_i^{mc} p^m p^c a_i^c}{\sigma_i^c \sigma_i^m} - \frac{p^m a_i^m p^f a_i^f}{\sigma_i^f \sigma_i^m}) = 0$$

then

$$\mathcal{R}_i = \sqrt{\frac{a_i^{mc} a_i^c p^m p^c \sigma_i^f + a_i^m a_i^f p^f p^m \sigma_i^c}{\sigma_i^f \sigma_i^m \sigma_i^c}}.$$

Example 6. Dengue is vector-transmitted disease that exhibits strain heterogeneity. Furthermore, a host's prior immunological history with Dengue strains can have a critical impact on the probability of host survival to infections from other strains. The model below was used to study the dynamics of two strains of Dengue (see Feng and Velasco-Hernandez, 1997) on a human population. Secondary infections were only allowed to be experienced by human hosts, that is, It was assumed infected mosquitos never recovered and could not be infected by additionals strains. The situation for human hosts was assumed to be different. Two scenarios were possible: either an I_1 *previously* infected individual who became now infected with strain 2 (through contact with V_2, infected mosquitoes) became a Y_2 infected host or a *previously* I_2 infected individual who become now infected with strain 1 (through contact with V_1 mosquitoes) became a Y_1 infected-host. The rates at which these two forms of host infection occur are given by $\sigma_1 B_1 I_2$ and $\sigma_2 B_2 I_1$, respectively. Here σ_i is a positive real number used to model either cross-immunity ($\sigma_i < 1$) or increased susceptibility ($\sigma_i > 1$). The model is given by the following set of equations:

$$\begin{aligned}
\frac{dS}{dt} &= \Lambda - (B_1 + B_2)S - \mu S, \\
\frac{dI_1}{dt} &= B_1 S - \sigma_2 B_2 I_1 - \mu I_1, \\
\frac{dI_2}{dt} &= B_2 S - \sigma_1 B_1 I_2 - \mu I_2, \\
\frac{dY_1}{dt} &= \sigma_1 B_1 I_2 - (e_1 + \mu + r)Y_1, \\
\frac{dY_2}{dt} &= \sigma_2 B_2 I_1 - (e_2 + \mu + r)Y_2, \\
\frac{dR}{dt} &= r(Y_1 + Y_2) - \mu R,
\end{aligned}$$

and

$$\begin{aligned}\frac{dW}{dt} &= q - (A_1 + A_2)W - \delta W,\\ \frac{dV_1}{dt} &= A_1 W - \delta V_1,\\ \frac{dV_2}{dt} &= A_2 W - \delta V_2,\end{aligned}$$

where

$$B_i = \frac{\beta_i V_i}{c + w_h N}, \quad A_i = \frac{\alpha_i (I_i + Y_i)}{c + w_v N}. \quad i = 1, 2.$$

$N = S + I_1 + I_2 + Y_1 + Y_2 + R$ and W is the number of susceptible mosquitoes. If we let $X = (S, R, W)$, and $Z = (I_1, I_2, Y_1, Y_2, V_1, V_2)$ then $\mathbf{U}_0 = (\Lambda/\mu, 0, q/\delta, 0, 0, 0, 0, 0, 0)$,

$$M = \begin{pmatrix} 0 & 0 & 0 & 0 & \beta_1 C_h & 0 \\ 0 & 0 & 0 & 0 & 0 & \beta_2 C_h \\ 0 & 0 & 0 & 0 & 0 & 0 \\ 0 & 0 & 0 & 0 & 0 & 0 \\ \alpha_1 C_\nu & 0 & 0 & 0 & 0 & 0 \\ 0 & \alpha_2 C_\nu & 0 & 0 & 0 & 0 \end{pmatrix},$$

and

$$D = \begin{pmatrix} \mu & 0 & 0 & 0 & 0 & 0 \\ 0 & \mu & 0 & 0 & 0 & 0 \\ 0 & 0 & e_1 + \mu + r & 0 & 0 & 0 \\ 0 & 0 & 0 & e_2 + \mu + r & 0 & 0 \\ 0 & 0 & 0 & 0 & \delta & 0 \\ 0 & 0 & 0 & 0 & 0 & \delta \end{pmatrix},$$

where $C_h = S^*/(c + w_h N^*)$, $C_\nu = S^*/(c + w_h N^*)$ and $S^* = N^* = \Lambda/\mu$. Hence

$$MD^{-1} = \begin{pmatrix} 0 & 0 & 0 & 0 & \frac{\beta_1}{\mu} C_h & 0 \\ 0 & 0 & 0 & 0 & 0 & \frac{\beta_2}{\mu} C_h \\ 0 & 0 & 0 & 0 & 0 & 0 \\ 0 & 0 & 0 & 0 & 0 & 0 \\ \frac{\alpha_1}{\delta} C_v & 0 & 0 & 0 & 0 & 0 \\ 0 & \frac{\alpha_2}{\delta} C_v & 0 & 0 & 0 & 0 \end{pmatrix},$$

with eigenvalues:

$$\lambda_{1,2} = 0, \quad \lambda_{3,4} = \pm\sqrt{\frac{\alpha_1 \beta_1 C_h C_v}{\delta \mu}} \quad \textit{and} \quad \lambda_{5,6} = \pm\sqrt{\frac{\alpha_2 \beta_2 C_h C_v}{\delta \mu}}.$$

Consequently

$$\mathcal{R}_0 = \max\left\{\sqrt{\frac{\alpha_1\beta_1 C_h C_v}{\delta\mu}},\ \sqrt{\frac{\alpha_2\beta_2 C_h C_v}{\delta\mu}}\right\}.$$

Example 7. Huang, Cooke, & Castillo-Chavez (1992) studied the sexual-transmission of HIV in a homosexually active population stratified by degree of sexual activity and (implicitly) sexual practices. Their model showed that asymmetric transmission rates between groups were capable of generating multiple endemic equilibria via a backward bifurcation. Their model is given by the following set of equations:

$$\begin{aligned}
\frac{dS_i(t)}{dt} &= \Lambda_i - B_i(t) - \mu S_i(t),\\
\frac{dI_i(t)}{dt} &= B_i(t) - (\alpha_i + \mu)I_i(t),\\
\frac{dA_i(t)}{dt} &= \alpha_i I_i(t) - (d_i + \mu)A_i(t),\\
B_i(t) &= S_i(t)c_i \sum_{j=1}^{n} \lambda_{ij} p_{ij}(t)\frac{I_j(t)}{T_j(t)}, \qquad i = 1,\cdots,n,
\end{aligned} \tag{2.4}$$

where A denotes number of individuals with AIDS, $T_j = S_j + I_j$, and c_i, λ_{ij}, and $p_{ij}(t)$ denotes the mixing matrix. Proportionate mixing was assumed, that is they took $p_{ij} = p_j = c_j T_j / N$ where $N = \sum_{k=1}^{n} c_k T_k$. The constants α_i and d_i denote the per capita disease-induced death rates. The notation $\theta_i = \eta_i \lambda_{ii} c_i$, and $l_{ij} = c_i c_j \lambda_{ij}$ used in Huang et al. (1992) helps rewrite System (2.4) (without the A equation) in the form:

$$\begin{aligned}
\frac{dS_i}{dt} &= \Lambda_i - S_i\left(\frac{\theta_i I_i}{T_i} + \frac{1}{N}\sum_{j=1}^{n} l_{ij} I_j\right) - \mu S_i,\\
\frac{dI_i}{dt} &= S_i\left(\frac{\theta_i I_i}{T_i} + \frac{1}{N}\sum_{j=1}^{n} l_{ij} I_j\right) - (\alpha_i + \mu)I_i. \quad i = 1,\cdots,n.
\end{aligned} \tag{2.5}$$

Note that at the disease-free state of (2.5) $S_i^* = T_i^* = \frac{\Lambda_i}{\mu}$ and $N^* = \sum_{k=1}^{n} c_k T_k^*$. Hence, under proportionate mixing with $Z = (I_1, I_2, \cdots, I_n)$ one gets

$$M = \begin{pmatrix}
\theta_1 + \frac{S_1^* l_{11}}{N^*} & \frac{S_1^* l_{12}}{N^*} & \cdots & \frac{S_1^* l_{1n}}{N^*}\\
\frac{S_2^* l_{21}}{N^*} & \theta_2 + \frac{S_2^* l_{22}}{N^*} & \cdots & \frac{S_2^* l_{2n}}{N^*}\\
\cdot & \cdot & & \cdot\\
\cdot & \cdot & & \cdot\\
\cdot & \cdot & & \cdot\\
\frac{S_n^* l_{n1}}{N^*} & \frac{S_n^* l_{n2}}{N^*} & \cdots & \theta_n + \frac{S_n^* l_{nn}}{N^*}
\end{pmatrix}$$

and

$$D = \begin{pmatrix} \alpha_1 + \mu & 0 & & \cdots & 0 \\ 0 & \alpha_2 + \mu & 0 & \cdots & 0 \\ \cdot & \cdot & & & \cdot \\ \cdot & \cdot & & & \cdot \\ \cdot & \cdot & & & \cdot \\ 0 & \cdots & & 0 & \alpha_n + \mu \end{pmatrix}.$$

M and D can be rewritten as:

$$M = \text{diag}(\theta_i) + \frac{1}{K}\text{diag}(\Lambda_i)L, \quad D = \text{diag}(\mu(\sigma_i + 1)),$$

where $K = \sum_{k=1}^{n} c_k \Lambda_k$, $L = (l_{ij})_{n\times n}$, and $\sigma_i = \alpha_i/\mu$.

Clearly

$$MD^{-1} = \frac{1}{\mu}\text{diag}\left(\frac{\theta_i}{\sigma_i + 1}\right) + \frac{1}{\mu}\text{diag}\left(\frac{\Lambda_i}{K(\sigma_i + 1)}\right)L.$$

If μ_0 (notation used by Huang et al.) denotes the spectral radius of the matrix

$$\text{diag}\left(\frac{\theta_i}{\sigma_i + 1}\right) + \text{diag}\left(\frac{\Lambda_i}{K(\sigma_i + 1)}\right)L,$$

then

$$R_0 = \frac{\mu_0}{\mu}.$$

Example 8. There is a vaccine for TB that is widely used around the world. A model was developed and analyzed by Castillo-Chavez and Feng (1997) to help determine the optimal (according to some appropriate set of criteria) vaccination age. The role of $\mathcal{R}_0$ was also critical in establishing of a useful concept of optimality. Hence, its explicit computation was critical to the analysis. Let's introduce this model and compute its $\mathcal{R}_0$. We let $s(t,a)$ denote the density function of the susceptible class ($S(t) = \int_0^\infty s(t,a)da$ gives the number of susceptibles at t) and let $v(t,a)$, $l(t,a)$, $i(t,a)$, and $j(t,a)$ denote the density functions of the vaccinated, latent, infectious, and treated classes, respectively. The model reads

$$
\begin{aligned}
(\frac{\partial}{\partial t}+\frac{\partial}{\partial a})s &= -\beta(a)c(a)B(t)s-\mu(a)s-\psi(a)s,\\
(\frac{\partial}{\partial t}+\frac{\partial}{\partial a})v &= \psi(a)s-\mu(a)v-\delta\beta(a)c(a)B(t)v,\\
(\frac{\partial}{\partial t}+\frac{\partial}{\partial a})l &= \beta(a)c(a)B(t)\big(s+\sigma j+\delta v\big)-(k+\mu(a))l,\\
(\frac{\partial}{\partial t}+\frac{\partial}{\partial a})i &= kl-(r+\mu(a))i,\\
(\frac{\partial}{\partial t}+\frac{\partial}{\partial a})j &= ri-\sigma\beta(a)c(a)B(t)j-\mu(a)j,\\
B(t) &= \int_0^\infty \frac{i(t,a')}{n(t,a')}p(t,a')da',\\
p(t,a') &= \frac{c(a')n(t,a')}{\int_0^\infty c(u)n(t,u)du},\\
s(t,0) &= \Lambda,\quad v(t,0)=l(t,0)=i(t,0)=j(t,0)=0,\\
s(0,a)=s_0(a),\ v(0,a) &= v_0(a),\ l(0,a)=l_0(a),\\
i(0,a) &= i_0(a),\ j(0,a)=j_0(a),
\end{aligned}
$$

where $n=s+v+l+i+j$; Λ is the birth rate; $\mu(a)$ is the age specific per capita natural death rate; $\beta(a)$ is the age specific (average) probability of becoming infected through contacts with infectious individuals; $c(a)$ is the age specific per capita contact/activity rate; σ and δ represent the reduction in risk of infection due to treatment and vaccination, respectively, $0\le\sigma,\ \delta\le 1$; k is the per capita rate of progression to active TB; r is the per capita treatment rate; $\psi(a)$ is the per capita vaccination rate. In addition, $p(t,a,a')$ gives the "probability" that an individual of age a has a contact with an individual of age a' given that the individual had a contact with a member of the population. Again, we assume proportionate mixing (otherwise the explicit computation of R_0 is impossible), that is, we take $p(t,a,a')=p(t,a')$ (as already defined above).

The steady demographic state (that is, the state where the infection is absent) of the system is given by the following nonuniform age-distribution:

$$
\begin{aligned}
n(a) &= \Lambda e^{-\mu a}, & s(a) &= \Lambda e^{-\mu a}\mathcal{F}_\psi(a),\\
v(a) &= \Lambda e^{-\mu a}\big(1-\mathcal{F}_\psi(a)\big), & l &= i=j=0,
\end{aligned}
$$

where

$$
\mathcal{F}(a)=e^{-\int_0^a \mu(s)ds},\quad \mathcal{F}_\psi(a)=e^{-\int_0^a \psi(b)db}.
$$

The probability that an individual of age $\alpha+\tau$, who was infected τ units of time ago, is still in class i, is given by

$$
\gamma(\tau,\alpha)=\int_0^\tau ke^{-(\mu+k)u}e^{-(r+\mu)(\tau-u)}du=:\mathcal{K}(\tau)e^{-\mu\tau}
$$

where

$$\mathcal{K}(\tau) = \frac{k}{r-k}(e^{-k\tau} - e^{-r\tau}). \tag{2.6}$$

Thus the expected infectivity is given by

$$A(\tau, a, \alpha) = \beta(a)c(a)p(\alpha+\tau)\frac{\gamma(\tau,\alpha)}{n(\alpha+\tau)},$$

where $p(a) = c(a)n(a)/\int_0^\infty c(u)n(u)du$. Letting $A(\tau, a, \alpha) = f(a)g(\tau, \alpha)$ where $f(a) = \beta(a)c(a)$ and $g(\tau, \alpha) = p(\alpha+\tau)\gamma(\tau, \alpha)/n(\alpha+\tau)$ and Formula (1.3) leads to the computation of the reproductive number associated with the vaccination strategy ψ. Namely,

$$\mathcal{R}(\psi) = \int_0^\infty \int_0^\infty p(\alpha+\tau)\beta(\alpha)c(\alpha)\mathcal{K}(\tau)\mathcal{V}_\psi(\alpha)d\tau d\alpha,$$

where $\mathcal{V}_\psi(a) = \mathcal{F}_\psi(a) + \delta(1 - \mathcal{F}_\psi(a)) < 1$ ($\mathcal{K}(\tau)$ is given by (2.6)). Hence, in the absence of a vaccine, that is, whenever, $\psi(a) = 0$, the above formula reduces to the basic reproductive number

$$\mathcal{R}_0 = \int_0^\infty \int_0^\infty p(\alpha+\tau)\beta(\alpha)c(\alpha)\mathcal{K}(\tau)d\tau d\alpha.$$

An alternative method for computing $\mathcal{R}_0$ can be found in Castillo-Chavez and Feng (1997).

Example 9. The following model was introduced and partially analyzed in Busenberg and Castillo-Chavez (1991). The focus of their paper was not the study of the transmission dynamics of HIV/AIDS per se but rather the development of general methods for modeling the mixing structure of a population. This paper focussed on the modeling of social structures since they often play a critical role in the study of the spread of disease. A model for the transmission dynamics of HIV/AIDS in a homosexually-active population stratified by risk and age was used to illustrate their approach. In order to introduce this model, we let $S(r, a, t)$, $I(r, a, \tau, t)$ and $A(r, a, \tau, t)$ denote the density functions of susceptible, infectious, and AIDS classes, respectively. Here, a denotes chronological age; τ is the age of infection for the I and A groups; and r denotes the sexual activity level. The model reads:

$$\begin{aligned}
\frac{\partial S}{\partial t} &+ \frac{\partial S}{\partial a} = \Lambda(r, a, t, T(r, a, t)) - B(r, a, t) - \mu(a)S, \\
\frac{\partial I}{\partial t} &+ \frac{\partial I}{\partial a} + \frac{\partial I}{\partial \tau} = -\big(\mu(a) + \nu(a, \tau) + \gamma(a, \tau)\big)I, \\
\frac{\partial A}{\partial t} &+ \frac{\partial A}{\partial a} + \frac{\partial A}{\partial \tau} = \gamma(a, \tau)I - \big(\mu(a) + \delta(a, \tau)\big)A,
\end{aligned}$$

where at $a = 0$, $S = I = A = 0$, and $I(r,a,0,t) = B(r,a,t)$,

$$\begin{aligned} B(r,a,t) = {} & c(r,a) \int_0^\infty \int_0^\infty \int_0^\infty \beta(r,a,\tau,r',a')\rho(r,a,r',a') \\ & \times \frac{I(r',a',\tau,t)}{T(r',a',t)} dr'da'd\tau, \\ T(r,a,t) = {} & S(r,a,t) + \int_0^\infty I(r,a,\tau,t)d\tau. \end{aligned}$$

At the steady demographic state

$$T(r,a) = \tilde{S}(r,a) = \int_0^a e^{-\int_x^a \mu(y)dy} \Lambda(r,x)dx. \tag{2.7}$$

Under the assumption of proportionate mixing, that is, with the use of

$$\begin{aligned} \rho(r,a,r',a') = {} & \frac{c(r',a')T(r',a')}{\int_0^\infty \int_0^\infty c(r',a')T(r',a')dr'da'}, \\ \beta(r,a,r',a',\tau) = {} & \beta(r',a',\tau), \end{aligned}$$

one finds that the infectivity function is given by

$$\begin{aligned} A(r,a,r',a'-\tau,\tau) & = \beta(r',a',\tau)c(r,a)\rho(r',a')\frac{\mathcal{F}(a',\tau)}{T(r',a')} \\ & =: f(r,a)g(r',a'-\tau,\tau), \qquad 0 \le \tau \le a', \end{aligned}$$

where

$$\mathcal{F}(a',\tau) = e^{-\int_0^\tau \left(\mu(a'-\tau+s)+\nu(a'-\tau+s,\tau)+\gamma(a'-\tau+s,\tau)\right)ds}, \tag{2.8}$$

and

$$f(r,a) = c(r,a), \qquad g(r',a'-\tau,\tau) = \frac{\beta(r',a',\tau)c(r',a')\mathcal{F}(a',\tau)}{\int_0^\infty \int_0^\infty c(r',a')T(r',a')dr'da'}.$$

We again compute the basic reproductive number using (1.3)

$$\begin{aligned} R_0 & = \int_0^\infty \int_0^\infty \int_0^{a'} f(r',a'-\tau)\tilde{S}(r',a'-\tau)g(r',a'-\tau,\tau)d\tau dr'da' \\ & = \int_0^\infty \int_0^\infty \int_0^{a'} c(r',a'-\tau)\left(\int_0^{a'-\tau} e^{-\int_x^{a'-\tau} \mu(y)dy}\Lambda(r',x)dx\right) \\ & \quad \times \frac{\beta(r',a',\tau)c(r',a')\mathcal{F}(a',\tau)}{\int_0^\infty \int_0^\infty c(r',a')T(r',a')dr'da'} d\tau dr'da' \\ & = \frac{1}{\int_0^\infty \int_0^\infty c(r',a')T(r',a')dr'da'} \\ & \quad \times \int_0^\infty \int_0^\infty c(r',a')\left\{\int_0^{a'} \beta(r',a',\tau)c(r',a'-\tau)\mathcal{F}(a',\tau)\right. \\ & \quad \times \left.\left(\int_0^{a'-\tau} e^{-\int_x^{a'-\tau} \mu(y)dy}\Lambda(r',x)dx\right)d\tau\right\}dr'da', \end{aligned}$$

where $T(r,a)$ and $\mathcal{F}(a',\tau)$ are given in (2.7), (2.8).

Example 10. The model of this last example was develop to determine optimal vaccination policies for models for infectious diseases (see Hadeler and Müller, 1995). The "general" age structure model for communicable diseases is typically given by the following system of three partial differential equations:

$$\begin{aligned} u_t + u_a &= -\mu(a)u - \psi(a)u + \gamma(a)w - \beta(a)u\frac{V}{N}, \\ w_t + w_a &= -\mu(a)w + \psi(a)u + \alpha(a)v - \gamma(a)w - \tilde{\beta}(a)w\frac{V}{N} \\ v_t + v_a &= -\tilde{\mu}(a)v - \alpha(a)v + (\beta(a)u + \tilde{\beta}(a)w)\frac{V}{N}, \end{aligned}$$

with boundary conditions

$$u(t,0) = \int_0^L [b(a)(u(t,a) + w(t,a)) + \tilde{b}(a)v(t,a)]da,$$
$$w(t,0) = 0, \quad v(t,0) = 0.$$

Here, $N(t) = \int_0^L [(u(t,a) + w(t,a)) + v(t,a)]da$ denotes the total population size while $V(t) = \int_0^L k(a)v(t,a)da$ gives the average number of contacts per unit of time of infectious with susceptible individuals. Furthermore, L represents maximum age; $\psi(a)$ denotes the age dependent vaccination rate; $k(a)$ the age specific contact distribution; $\alpha(a)$ denotes the age dependent recovery rate; and $\gamma(a)$ is the age specific loss of immunity.

The steady demographic state, in the presence of an age specific vaccination policy $\psi(a)$, is $(\bar{u}(a), \bar{w}(a), \bar{v}(a))$ where

$$\bar{u}(a) = P(a)D(a), \quad \bar{w}(a) = P(a) - \bar{u}(a), \quad \bar{v}(a) = 0,$$

and

$$\begin{aligned} P(a) &= e^{-\int_0^a \mu(s)ds}, \\ D(a) &= e^{-\int_0^a (\gamma(s)+\psi(s))ds} + \int_0^a e^{-\int_s^a (\gamma(\tau)+\psi(\tau))d\tau}\gamma(s)ds. \end{aligned}$$

If $A_u(\tau,\xi,\eta)$ and $A_v(\tau,\xi,\eta)$ denote the infectivity functions corresponding to susceptibles $\bar{u}(\xi)$ and vaccinated individuals $\bar{v}(\xi)$, respectively, then

$$A_u(\tau,\xi,\eta) = f_u(\xi)g(\tau,\eta), \quad A_v(\tau,\xi,\eta) = f_v(\xi)g(\tau,\eta),$$

where

$$f_u(\xi) = \beta(\xi), \quad f_v(\xi) = \tilde{\beta}(\xi), \quad g(\tau,\eta) = k(\eta+\tau)\frac{e^{-\int_0^\tau [\tilde{\mu}(\eta+s)+\alpha(\eta+s)]ds}}{N}.$$

Using Formula (1.3) again, we compute the basic reproductive number:

$$\begin{aligned} R(\psi) &= \int_0^L \int_0^L f_u(\eta)\bar{u}(\eta)g(\tau,\eta)d\tau d\eta + \int_0^L \int_0^L f_v(\eta)\bar{w}(\eta)g(\tau,\eta)d\tau d\eta \\ &= \frac{1}{N}\int_0^L \int_0^L k(\eta+\tau)e^{-\int_0^\tau [\tilde{\mu}(\eta+s)+\alpha(\eta+s)]ds}(\beta(\eta)\bar{u}(\eta) + \tilde{\beta}(\eta)\bar{w}(\eta))d\tau d\eta. \end{aligned}$$

Some changes of variables and exchanges in the order of integrations leads to

$$R(\psi) =$$

$$\frac{\int_0^L\int_0^\theta k(\theta)P(\eta)e^{-\int_\eta^\theta(\tilde{\mu}(r)+\alpha(r))dr}\Big(\beta(\eta)D(\eta)+\tilde{\beta}(\eta)(1-D(\eta))\Big)\,d\eta d\theta}{\int_0^L P(a)da}. \tag{2.9}$$

Note that $P(\eta)P(\tau) = P(\eta+\tau)$ and $\delta(a) = \tilde{\mu}(a) - \mu(a)$. It can be checked that (2.9) gives the same formula for $\mathcal{R}(\psi)$ as that found in the paper by Hadeler and Müller (Formula (3.20)).

3. Global stability conditions for the disease-free equilibrium when $\mathcal{R}_0 < 1$. For all the differential equation examples of Section 2, it can be established that the disease-free equilibrium is locally asymptotic stable (l.a.s.) whenever $\mathcal{R}_0 < 1$ and unstable when $\mathcal{R}_0 > 1$. In this section, we list two conditions that if met, also guarantee the global asymptotic stability of the disease-free state. First, System (1.1) must be written in the form:

$$\begin{aligned} \frac{dX}{dt} &= F(\mathbf{x}, Z), \\ \frac{dZ}{dt} &= G(X, Z), \qquad G(\mathbf{x}, 0) = 0, \end{aligned} \tag{3.1}$$

where $X \in \mathbb{R}^m$ denotes (its components) the number of uninfected individuals and $Z \in \mathbb{R}^n$ denotes (its components) the number of infected individuals including latent, infectious, etc. $\mathbf{U}_0 = (x^*, 0)$ denotes the disease-free equilibrium of this system.

The conditions (H1) and (H2) below must be met to guarantee local asymptotic stability.

(H1) For $\frac{dX}{dt} = F(X, 0)$, X^* is globally asymptotically stable (g.a.s.),

(H2) $G(X, Z) = AZ - \widehat{G}(X, Z)$, $\widehat{G}(X, Z) \geq 0$ for $(X, Z) \in \Omega$,

where $A = D_Z G(X^*, 0)$ is an M-matrix (the off diagonal elements of A are nonnegative) and Ω is the region where the model makes biological sense.

If System (3.1) satisfies the above two conditions then the following theorem holds:

Theorem. The fixed point $\mathbf{U}_0 = (x^*, 0)$ *is a globally asymptotic stable (g.a.s.) equilibrium of (3.1) provided that* $\mathcal{R}_0 < 1$ *(l.a.s.) and that assumptions (H1) and (H2) are satisfied*

Proof. Let $I_0 = I(0)$, observe that $I(t) \geq 0$ if $I_0 > 0$ and that e^{At} is a positive semigroup (since A is an M-matrix). Hence, using the variation-of-constant formula, we have

$$\begin{aligned} 0 \leq I(t) &= e^{At}I_0 - \int_0^t e^{A(t-s)}\widehat{G}\big(X(s), Z(s)\big)ds \\ &\leq e^{At}I_0. \end{aligned}$$

Since A is an M-matrix, A has a dominant eigenvalue $m(A)$ with $m(A) < 0$ for $\mathcal{R}_0 < 1$. Thus

$$\lim_{t\to\infty} \|e^{At}\| = 0, \implies \lim_{t\to\infty} I(t) = 0.$$

Note that X^* is a g.a.s. equilibrium of $\frac{dX}{dt} = F(X,0)$, a limiting system of $\frac{dX}{dt} = F(X(t), Z(t))$. Thus,

$$\lim_{t\to\infty} X(t) = X^*.$$

Remark. If A is irreducible and some additional conditions on $\widehat{G}(X,Z)$, then the theorem remains true for $\mathcal{R}_0 \leq 1$.

Rewrite Example 2 in the form of (3.1, then $X = (S,R)$, $Z = (E,I)$, $F(X,0) = \begin{pmatrix} \Lambda - \mu S \\ 0 \end{pmatrix}$, and

$$A = \begin{pmatrix} -(\mu+k) & \beta \\ k & -(\mu+\gamma) \end{pmatrix}, \qquad \widehat{G}(X,Z) = \begin{pmatrix} \beta I(1-\frac{S}{N}) \\ 0 \end{pmatrix}.$$

Since $0 \leq S \leq N$, it is clear that $\widehat{G}(X,Z) \geq 0$. It is also clear that $X^* = (\Lambda/\mu, 0)$ is a g.a.s equilibrium of $\frac{dX}{dt} = F(X,0)$. Hence, by the above theorem $\mathbf{U}_0$ is g.a.s.

If the model in Example 3 is re-written in the form of (3.1) then $X = (S,T)$, $Z = (E_1, I_1, E_2, I_2)$, $F(X,0) = (\,\Lambda - \mu S 0\,)$,

$$A = \begin{pmatrix} -(\mu+k_1+r) & \beta_1 + p\tilde{r} & 0 & 0 \\ k & -(\mu+d_1+\tilde{r}) & 0 & 0 \\ 0 & q\tilde{r} & -(\mu+k_2) & \beta_2 \\ 0 & 0 & k_2 & -(\mu+d_2) \end{pmatrix},$$

and

$$\widehat{G}(X,Z) = \begin{pmatrix} \beta_1 I_1(1-\frac{S+\sigma T}{N}) + \beta_2 E_1 \frac{I_2}{N} \\ 0 \\ \beta_2 I_2(1-\frac{S+E_1+T}{N}) \\ 0 \end{pmatrix}.$$

Since $\sigma \leq 1$ and $0 \leq S + \sigma T \leq S + E_1 + T \leq N$ then $\widehat{G}(X,Z) \geq 0$. The global stability of $X^* = (\Lambda/\mu, 0)$ of the system $\frac{dX}{dt} = F(X,0)$ is easy to check. Hence, $\mathbf{U}_0$ is g.a.s.

The next example illustrates a case in which one of the assumptions of the theorem is violated. For this model, it was shown that a backward bifurcation occurs at $\mathcal{R}_0 = 1$, that is , it was shown that multiple endemic equilibria can exist even though $\mathcal{R}_0 < 1$. Consider the TB model with reinfection studied in Feng, Castillo-Chavez, and Capurro (2000):

$$\begin{aligned}
\frac{dS}{dt} &= \Lambda - \beta S\frac{I}{N} - \mu S,\\
\frac{dE}{dt} &= \beta S\frac{I}{N} - p\beta E\frac{I}{N} - (\mu + k)E + \sigma\beta T\frac{I}{N},\\
\frac{dI}{dt} &= p\beta E\frac{I}{N} + kE - (\mu + r + d)I,\\
\frac{dT}{dt} &= rI - \sigma\beta T\frac{I}{N} - \mu T,\\
N &= S + E + I + T.
\end{aligned}$$

Here, $p\beta E\frac{I}{N}$ denotes the reinfection rate, $0 \leq p < 1$. Whenever $p = 0$ the model becomes equivalent to the model in Example 2.

If $0 < p < 1$ then $X = (S, T)$, $Z = (E, I)$, $\mathbf{U}_0 = (S^*, T^*, E^*, I^*) = (\Lambda/\mu, 0, 0, 0,)$ and

$$\widehat{G}(X, Z) = \begin{pmatrix} \widehat{G}_1(X, Z) \\ \widehat{G}_2(X, Z) \end{pmatrix} = \begin{pmatrix} \beta I(1 - \frac{S+\sigma T}{N}) + p\beta E\frac{I}{N} \\ -p\beta E\frac{I}{N} \end{pmatrix}.$$

Hence $\widehat{G}_2(X, Z) < 0$, that is, (H2) is not satisfied. Consequently, $\mathbf{U}_0$ may not be globally asymptotic stable. It was proved in Feng, Castillo-Chavez, and Capurro (2000) that a backward bifurcation occurs at $\mathcal{R}_0 = 1$ and that two endemic equilibria can be supported as long as $\mathcal{R}_c < \mathcal{R}_0 < 1$ (where $\mathcal{R}_c$ is an appropriate positive constant).

4. Conclusions. For a long period of time $\mathcal{R}_0 < 1$ was considered the key to understanding the dynamics of epidemiological models. This view arose from the work of Lajmanovich and Yorke (1976) on gonorrhea transmission (these authors studied what appeared to be quite a general epidemiological model) and from relationship of many epidemic models to monotone systems. Recent work (beginning with Castillo-Chavez et al. (1989) and Huang et al. (1992)) showed that this was not the case. Their work arose in the context of the study of HIV/AIDS dynamics, that is from models that had to incorporate selection (differential mortality). The incorporation of differential mortality has had a dramatic impact in the field of theoretical and mathematical epidemiology (see Hadeler and Castillo-Chavez (1995) and Feng et al. (2000), for applications to HIV and TB, respectively). The theorem in the last section not only connects $\mathcal{R}_0$ to the concept of global asymptotic stability but also identifies some mathematical conditions that must be met for a transcritical bifurcation (with transfer of stability and "boring" (predictable) dynamics) to occur.

Acknowledgments. This research was partially supported by NSF grant DEB-925370 (Presidential Faculty Fellowship Award) to Carlos Castillo-Chavez and by NSF grant DMS-9974389 to Zhilan Feng. This work was completed while CCC and ZF visited the IMA in Minnesota. We thank Baojun Song for his comments.

REFERENCES

ANDERSON, R.M. AND R.M. MAY, Eds. (1982), *Population Biology of Infectious Diseases*, Springer-Verlag, Berlin, Heidelberg, New York.

BUSENBERG, S. AND C. CASTILLO-CHAVEZ (1991), *A general solution of the problem of mixing subpopulations, and its application to risk- and age-structure epidemic models for the spread of AIDS,* IMA J. of Math. Appl. Med. Biol. **8**:1–29.

BUSENBERG, S. AND K. COOK (1993), Vertically Transmitted Diseases: Models and Dynamics Biomathemtics **23**, Springer-Verlag, New York.

CASTILLO-CHAVEZ, C., K. COOK, W. HUANG, AND S.A. LEVIN (1989), Results on the dynamics for models for the sexual transmission of human immunodeficiendy virus. Appl. Math. Lett. **2(4)**:327–331.

CASTILLO-CHAVEZ, C. AND Z. FENG (1997), *To treat or not to treat: the case of tuberculosis,* J. Math. Biol. **35**:629–656.

CASTILLO-CHAVEZ, C. AND Z. FENG (1998), *Global stability of an age-structure model for TB and its applications to optimal vaccination strategies*, Math. Biosc. **151**:135–154.

CASTILLO-CHAVEZ, C., J.X. VELASCO-HERNANDEZ, AND S. FRIDMAN (1994), *Modeling contact structures in Biology.* In: *Frontiers of Theoretical Biology,* S.A. Levin (ed.), Lecture notes in Biomathematics, 100. Spring-Verlag, New York.

CASTILLO-CHAVEZ, C., W. HUANG, AND J. LI (1997), *The effects of females' susceptibility on the coexistence of multiple pathogen strains of sexually transmitted diseases,* J. Math. Biol. **35**:503–522.

DIEKMANN, O., J.A.P. HEESTERBEEK, AND J.A.J. METZ (1990), *On the definition and the computation of the basic reproduction ratio $\mathcal{R}_0$ in models for infectious diseases in heterogeneous population,* J. Math. Biol. **28**:365–382.

DIEKMANN, O. AND J.A.P. HEESTERBEEK (2000), *Mathematical Epidemiology of Infectious Diseases*: Model Building, Analysis and Interpretation. Wiley, New York.

FENG, Z., C. CASTILLO-CHAVEZ, AND A. CAPURRO (2000), *A model for TB with exogenous reinfection*, Theo. Pop. Biol. **578**:237–247.

FENG, Z., W. HUANG, AND C. CASTILLO-CHAVEZ (2001), *On the role of variable latent periods in mathematical models for tuberculosis*, J. Dyn. Diff. Eq. (to appear).

FENG, Z. AND J. X. VELASCO-HERNANDEZ (1997), *Competitive exclusion in a vector-host model for the dengue fever*, J. Math. Biol. **35**:523–544.

HADELER, K.P. AND J. MÜLLER (1995), *Vaccination in age structured population I: The reproduction number*, In Models for Infectious Human Diseases: Their Structure and Relation to Data, V. Isham and G. Medley, eds., Cambridge University Press.

HADELER, K.P. AND C. CASTILLO-CHAVEZ (1995), *A core group model for disease transmission* , Math. Biosci. **128**:41–55.

HUANG, W., K.L. COOKE AND C. CASTILLO-CHAVEZ (1992), *Stability and Bifurcation for a multiple-group model for the dynamics of HIV-AIDS transmission*, SIAM J. Appl. Math. **52**:835–854.

KERMACK, W.O. AND A.G. MCKENDRICK (1927), *Contributions to the mathematical theory of epidemics, Part 1,* Proc. Roy. Soc. London Ser. **A, 115**: 700–721.

LAJMANOVICH, A. AND J.A. YORK (1976), *A deterministic model for gonorrehea in a nonhomogeneous population*, Math. Biosci. **28**:221–236.

MACDONALD, G. (1957), The epidemiology and control of malaria. Oxford University Press.

SONG, B., C. CASTILLO-CHAVEZ, AND J.P. APARICIO (2001), *Global dynamics of TB models with density-dependent demography* (this volume).

ROSS, R. (1911), The Prevention of Malaria (2nd edition, with addendum) John Murray, London 1911.

ZHOU, Y., B. SONG, AND Z. MA (2001), *The global stability analysis for an SIS model with age and infection age structures* (this volume).

NONLINEAR MATING MODELS FOR POPULATIONS WITH DISCRETE GENERATIONS

CARLOS CASTILLO-CHAVEZ*, ABDUL-AZIZ YAKUBU†, HORST THIEME‡, AND MAIA MARTCHEVA§

Abstract. Extensions of the discrete Malthus model are carried out to include males, females and various forms of mating. The resulting discrete nonlinear homogeneous pair-formation model parallels those of Kendall [25], Keyfitz [26], Fredrickson [12], Pollard [37] and Hadeler *et al.'s* [14–19]. Consequently, they provide an appropriate framework for the study of sexually-transmitted diseases (STDs) in the wild. The analysis of Hadeler *et al.* goes through even when the mating function depends on the number of females or males in pairs, that is, in the presence of interference competition for the search of single individuals. This framework and analysis should be useful to those interested in the study of STDs in animal populations with complex mating systems.

1. Introduction. The discrete-time analogue of the Malthus model is given by

$$(DM) \qquad P(t+1) = \lambda P(t), \qquad P(0) = P_0,$$

where $P(t)$ is the population at generation t and λ is the multiplicative growth factor per generation [29, 31–33, 38]. Hence, for the initial population size $P_0 > 0$ the model predicts unbounded geometric growth if $\lambda > 1$; geometric decline to extinction if $\lambda < 1$; and no growth ($P(t) = P_0$) if $\lambda = 1$.

Two-sex models with various mating strategies have been developed but mostly at the level of the gene (see [11, 13, 20, 27]). Developing useful mating models at the level of the individual has proved difficult. Nevertheless, successful first-level approaches have been developed for continuous-time models that include interference competition of single females and males by Kendall [25], Keyfitz [26], McFarland [34], Fredrickson [12], Pollard [37], Hoppensteadt [20], Waldstätter [39], and more recently by Castillo-Chavez *et al.* [1–8], Caswell [10], Hadeler *et al.* [14–19], Hsu [21–23], Martcheva [30]; to name a few). Analogue stochastic pair-formation models have also been developed (see Luo and Castillo-Chavez [28]). The work of these researchers has been driven by either demographic considerations or by efforts to understand the role of complex mating strategies on HIV dynamics.

In this article we reformulate the continuous-time pair formation models of Kendall [25], Keyfitz [26], Fredrickson [12], Pollard [37] and Hadeler

*Biometrics, Statistics and Theoretical & Applied Mechanics Departments, Cornell University, Ithaca, New York 14853.

†Department of Mathematics, Howard University, Washington, DC 20059.

‡Department of Mathematics, University of Arizona, Tempe, AZ 85787.

§Department of Mathematics, Polytechnic University, Brooklyn, NY 11201.

et al.'s [14–19] for populations with discrete generations. Specifically, we expand from first principles the discrete-time Malthus model into a nonlinear homogeneous model that includes males, females, and couples. This discrete-time pair-formation model is capable of supporting geometric solutions, and hence, it can be extended to heterogeneous mixing populations that support stable pair distributions (see Castillo-Chavez *et al.* [4–9], Luo and Castillo-Chavez [28]). Our model is not a discretization of continuous-time models but rather a truly discrete-time version based on population principles [9]. Consequently, our framework may be useful in the study of mating systems (at the level of the individual) for animal populations in the wild.

The paper is organized as follows: Section 2 introduces the basic two-sex discrete-time model; Sections 3 explores the possibilities of constant solutions and sets conditions for the existence of geometric solutions; Section 4 examines stability of solutions; Section 5 gives an illustrative example; Section 6 discusses some of the implications of our work and outlines some future work; and Section 7 is the Appendix section.

2. Homogeneous discrete-time pair-formation model. At generation t, we let $x(t)$ denote the population size of single females; $y(t)$ denote the population size of single males; $p(t)$ denote the population size of pairs (couples); $p_x(t)$ denote the population size of coupled females; and $p_y(t)$ denote the population size of coupled males. We will require serial monogamy, that is, we will make the necessary assumptions so that $p(t) = p_x(t) = p_y(t)$. Hence, the total population size at generation t, $T(t)$, will be given by $T(t) \equiv x(t) + y(t) + 2p(t)$. The model is built assuming an implicit serial process which is typical of many discrete-time models (see Caswell [10]) but not essential. Its use clarifies the underlying modeling assumptions and facilitates the formulation of natural extensions. Hence, only the proportion of surviving females (μ_x), males (μ_y) or pairs ($\mu_x\mu_y$) can find a partner, and, only surviving pairs can reproduce or separate ($0 \leq \mu_x, \mu_y \leq 1$). This set up simplifies the governing equation for the dynamics of the total population. At the end of each generation, new females [respectively, males] are born, from surviving pairs at the per-capita production rate of β_x [respectively, β_y] per generation; the fraction $(1-\mu_x)$ [respectively, $(1-\mu_y)$] of females [respectively, males] are removed (death or retirement from mating activities); and, couples may separate independently with probability $(1-\sigma)$.

The populations of single females and single males increase by the death of a partner (widows become single), separation of couples ("divorcees" become single) or birth. Individuals are removed from the single classes by mating (pair-formation) or death. The functions $G : [0,\infty) \times [0,\infty) \times [0,\infty) \times [0,\infty) \to [0,1]$ and $H : [0,\infty) \times [0,\infty) \times [0,\infty) \times [0,\infty) \to [0,1]$ denote the state-dependent "probability" functions that model the proportion of individuals who were not capable of finding a partner at generation t, given that they had a contact with a potential partner, that is, a single female (if you are a male) or a single male (if you are a female). G and H are assumed to be functions of the population vectors at generation t, $(x(t), y(t), p_x(t), p_y(t))$. The pair-formation (marriage) function has been typically modeled as a function of the population vector of singles $(x(t), y(t))$ [36]. Fredrickson [12], Hadeler et al.[14–19], Kendall [25], Keyfitz [26], McFarland [34] and Pollard [37] have proposed various functional forms for ϕ. Fredrickson [12] postulated the following properties for ϕ (a function from $[0,\infty) \times [0,\infty) \to [0,\infty)$) : (i) $\phi(x,y) \geq 0$ (ii) $\phi(x+u, y+v) \geq \phi(x,y)$ (iii) $\phi(kx, ky) = k\phi(x,y)$ (iv) $\phi(x,0) = \phi(0,y) = 0$, for all $(x,y) \in [0,\infty) \times [0,\infty)$ and $u, v, k \in [0,\infty)$.

It is clearly reasonable to assume that the marriage functions are also functions of (x, y, p_x, p_y). This would be applicable for situations in which paired individuals cannot be clearly identified. Since $p_x = p_y = p$, we let $\phi = \phi(x,y,p)$ in populations where the search for a partner requires some effort (interference competition) before the real status (single or paired) of an individual can be determined. In general, $\phi(x,y,0) > 0$ whenever $x > 0$ and $y > 0$, that is, in the absence of competition the rate of pair-formation should be positive provided that $x > 0$ and $y > 0$. Hence, $\phi(x,y,p)$ would be required to satisfy initially the following properties: (i) $\phi(x,y,p) \geq 0$ (ii) $\phi(kx,ky,kp) = k\phi(x,y,p)$ (iii) $\phi(x,0,p) = \phi(0,y,p) = 0$ (iv) $\phi_x(x,y,p) > 0$, $\phi_y(x,y,p) > 0$ and $\phi_p(x,y,p) \leq 0$ whenever $x > 0$, $y > 0$ and $p > 0$. Our assumptions and definitions lead to the following discrete-time pair-formation nonlinear homogeneous model:

$$
(1) \qquad \left.\begin{aligned}
x(t+1) &= (\beta_x \mu_x \mu_y + (1-\mu_y)\mu_x + (1-\sigma)\mu_x\mu_y)p(t) + \mu_x x(t) \\
&\quad - \rho_G(x(t), y(t), p_x(t), p_y(t)), \\
y(t+1) &= (\beta_y \mu_y \mu_x + (1-\mu_x)\mu_y + (1-\sigma)\mu_x\mu_y)p(t) + \mu_y y(t) \\
&\quad - \rho_H(x(t), y(t), p_x(t), p_y(t)), \\
p_x(t+1) &= \sigma\mu_x\mu_y p(t) + \rho_G(x(t), y(t), p_x(t), p_y(t)), \\
p_y(t+1) &= \sigma\mu_x\mu_y p(t) + \rho_H(x(t), y(t), p_x(t), p_y(t)),
\end{aligned}\right\}
$$

where $\rho_G(x,y,p_x,p_y) = \mu_x x(1 - G(x,y,p_x,p_y))$ and $\rho_H(x,y,p_x,p_y) = \mu_y y(1 - H(x,y,p_x,p_y))$.

We observe that any set of initial conditions $(x(0), y(0), p_x(0), p_y(0))$ in $\mathbb{R}^4_+$ will generate orbits in $\mathbb{R}^4_+$ provided that the real valued nonnegative functions ρ_G and ρ_H satisfy $\rho_G(x,y,p_x,p_y) \leq \mu_x x$ and $\rho_H(x,y,p_x,p_y) \leq \mu_y y$, that is, the number of males and females who find partners at generation t does not exceed the number of single males or females available at time t.

If ρ_G and ρ_H are replaced by the nonnegative function ϕ satisfying $\phi \leq \rho_G$ and $\phi \leq \rho_H$ then we have monogamy. Serial monogamy results whenever the total nonnegative functions that model the rates of pair-formation of males and females per-generation $\rho_G(x,y,p_x,p_y) = \mu_x x(1-G(x,y,p_x,p_y))$ and $\rho_H(x,y,p_x,p_y) = \mu_y y(1-H(x,y,p_x,p_y))$ match, where $p_x(0) = p_y(0)$. Hence, it is assumed throughout that at each point (x, y, p_x, p_y) in $\mathbb{R}^4_+$

$$(*)\qquad \left.\begin{array}{l} p_x(0) = p_y(0), \\ \rho_G(x, y, p_x, p_y) = \rho_H(x, y, p_x, p_y) \equiv \phi(x, y, p), \\ \text{and that } \phi(x, y, p) \leq \min\{\mu_x x, \mu_y y\}. \end{array}\right\}$$

Condition (*) implies that the prior specification of the function G defines H uniquely.

If you are a single female there is a "probability" G of remaining single and a "probability" $1-G$ of finding a partner per-generation. These probabilities are in general different for males and females. If G is given so is $1 - G$ is and (*) defines H and $1 - H$. Note that, $G = H$ implies $\mu_x x = \mu_y y$ or $\frac{x}{y} = \frac{\mu_y}{\mu_x}$ or $\frac{\mu_x x}{\mu_y y} = 1$, that is, (*) requires that the single sex-ratio be given by the ratios of the average life-spans of single individuals or equivalently the effective sex ratio must be equal to 1 for all t.

Let $G(x, y, p, p) \equiv g(x, y, p)$ and $H(x, y, p, p) \equiv h(x, y, p)$. If g is given then the requirement $\rho_G = \rho_H$ implies that h is completely determined. In fact,

$$h(x, y, p) = 1 - (\frac{\mu_x x}{\mu_y y})(1 - g(x, y, p)) = 1 - \frac{\phi(x, y, p)}{\mu_y y}.$$

The assumption that $\phi(x, y, p) \leq \min\{\mu_x x, \mu_y y\}$ implies that h is well defined.

A specific example that incorporates interference competition by all individuals is given by

$$g(x, y, p) = 1 - \frac{\mu_y y}{\mu_x x + \mu_y y}(\frac{\epsilon x + y}{\epsilon x + y + p})$$

where the constant $\epsilon \in [0, \infty)$ is a measure of interference competition from single females. Therefore, the probability of finding a male partner when $p = 0$ is given by $1 - g(x, y, 0) = \frac{\mu_y y}{\mu_x x + \mu_y y}$. That is, the ratio of surviving single males to surviving singles. Hence,

$$\phi(x, y, p) = \frac{\mu_y y \mu_x x}{\mu_x x + \mu_y y}(\frac{\epsilon x + y}{\epsilon x + y + p}),$$

$$h(x, y, p) = 1 - \frac{\mu_y x}{\mu_x x + \mu_y y}(\frac{\epsilon x + y}{\epsilon x + y + p}),$$

and $1 - h(x, y, 0) = \frac{\mu_x x}{\mu_x x + \mu_y y}$, that is, the probability of finding a female partner when $p = 0$ is given by the ratio of surviving single females to surviving singles. Notice that $h \neq g$ and ϕ satisfies all the specified properties.

3. Geometric solutions. Since $p_x(t) = p_y(t) \equiv p(t)$, we can focus on only the first three equations in System (1). Hence, the fixed points satisfy the equation $(x(t+1), y(t+1), p(t+1)) = (x(t), y(t), p(t))$, that is, the fixed points are solutions of the following:

$$(\beta_x\mu_x\mu_y + (1-\mu_y)\mu_x + (1-\sigma)\mu_x\mu_y)p - x + \mu_x x G(x,y,p,p) = 0 \tag{2}$$

$$(\beta_y\mu_y\mu_x + (1-\mu_x)\mu_y + (1-\sigma)\mu_x\mu_y)p - y + \mu_y y H(x,y,p,p) = 0 \tag{3}$$

$$-p + \sigma\mu_x\mu_y p + \mu_x x - \mu_x x G(x,y,p,p) = 0 \tag{4}$$

where $(x(t), y(t), p(t), p(t)) = (x, y, p, p)$. Using Equation (2), (3) and (4) together with the fact that $\mu_x x(t)(1 - G(x(t), y(t), p(t), p(t))) = \mu_y y(t)(1 - H(x(t), y(t), p(t), p(t))) \equiv \phi(x(t), y(t), p(t))$ we obtain that

$$\left.\begin{aligned} \frac{x}{p} &= \frac{\beta_x\mu_x\mu_y + \mu_x - 1}{1-\mu_x}, \\ \frac{y}{p} &= \frac{\beta_y\mu_y\mu_x + \mu_y - 1}{1-\mu_y}. \end{aligned}\right\} \tag{5}$$

Equation (4) implies that $\phi(x, y, p, p) = p(1 - \sigma\mu_x\mu_y)$. Consequently, System (5) and the homogeneity condition on ϕ imply that

$$(1-\sigma\mu_x\mu_y)p = p\phi\left(\frac{\beta_x\mu_x\mu_y + \mu_x - 1}{1-\mu_x}, \frac{\beta_y\mu_y\mu_x + \mu_y - 1}{1-\mu_y}, 1\right). \tag{6}$$

Parameters in System (1) are not likely to satisfy Equation (6). Hence constant solutions rarely exist, that is, they are not generic. We therefore focus on a search for geometric solutions, that is solutions of the form

$$\left.\begin{aligned} x(t) &= \lambda^t x_0, \\ y(t) &= \lambda^t y_0, \\ p(t) &= \lambda^t p_0. \end{aligned}\right\} \tag{7}$$

Substituting (7) in System (1), leads to the following nonlinear eigenvalue problem:

$$\left.\begin{aligned} \lambda x_0 &= (\beta_x\mu_x\mu_y + (1-\mu_y)\mu_x + (1-\sigma)\mu_x\mu_y)p_0 + \mu_x x_0 - \phi(x_0, y_0, p_0), \\ \lambda y_0 &= (\beta_y\mu_y\mu_x + (1-\mu_x)\mu_y + (1-\sigma)\mu_x\mu_y)p_0 + \mu_y y_0 - \phi(x_0, y_0, p_0), \\ \lambda p_0 &= \sigma\mu_x\mu_y p_0 + \phi(x_0, y_0, p_0). \end{aligned}\right\} \tag{8}$$

From (8) we see that,

$$\left.\begin{aligned} \phi(x_0, y_0, p_0) &= (\beta_x\mu_x\mu_y + (1-\mu_y)\mu_x + (1-\sigma)\mu_x\mu_y)p_0 + (\mu_x - \lambda)x_0, \\ \phi(x_0, y_0, p_0) &= (\beta_y\mu_y\mu_x + (1-\mu_x)\mu_y + (1-\sigma)\mu_x\mu_y)p_0 + (\mu_y - \lambda)y_0, \\ \phi(x_0, y_0, p_0) &= (-\sigma\mu_x\mu_y + \lambda)p_0. \end{aligned}\right\} \tag{9}$$

There are two trivial solutions.

$$\left.\begin{aligned} &(1,0,0) \quad \text{with} \quad \lambda = \mu_x, \\ &(0,1,0) \quad \text{with} \quad \lambda = \mu_y. \end{aligned}\right\} \tag{10}$$

Consequently, $[(\mu_x)^t, 0, 0]$ and $[0, (\mu_y)^t, 0]$ are the trivial geometric solutions of System (1). Since there are no pairs then the population eventually becomes extinct whenever $0 \leq \mu_x, \mu_y < 1$. We now look for nontrivial solutions, that is, solutions where $x_0 > 0, y_0 > 0$ and $p_0 > 0$. From System (9) we find that

$$\left.\begin{aligned}(-\sigma\mu_x\mu_y+\lambda)p_0 &= (\beta_x\mu_x\mu_y+(1-\mu_y)\mu_x+(1-\sigma)\mu_x\mu_y)p_0+(\mu_x-\lambda)x_0,\\ (-\sigma\mu_x\mu_y+\lambda)p_0 &= (\beta_y\mu_y\mu_x+(1-\mu_x)\mu_y+(1-\sigma)\mu_x\mu_y)p_0+(\mu_y-\lambda)y_0.\end{aligned}\right\} \tag{11}$$

Hence,

$$\begin{cases} \dfrac{x_0}{p_0} = \dfrac{\beta_x\mu_x\mu_y + \mu_x - \lambda}{\lambda - \mu_x} \\ \dfrac{y_0}{p_0} = \dfrac{\beta_y\mu_y\mu_x + \mu_y - \lambda}{\lambda - \mu_y}, \end{cases}$$

and, $\phi(\frac{x_0}{p_0}, \frac{y_0}{p_0}, 1) = (-\sigma\mu_x\mu_y + \lambda)$. Substituting the above expressions for $\frac{x_0}{p_0}, \frac{y_0}{p_0}$ leads to the characteristic equation of System (1):

$$-\sigma\mu_x\mu_y + \lambda = \phi\left(\frac{\beta_x\mu_x\mu_y}{\lambda - \mu_x} - 1, \frac{\beta_y\mu_y\mu_x}{\lambda - \mu_y} - 1, 1\right), \tag{12}$$

therefore, the existence of geometric solutions depends on proving the existence of positive λ–solutions to (12) with initial condition (x_0, y_0, p_0). This is established in Proposition 1. Note that if Equation (12) has a solution then it is positive.

PROPOSITION 1. *System (9) has two trivial solutions (10) and possibly, a unique nontrivial solution (x^*, y^*, p^*) with $x^* > 0, y^* > 0, p^* > 0$. The nontrivial solution exists provided that either $\mu_x = \mu_y$ or that the following inequalities,*

(i) $\left(\dfrac{\beta_y\mu_y\mu_x}{\mu_x - \mu_y} - 1\right)\phi_y(1, 0, 0) > -\sigma\mu_x\mu_y + \mu_x$ where $\mu_x > \mu_y$,

(ii) $\left(\dfrac{\beta_x\mu_x\mu_y}{\mu_y - \mu_x} - 1\right)\phi_x(0, 1, 0) > -\sigma\mu_x\mu_y + \mu_y$ where $\mu_x < \mu_y$,

are satisfied.

The proof outline of Proposition 1 is in the Appendix.

The matrix equation for the first three equations of System (1) is

$$u(t+1) = Au(t) + f(u(t)), \tag{14}$$

where

$$A = \begin{bmatrix} \mu_x & 0 & \mu_x + \beta_x\mu_x\mu_y - \sigma\mu_x\mu_y \\ 0 & \mu_y & \mu_y + \beta_y\mu_x\mu_y - \sigma\mu_x\mu_y \\ 0 & 0 & \sigma\mu_x\mu_y \end{bmatrix}, \quad u = [x, y, p]' \in \mathbb{R}^3_+$$

and

$f(u) = [-\phi(x, y, p), -\phi(x, y, p), \phi(x, y, p)]'$ is homogeneous ($'$ = transpose).

To establish conditions for the stability of geometric solutions, we let $L : \mathbb{R}^3_+ \to \mathbb{R}_+$ be a linear functional. Observe that $L(\lambda^t u_0) = \lambda^t L(u_0)$. The introduction of the new variable $w(t) = \frac{u(t)}{L(u(t))}$ implies that the geometric solution $u(t) = \lambda^t u_0$ corresponds to $w(t) = \frac{\lambda^t u_0}{\lambda^t L(u_0)} = \frac{u_0}{L(u_0)}$, that is, to a constant solution in $\mathbb{R}^3_+$.

A simple computation transforms System (14) into the following nonlinear system of equations for the new variable $w(t)$:

$$
\left.\begin{array}{rcl} w(t+1) & = & \dfrac{Aw(t)+f(w(t))}{L(Aw(t)+f(w(t)))} \\ L(w(t)) & = & 1. \end{array}\right\} \tag{15}
$$

System (15) is a nonhomogeneous system of difference equations and its fixed points, w_∞, satisfy the equation

$$
w_\infty = \frac{Aw_\infty + f(w_\infty)}{L(Aw_\infty + f(w_\infty))} = \frac{Aw_\infty + f(w_\infty)}{\lambda^*}
$$

where $L(Aw_\infty + f(w_\infty)) \equiv \lambda^*$ is a number (due to the homogeneity of L) and $L(w_\infty) = 1$. Consequently, the fixed points or constant solutions of Equation (15) satisfy the nonlinear eigenvalue problem

$$
\lambda^* w_\infty = Aw_\infty + f(w_\infty). \tag{16}
$$

Equation (16) is equivalent to Equation (8).

If $u(t)$ is a solution of System (14) then $w(t)$ is a solution of System (15). Conversely, if we assume that $\overline{w}$ is a constant solution of System (15) then $u(t) = \overline{w}(\overline{\lambda}^*)^t L(u_0)$ is a solution of System (14) provided that the vector $\overline{w}$ and the number $\overline{\lambda}^*$ form a solution of Equation (16). Hence, System (14) and System (15) are equivalent in the sense that if a solution to System (14) is found then a solution of the other can be immediately determined and vice versa.

4. Local stability of homogeneous systems. Consider a general discrete dynamical system

$$
u(t+1) = F(u(t)) \tag{17}
$$

where $u(t) \in \mathbb{R}^m$ and $F : \mathbb{R}^m \to \mathbb{R}^m$ is a differentiable function satisfying

$$
F(au) = aF(u) \text{ for all } u \in \mathbb{R}^m. \tag{18}
$$

Equation (18) implies that

$$
F(u) = F'(u)u \text{ for all } u \in \mathbb{R}^m. \tag{19}
$$

Notice that $L(w(t)) \equiv 1$ whenever $w(t) = \frac{u(t)}{L(u(t))}$. In the new variable, Equation (17) becomes

$$w(t+1) = \frac{F(w(t))}{L(F(w(t)))} \tag{20}$$

If w_∞ is an equilibrium solution of Equation (20), then

$$w_\infty = \frac{F(w_\infty)}{L(F(w_\infty))} = \frac{F(w_\infty)}{\lambda^*} \tag{21}$$

where $L(w_\infty) = 1$, $L(F(w_\infty)) = \lambda^*$ and $F(w_\infty) = \lambda^* w_\infty$.

Now, let $w(t) = v(t) + w_\infty$. Then the perturbations, $v(t)$, satisfy the equation

$$v(t) = \frac{F'(w_\infty)}{\lambda^*} v(t) - \frac{L(F'(w_\infty)v(t))}{\lambda^*} w_\infty \tag{22}$$

where $v(t) \in \ker L$. Using the following linear operator

$$g'(w_\infty)y = \frac{F'(w_\infty)}{\lambda^*} y - \frac{L(F'(w_\infty)y)}{\lambda^*} w_\infty \tag{23}$$

we obtain the following result (the proof is similar to that of Theorem 2.1 in [24]).

THEOREM 1. (1) *Zero is an eigenvalue of* $g'(w_\infty)$ *with corresponding eigenvector* w_∞.

(2) *If* $\lambda \neq \lambda^*$ *is an eigenvalue of* $F'(w_\infty)$ *with corresponding eigenvector* w, *then* $\frac{\lambda}{\lambda^*}$ *is an eigenvalue of* $g'(w_\infty)$ *with corresponding eigenvector* $w - L(w)w_\infty$ *and* $w - L(w)w_\infty \in \ker L$.

(3) *If* $\lambda \neq \lambda^*$ *is an eigenvalue of* $g'(w_\infty)$ *with corresponding eigenvector* y, *then* λ *is an eigenvalue of* $F'(w_\infty)$ *with corresponding eigenvector* $y + \frac{L(F'(w_\infty)y)}{(\lambda-\lambda^*)} w_\infty$.

Proof. For the proof of (1) proceed using direct substitution. To prove (2), assume that $F'(w_\infty)w = \lambda w$ where $\lambda \neq \lambda^*$. Then

$$\begin{aligned} g'(w_\infty)(w - L(w)w_\infty) &= \frac{F'(w_\infty)w}{\lambda^*} - \frac{L(w)F'(w_\infty)w_\infty}{\lambda^*} - \frac{L(F'(w_\infty)w)w_\infty}{\lambda^*} \\ &\quad + \frac{L(w)L(F'(w_\infty)w_\infty)w_\infty}{\lambda^*} \\ &= \frac{F'(w_\infty)w}{\lambda^*} - \frac{L(F'(w_\infty)w)w_\infty}{\lambda^*} \\ &= \frac{\lambda w}{\lambda^*} - \frac{\lambda L(w)w_\infty}{\lambda^*} \\ &= \frac{\lambda}{\lambda^*}(w - L(w)w_\infty). \end{aligned}$$

To prove (2), assume that $\frac{F'(w_\infty)y}{\lambda^*} - \frac{L(F'(w_\infty)y)w_\infty}{\lambda^*} = \frac{\lambda}{\lambda^*}y$. Then,

$$
\begin{aligned}
F'(w_\infty)(y + \frac{L(F'(w_\infty)y)w_\infty}{(\lambda-\lambda^*)})
&= F'(w_\infty)y + \frac{\lambda^* L(F'(w_\infty)y)w_\infty}{(\lambda-\lambda^*)} \\
&= F'(w_\infty)y - \frac{\lambda L(F'(w_\infty)y)w_\infty}{(\lambda-\lambda^*)} \\
&\quad + \frac{\lambda L(F'(w_\infty)y)w_\infty}{(\lambda-\lambda^*)} + \frac{\lambda^* L(F'(w_\infty)y)w_\infty}{(\lambda-\lambda^*)} \\
&= F'(w_\infty)y - L(F'(w_\infty)y)w_\infty + \frac{\lambda L(F'(w_\infty)y)w_\infty}{(\lambda-\lambda^*)} \\
&= \lambda y + \frac{\lambda L(F'(w_\infty)y)w_\infty}{(\lambda-\lambda^*)} = \lambda(y + \frac{L(F'(w_\infty)y)w_\infty}{(\lambda-\lambda^*)}).
\end{aligned}
$$

□

The following result, Corollary (1), is an immediate consequence of Theorem (1).

COROLLARY 1. *Let $\lambda^*, \lambda_1, ..., \lambda_{m-1}$ be the eigenvalues of $F'(w_\infty)$. Then the geometric solution of System (17) is locally stable if*

$$
\left| \frac{\lambda_i}{\lambda^*} \right| < 1 \text{ for all } i \in \{1, 2, ..., m-1\}
$$

or equivalently,

$$
| \lambda_i | < \lambda^* \text{ for all } i \in \{1, 2, ..., m-1\}.
$$

5. Stability of nontrivial equilibrium. We now investigate the stability of the nontrivial geometric solution $((\lambda^*)^t x_0, (\lambda^*)^t y_0, (\lambda^*)^t p_0)$ of System (1). If we divide by $L(u(t)) \equiv p(t)$ in System (1) and use homogeneity then $\xi(t) = \frac{x(t)}{p(t)}$, $\eta(t) = \frac{y(t)}{p(t)}$ and $\varsigma(t) = \frac{p(t)}{p(t)}$ satisfy the following equations:

$$
\left.
\begin{aligned}
\xi(t+1) &= \frac{\beta_x \mu_x \mu_y + \mu_x + \mu_x \xi(t)}{\sigma \mu_x \mu_y + \phi(\xi(t), \eta(t), 1)} - 1, \\
\eta(t+1) &= \frac{\beta_y \mu_x \mu_y + \mu_y + \mu_y \eta(t)}{\sigma \mu_x \mu_y + \phi(\xi(t), \eta(t), 1)} - 1, \\
\varsigma(t+1) &= 1.
\end{aligned}
\right\} \tag{24}
$$

If $(\xi_0, \eta_0, 1) = (\frac{x_0}{p_0}, \frac{y_0}{p_0}, 1)$ is a positive fixed point of System (24) then the Jacobian matrix at this fixed point is $J(\xi_0, \eta_0, 1) =$

$$
\begin{bmatrix}
\frac{(\sigma\mu_x\mu_y + \phi(\xi_0,\eta_0,1))\mu_x - (\beta_x\mu_x\mu_y + \mu_x + \mu_x\xi_0)\phi_\xi(\xi_0,\eta_0,1)}{(\sigma\mu_x\mu_y + \phi(\xi_0,\eta_0,1))^2} & \frac{-(\beta_x\mu_x\mu_y + \mu_x + \mu_x\xi_0)\phi_\eta(\xi_0,\eta_0,1)}{(\sigma\mu_x\mu_y + \phi(\xi_0,\eta_0,1))^2} & 0 \\
\frac{-(\beta_y\mu_x\mu_y + \mu_y + \mu_y\eta_0)\phi_\xi(\xi_0,\eta_0,1)}{(\sigma\mu_x\mu_y + \phi(\xi_0,\eta_0,1))^2} & \frac{(\sigma\mu_x\mu_y + \phi(\xi_0,\eta_0,1))\mu_y - (\beta_y\mu_x\mu_y + \mu_y + \mu_y\eta_0)\phi_\eta(\xi_0,\eta_0,1)}{(\sigma\mu_x\mu_y + \phi(\xi_0,\eta_0,1))^2} & 0 \\
0 & 0 & 0
\end{bmatrix}
$$

$$= \begin{bmatrix} \frac{(1+\xi_0)(\mu_x-(1+\xi_0)\phi_\xi(\xi_0,\eta_0,1))}{\mu_x(\beta_x\mu_y+1+\xi_0)} & \frac{-(1+\xi_0)^2\phi_\eta(\xi_0,\eta_0)}{\mu_x(\beta_x\mu_y+1+\xi_0)} & 0 \\ \frac{-(1+\eta_0)^2\phi_\xi(\xi_0,\eta_0,1)}{\mu_y(\beta_y\mu_x+1+\eta_0)} & \frac{(1+\eta_0)(\mu_y-(1+\eta_0)\phi_\eta(\xi_0,\eta_0,1))}{\mu_y(\beta_y\mu_x+1+\eta_0)} & 0 \\ 0 & 0 & 0 \end{bmatrix}.$$

Naturally, due to the rescaling $\lambda = 0$, is an eigenvalue of J. Applying the Jury test on the remaining 2 by 2 submatrix with nonzero entries one has that $(\xi_0, \eta_0, 1)$ is asymptotically stable provided that $| \, tra(J(\xi_0, \eta_0, 1)) \, | < 1 + \det(J(\xi_0, \eta_0, 1)) < 2$ where

$$tra(J(\xi_0,\eta_0,1)) = \frac{(1+\xi_0)(\mu_x - (1+\xi_0)\phi_\xi(\xi_0,\eta_0,1))}{\mu_x(\beta_x\mu_y+1+\xi_0)} + \frac{(1+\eta_0)(\mu_y - (1+\eta_0)\phi_\eta(\xi_0,\eta_0,1))}{\mu_y(\beta_y\mu_x+1+\eta_0)}$$

and

$$\det(J(\xi_0,\eta_0,1)) = \left(\frac{(1+\xi_0)(\mu_x - (1+\xi_0)\phi_\xi(\xi_0,\eta_0,1))}{\mu_x(\beta_x\mu_y+1+\xi_0)}\right) \times \left(\frac{(1+\eta_0)(\mu_y - (1+\eta_0)\phi_\eta(\xi_0,\eta_0,1))}{\mu_y(\beta_y\mu_x+1+\eta_0)}\right) - \left(\frac{(1+\eta_0)^2\phi_\xi(\xi_0,\eta_0,1)}{\mu_y(\beta_y\mu_x+1+\eta_0)}\right)\left(\frac{(1+\xi_0)^2\phi_\eta(\xi_0,\eta_0,1)}{\mu_x(\beta_x\mu_y+1+\xi_0)}\right).$$

In fact,

$$tra(J(\xi_0,\eta_0,1)) = \frac{(1+\xi_0)(\mu_x - (1+\xi_0)\phi_\xi(\xi_0,\eta_0,1) + \mu_y - (1+\eta_0)\phi_\eta(\xi_0,\eta_0,1))}{\mu_x\beta_x\mu_y + \mu_x + \mu_x\xi_0}$$

and

$$\det(J(\xi_0,\eta_0,1)) = \frac{(1+\xi_0)^2(\mu_x\mu_y - \mu_y(1+\xi_0)\phi_\xi(\xi_0,\eta_0,1) - \mu_x(1+\eta_0)\phi_\eta(\xi_0,\eta_0,1))}{(\mu_x\beta_x\mu_y + \mu_x + \mu_x\xi_0)^2}.$$

If $tra(J(\xi_0,\eta_0,1)) > 0$, then $| \, tra(J(\xi_0,\eta_0,1)) \, | < 1 + \det(J(\xi_0,\eta_0,1)) < 2$. Moreover, if $\mu_y < (1+\eta_0)\phi_\eta(\xi_0,\eta_0,1)$ or $\mu_x < (1+\xi_0)\phi_\xi(\xi_0,\eta_0,1)$ or $\mu_x\mu_y < (1+\xi_0)(1+\eta_0)\phi_\eta(\xi_0,\eta_0,1)\phi_\xi(\xi_0,\eta_0,1)$, then $(tra(J(\xi_0,\eta_0,1)))^2 - 4\det(J(\xi_0,\eta_0,1)) > 0$ and J has three real eigenvalues: $\lambda = 0$ and

$$\frac{tra(J(\xi_0,\eta_0,1)) \pm \sqrt{(tra(J(\xi_0,\eta_0,1)))^2 - 4\det(J(\xi_0,\eta_0,1))}}{2}.$$

In this situation, the dominant positive eigenvalue is either

$$\left| \frac{tra(J(\xi_0,\eta_0,1)) + \sqrt{(tra(J(\xi_0,\eta_0,1)))^2 - 4\det(J(\xi_0,\eta_0,1))}}{2} \right|$$

or

$$\left| \frac{tra(J(\xi_0,\eta_0,1)) - \sqrt{(tra(J(\xi_0,\eta_0,1)))^2 - 4\det(J(\xi_0,\eta_0,1))}}{2} \right|$$

and the following result is immediate (Corollary 1).

PROPOSITION 2. *In System (24), the nontrivial equilibrium* $(\xi_0, \eta_0, 1)$ *is locally asymptotically stable whenever at least one of the following two conditions is satisfied:*

(1) $tra(J(\xi_0,\eta_0,1)) > 0$

(2) $\mu_x < (1+\xi_0)\phi_\xi(\xi_0,\eta_0,1)$ or $\mu_y < (1+\eta_0)\phi_\eta(\xi_0,\eta_0,1)$ or $\mu_x\mu_y < (1+\xi_0)(1+\eta_0)\phi_\eta(\xi_0,\eta_0,1)\phi_\xi(\xi_0,\eta_0,1)$ and

$$\left| \frac{tra(J(\xi_0,\eta_0,1)) \pm \sqrt{(tra(J(\xi_0,\eta_0,1)))^2 - 4\det(J(\xi_0,\eta_0,1))}}{2} \right| < 1.$$

6. Stability: Original system versus re-scaled system. Now, we use the stability criteria of the previous section to determine the stability of trivial equilibrium solutions. Our results are summarized in the following theorem:

THEOREM 2. *System (1) always has two geometric trivial solutions at*

$$((\mu_x)^t, 0, 0)\, and \quad (0, (\mu_y)^t, 0).$$

If $\mu_x = \mu_y$ *or if the following two sets of inequalities,*

$$(i)\ \left(\frac{\beta_y\mu_y\mu_x}{\mu_x - \mu_y} - 1\right)\phi_y(1,0,0) > -\sigma\mu_x\mu_y + \mu_x \text{ where } \mu_x > \mu_y,$$

$$(ii)\ \left(\frac{\beta_x\mu_x\mu_y}{\mu_y - \mu_x} - 1\right)\phi_x(0,1,0) > -\sigma\mu_x\mu_y + \mu_y \text{ where } \mu_x < \mu_y,$$

are satisfied, then a positive nontrivial geometric solution exists. The nontrivial geometric solution is linearly stable whenever at least one of the following two conditions is satisfied:

(1) $tra(J(\frac{x_0}{p_0}, \frac{y_0}{p_0}, 1)) > 0$

(2) $\mu_x < (x_0 + p_0)\phi_x(x_0, y_0, p_0)$ or $\mu_y < (y_0 + p_0)\phi_y(x_0, y_0, p_0)$ or $\mu_x\mu_y < (x_0 + p_0)(y_0 + p_0)\phi_x(x_0, y_0, p_0)\phi_y(x_0, y_0, p_0)$ *where the nontrivial solution is at* $(\lambda^t x_0, \lambda^t y_0, \lambda^t p_0)$ and

$$\left| \frac{tra(J(\frac{x_0}{p_0}, \frac{y_0}{p_0}, 1)) \pm \sqrt{(tra(J(\frac{x_0}{p_0}, \frac{y_0}{p_0}, 1)))^2 - 4\det(J(\frac{x_0}{p_0}, \frac{y_0}{p_0}, 1))}}{2} \right| < 1.$$

If inequalities (i) and (ii) are satisfied then the two trivial solutions $((\mu_x)^t, 0, 0)$ *and* $(0, (\mu_y)^t, 0)$ are unstable. *Moreover, if*

$$\left(\frac{\beta_y\mu_y\mu_x}{\mu_x - \mu_y} - 1\right)\phi_y(1,0,0) < -\sigma\mu_x\mu_y + \mu_x \text{ where } \mu_x > \mu_y$$

and

$$(\frac{\beta_x \mu_x \mu_y}{\mu_y - \mu_x} - 1)\phi_x(0,1,0) > -\sigma\mu_x\mu_y + \mu_y \text{ where } \mu_x < \mu_y$$

then $((\mu_x)^t, 0, 0)$ *is stable,* $(0, (\mu_y)^t, 0)$ *is unstable and there is no positive nontrivial geometric solution. However, if*

$$(\frac{\beta_y \mu_y \mu_x}{\mu_x - \mu_y} - 1)\phi_y(1,0,0) > -\sigma\mu_x\mu_y + \mu_x \text{ where } \mu_x > \mu_y$$

and

$$(\frac{\beta_x \mu_x \mu_y}{\mu_y - \mu_x} - 1)\phi_x(0,1,0) < -\sigma\mu_x\mu_y + \mu_y \text{ where } \mu_x < \mu_y,$$

then $((\mu_x)^t, 0, 0)$ *is unstable,* $(0, (\mu_y)^t, 0)$ *is stable and there is no positive nontrivial geometric solution.*

Proof. If $\mu_x = \mu_y$ or if either inequality (i) or (ii) is satisfied and $\mu_y < (y_0 + p_0)\phi_y(x_0, y_0, p_0)$ or $\mu_x < (x_0 + p_0)\phi_x(x_0, y_0, p_0)$ or $\mu_x\mu_y < (x_0+p_0)(y_0+p_0)\phi_x(x_0, y_0, p_0)\phi_y(x_0, y_0, p_0)$ then Proposition 1, Proposition 2 and Theorem 1 guarantee the existence of a linearly stable nontrivial geometric solution. First, we show that if λ is any other eigenvalue of $J(1,0,0)$, then $\lambda < \mu_x$. If $\mu_x \neq \mu_y$ then the positive nontrivial geometric solution does not exist whenever either inequality (i) is not satisfied where $\mu_x > \mu_y$ or (ii) is not satisfied where $\mu_x < \mu_y$. Now, we prove the stability of the trivial solutions.

Recall that $(1,0,0)$ is a trivial solution of System (9) where $\lambda = \mu_x$. Notice that

$$\begin{aligned} \phi_x(1,0,0) &= \lim_{h\to 0} \tfrac{\phi(1+h,0,0)-\phi(1,0,0)}{h} \\ &= \lim_{h\to 0} \tfrac{(1+h-1)\phi(1,0,0)}{h} \\ &= \lim_{h\to 0} \phi(1,0,0) = 0. \end{aligned}$$

Consequently,

$$J(1,0,0) = \begin{vmatrix} \mu_x - \lambda & -\phi_y(1,0,0) & \mu_x + \beta_x\mu_x\mu_y - \sigma\mu_x\mu_y \\ 0 & \mu_y - \phi_y(1,0,0) - \lambda & \mu_y + \beta_y\mu_x\mu_y - \sigma\mu_x\mu_y \\ 0 & \phi_y(1,0,0) & \sigma\mu_x\mu_y - \lambda \end{vmatrix}.$$

It is easy to see that μ_x is an eigenvalue of $J(1,0,0)$. Next, we show that if λ is any other eigenvalue of $J(1,0,0)$, then $\lambda < \mu_x$.

$$\begin{vmatrix} \mu_y - \phi_y(1,0,0) - \lambda & \mu_y + \beta_y\mu_x\mu_y - \sigma\mu_x\mu_y \\ \phi_y(1,0,0) & \sigma\mu_x\mu_y - \lambda \end{vmatrix} =$$

$$(\mu_y - \phi_y(1,0,0) - \lambda)(\sigma\mu_x\mu_y - \lambda) - (\mu_y + \beta_y\mu_x\mu_y - \sigma\mu_x\mu_y)\phi_y(1,0,0).$$

Consequently, the other eigenvalues are roots of the characteristic equation

$$\lambda^2 - (\sigma\mu_x\mu_y + \mu_y - \phi_y(1,0,0))\lambda - (\mu_y + \beta_y\mu_x\mu_y - \sigma\mu_x\mu_y)\phi_y(1,0,0) = 0.$$

The discriminant $(\sigma\mu_x\mu_y + \mu_y - \phi_y(1,0,0))^2 + 4(\mu_y + \beta_y\mu_x\mu_y - \sigma\mu_x\mu_y)\phi_y(1,0,0) \geq 0$ implies that all the eigenvalues are real. Let $z = \lambda - \mu_x$. To show that $z < 0$, we first obtain the following characteristic polynomial in terms of the new variable, z :

$$(\mu_y - \phi_y(1,0,0) - z - \mu_x)(\sigma\mu_x\mu_y - z - \mu_x) - (\mu_y + \beta_y\mu_x\mu_y - \sigma\mu_x\mu_y)\phi_y(1,0,0).$$

This corresponds to the characteristic polynomial of the following 2×2 matrix:

$$\overline{J} = \begin{bmatrix} \mu_y - \phi_y(1,0,0) - \mu_x & \mu_y + \beta_y\mu_x\mu_y - \sigma\mu_x\mu_y \\ \phi_y(1,0,0) & \sigma\mu_x\mu_y - \mu_x \end{bmatrix}$$

Notice that the trace of $\overline{J}$ is $tr(\overline{J}) = \mu_y - \phi_y(1,0,0) - 2\mu_x + \sigma\mu_x\mu_y$ and $\det\overline{J} = (\mu_x - \mu_y)(-\sigma\mu_x\mu_y + \mu_x + \phi_y(1,0,0)) - \beta_y\mu_x\mu_y\phi_y(1,0,0)$. By the Routh-Hurwitz criteria, $z < 0$ if the trace is negative and the determinant is positive. If $\mu_x > \mu_y$ then $tr(\overline{J}) < 0$. However, $(\frac{\beta_y\mu_y\mu_x}{(\mu_x - \mu_y)} - 1)\phi_y(1,0,0) > \mu_x - \sigma\mu_x\mu_y$ and $\mu_x > \mu_y$ imply that $\det\overline{J} < 0$ and $z > 0$ while $(\frac{\beta_y\mu_y\mu_x}{(\mu_x - \mu_y)} - 1)\phi_y(1,0,0) < \mu_x - \sigma\mu_x\mu_y$ and $\mu_x > \mu_y$ imply that $\det\overline{J} > 0$ and $z < 0$. Consequently, $(\frac{\beta_y\mu_y\mu_x}{(\mu_x - \mu_y)} - 1)\phi_y(1,0,0) > \mu_x - \sigma\mu_x\mu_y$ and $\mu_x > \mu_y$ implies the instability of $(1,0,0)$ while $(\frac{\beta_y\mu_y\mu_x}{(\mu_x - \mu_y)} - 1)\phi_y(1,0,0) < \mu_x - \sigma\mu_x\mu_y$ and $\mu_x > \mu_y$ implies the stability of $(1,0,0)$. The constraint for ϕ forces $\phi_y(1,0,0) < \mu_y$. To show that $\lambda > -\mu_x$, notice that the variational two by two matrix has non-negative entries so $\max\{|\lambda| : \lambda \text{ is an eigenvalue}\}$ is an eigenvalue itself. For the stability of $(0,1,0)$ proceed exactly as above using inequality (ii). □

7. Application. In the pair-formation model of Kendall [25] and Keyfitz [26], and its subsequent generalizations described in the introduction, it is implicitly assumed that single females interfere with single females and males and that single males interfere with single females and males in their search for available partners. This can be seen immediately from their common use of the harmonic mean, that is, in continuous-time models

$$\phi(x,y) = \rho x(\frac{y}{x+y}) = \rho y(\frac{x}{x+y})$$

where ρx and ρy are the single rates of pair-formation and $\frac{y}{x+y}$ and $\frac{x}{x+y}$ represent the "probabilities" of finding a mate of the right gender (a process that one assumes to be obvious). Here, we assume that $\phi = \phi(x,y,p)$, that is, individuals experience interference competition from paired individuals of the same gender, a more likely possibility at least among humans. To illustrate this situation, we consider System (1) with no delay ($k = 0$) and with

$$g(x,y,p) = \frac{x + (1-\mu_y)y + p}{x+y+p}.$$

Then

$$h(x,y,p) = \frac{(1-\mu_x)x + y + p}{x+y+p}$$

and

$$\phi(x,y,p) = \frac{\mu_x \mu_y xy}{x+y+p}.$$

Consequently, $\phi_x(0,1,0) = \phi_y(1,0,0) = \mu_x\mu_y$.

If $(\frac{\beta_y\mu_y\mu_x}{\mu_x-\mu_y}-1)\mu_y > 1-\sigma\mu_y$ and $(\frac{\beta_x\mu_x\mu_y}{\mu_y-\mu_x}-1)\mu_x > 1-\sigma\mu_x$ then a positive nontrivial geometric solution exists and $((\mu_x)^t,0,0)$ and $(0,(\mu_y)^t,0)$ are unstable (Theorem 2). In this situation, the nontrivial equilibrium is stable whenever

$$1 < \frac{\mu_x x_0(x_0+p_0)(y_0+p_0)}{(x_0+y_0+p_0)^2} \quad \text{or} \quad 1 < \frac{\mu_y y_0(x_0+p_0)(y_0+p_0)}{(x_0+y_0+p_0)^2} \quad \text{or}$$

$$1 < \frac{\mu_x\mu_y x_0 y_0 (x_0+p_0)^2(y_0+p_0)^2}{(x_0+y_0+p_0)^4} \quad \text{and}$$

$$\left| \frac{tra(J(\frac{x_0}{p_0},\frac{y_0}{p_0},1)) \pm \sqrt{(tra(J(\frac{x_0}{p_0},\frac{y_0}{p_0},1)))^2 - 4\det(J(\frac{x_0}{p_0},\frac{y_0}{p_0},1))}}{2} \right| < 1.$$

Moreover, if $(\frac{\beta_y\mu_y\mu_x}{\mu_x-\mu_y} - 1)\mu_y < 1-\sigma\mu_y$ and $(\frac{\beta_x\mu_x\mu_y}{\mu_y-\mu_x} - 1)\mu_x > 1-\sigma\mu_x$ then $((\mu_x)^t,0,0)$ is stable, $(0,(\mu_y)^t,0)$ is unstable and there is no positive nontrivial geometric solution (Theorem 2). Also, if $(\frac{\beta_y\mu_y\mu_x}{\mu_x-\mu_y}-1)\mu_y > 1-\sigma\mu_y$ and $(\frac{\beta_x\mu_x\mu_y}{\mu_y-\mu_x} - 1)\mu_x < 1-\sigma\mu_x$ then $((\mu_x)^t,0,0)$ is unstable, $(0,(\mu_y)^t,0)$ is stable and there is no positive nontrivial geometric solution (Theorem 2).

8. Conclusion. In this article we extend the pair-formation models of Kendall [25], Keyfitz [26], Fredrickson [12], Pollard [37] and Hadeler et al.'s [14–19] to populations with discrete non-overlapping reproductive periods. Pair formation models are important in the study of the dynamics of sexually-transmitted diseases (STDs) but most of their applications have been for human populations ([1–5], [8], [14], [18], [19], [20–25], [28] and [39]). The model and the analysis in this paper provides a framework for the study of STDs in populations n the wild with "advanced" mating systems. The results on existence and stability of geometric solutions parallel those of

Hadeler et al. even for the case when the marriage function ϕ is a function of p, the population size of pairs. Our formalism also allows for the exploration of mating systems on population with complex (chaotic) dynamics. In fact, when $\mu = \mu_x = \mu_y$, the total population $T(t) \equiv x(t) + y(t) + 2p(t)$ satisfies

$$T(t+1) = F(p(t)) + \mu T(t).$$

The exploration of the role of various functional forms for F on the dynamics of a two-sex population leads to an interesting class of mathematical problems for systems of nonlinear difference equations [31–33, 35, 38].

Extensions of the models in this paper to include an integer delay in the recruitment of singles has been carried out by Castillo-Chavez and Yakubu in [9]. In fact, most of the results in this paper are included as a particular case in their paper.

APPENDIX

Proof outline of Proposition 1. To establish the result, we prove that Equation (12), the characteristic equation, has a unique real solution whenever the inequalities (hypothesis) are satisfied.

Let $E(\lambda) = -\sigma\mu_x\mu_y + \lambda$ and $F(\lambda) = \phi(\frac{\beta_x\mu_x\mu_y}{\lambda-\mu_x} - 1, \frac{\beta_y\mu_y\mu_x}{\lambda-\mu_y} - 1, 1)$. Both arguments of ϕ are positive provided that $\frac{\beta_x\mu_x\mu_y}{\lambda-\mu_x} > 1$ and $\frac{\beta_y\mu_y\mu_x}{\lambda-\mu_y} > 1$. Hence, both arguments of ϕ are positive provided that $\lambda > \lambda_{\min} \equiv \max\{\mu_x, \mu_y\}$ and $\lambda < \lambda_{\max} \equiv \min\{\beta_x\mu_x\mu_y + \mu_x, \beta_y\mu_y\mu_x + \mu_y\}$. We assume that $\lambda_{\min} < \lambda_{\max}$ and search for solutions λ in the open interval $(\lambda_{\min}, \lambda_{\max})$.

As λ increases, $E(\lambda)$ is increasing (the left-hand-side of Equation (12)) while $F(\lambda)$ is decreasing (the right-hand-side of Equation (12)). $E(\lambda_{\min}) > 0, F(\lambda_{\max}) = 0$ and $F(\lambda_{\min}^+) = C \leq \infty$. Hence, Equation (12) has a unique solution (unique intersection of $E(\lambda)$ and $F(\lambda)$) in $(\lambda_{\min}, \lambda_{\max})$, if and only if,

$$C > E(\lambda_{\min}) = -\sigma\mu_x\mu_y + \lambda_{\min} > 0. \tag{13}$$

Notice that $\phi(x, 0, p) = \phi(0, y, p) = 0$ and the homogeneity condition on ϕ imply that $\phi_p(1, 0, 0) = \phi_p(0, 1, 0) = 0$. For x large enough ($x \to \infty$), $\phi(x, y, 1) = x\phi(1, \frac{y}{x}, \frac{1}{x}) \approx x[\phi(1, 0, 0) + \phi_y(1, 0, 0)\frac{y}{x} + \phi_p(1, 0, 0)\frac{1}{x}] = y\phi_y(1, 0, 0)$. Therefore,

$$\phi(x, y, 1) \approx \begin{cases} y\phi_y(1, 0, 0) & \text{as } x \to \infty \\ x\phi_x(0, 1, 0) & \text{as } y \to \infty. \end{cases}$$

$$\text{As } \lambda \to \mu_x^+, \frac{\beta_x\mu_x\mu_y}{\lambda - \mu_x} - 1 \to +\infty$$

and

$$\phi(\frac{\beta_x\mu_x\mu_y}{\lambda-\mu_x}-1,\frac{\beta_y\mu_y\mu_x}{\lambda-\mu_y}-1,1)\approx(\frac{\beta_y\mu_y\mu_x}{\mu_x-\mu_y}-1)\phi_y(1,0,0).$$

Similarly,

$$\text{as } \lambda\to\mu_y^+,\ \frac{\beta_y\mu_y\mu_x}{\lambda-\mu_y}-1\to+\infty$$

and

$$\phi(\frac{\beta_x\mu_x\mu_y}{\lambda-\mu_x}-1,\frac{\beta_y\mu_y\mu_x}{\lambda-\mu_y}-1,1)\approx(\frac{\beta_x\mu_x\mu_y}{\mu_y-\mu_x}-1)\phi_x(0,1,0).$$

Therefore,

$$C\approx\begin{cases}\dfrac{\beta_y\mu_y\mu_x-\mu_x+\mu_y}{\mu_x-\mu_y}\phi_y(1,0,0) & \text{as } \lambda\to\mu_x^+,\\ \dfrac{\beta_x\mu_x\mu_y-\mu_y+\mu_x}{\mu_y-\mu_x}\phi_x(0,1,0) & \text{as } \lambda\to\mu_y^+.\end{cases}$$

If $\lambda\to\mu_x^+$ then Equation (13) implies that

$$(\frac{\beta_y\mu_y\mu_x}{\mu_x-\mu_y}-1)\phi_y(1,0,0)>-\sigma\mu_x\mu_y+\mu_x$$

where $\mu_x>\mu_y$.

Similarly, if $\lambda\to\mu_y^+$ then Equation (13) implies that

$$(\frac{\beta_x\mu_x\mu_y}{\mu_y-\mu_x}-1)\phi_x(0,1,0)>-\sigma\mu_x\mu_y+\mu_y$$

where $\mu_x<\mu_y$.

If $\mu_x=\mu_y$ then $\lambda_{\min}<\lambda_{\max}$ and the last two inequalities are satisfied.

Acknowledgments. This study was partially supported by grants from National Science Foundation (NSF Grant DMS 9977919); National Security Agency (NSA Grant MDA 9149710074); Presidential Mentoring Award (NSF Grant HRD 9724850) to Carlos Castillo-Chavez. We thank the office of the provost of Cornell University for its support, and, we thank the Intel Technology for Education 200 Equipment Grant. Abdul-Aziz Yakubu was supported in part by the NSF IGERT Program in Nonlinear Systems at Cornell University. This research was completed while Abdul-Aziz Yakubu was a Visiting Scientist at the Center for Applied Mathematics in Cornell University.

REFERENCES

[1] BUSENBERG, S. AND C. CASTILLO-CHAVEZ, Interaction, pair formation and force of infection terms in sexually-transmitted diseases. In: *C. Castillo-Chavez (ed.), Mathematical and statistical approaches to AIDS epidemiology, pp. 289–300. Lecture Notes in Biomathematics*, Vol. **83**, Springer-Verlag (1989).

[2] CASTILLO-CHAVEZ, C. AND BUSENBERG, S., On the solution of the two-sex problem. In: Proceeding (1991's of the International Conference on Differential Equations and Applications to Biology and Population Dynamics (S. Busenberg & M. Martelli, eds.), *Lecture Notes in Biomathematics*, 80–98, Springer-Verlag (1991).

[3] CASTILLO-CHAVEZ, C., S. BUSENBERG, AND K. GEROW, Pair formation in structured populations, In: J. Goldstein, F. Kappel, and W. Schappacher (eds.), *Differential Equations with Applications in Biology, Physics and Engineering*, 47–65, Marcel Dekker, New York (1991).

[4] CASTILLO-CHAVEZ, C. AND S-F. HSU SCHMITZ, The evolution of age-structured marriage functions: It takes two to tango. *In: Structured-Population models Marine, Terrestial, and Freshwater Systems.* Chapter 18 in S. Tuljapurkar and H. Caswell, eds., Chapman & Hall, New York, pp. 533–550 (1997).

[5] CASTILLO-CHAVEZ, C., S-F. SHYU, G. RUBIN, AND D. UMBAUCH, On the estimation problem of mixing/pair formation matrices with applications to models for sexually-transmitted diseases. In: N.P. Jewell, K. Dietz, and V.T. Farewell (eds.), *AIDS Epidemiology: Methodology Issues*, pp. 384–402. Birkhäuser: Boston (1992).

[6] CASTILLO-CHAVEZ, C. AND W. HUANG, The logistic equation revisited: *Math. Biosc.* **128**:299–316 (1995).

[7] CASTILLO-CHAVEZ, C., W. HUANG, AND J. LI, On the existence of stable pairing distributions, *J. Math. Biol.* **34**(4):413–441 (1996).

[8] CASTILLO-CHAVEZ, C., VELASCO-HERNÀNDEZ, J. X., AND FRIDMAN, S., Modeling Contact Structures in Biology. In *(S.A. Levin, ed.), Frontiers of Theoretical Biology, Lecture Notes in Biomathematics* **100**, *Springer-Verlag* (1994).

[9] CASTILLO-CHAVEZ, C. AND YAKUBU, A.-A., Discrete-time nonlinear pair-formation models with geometric solutions (submitted).

[10] CASWELL, H., Matrix population models: Construction, Analysis, and Interpretation (Second Edition). *Sinauer Associates, Sunderland, Mass* (2001).

[11] CROW, J.F. AND KIMURA, M., An introduction to population genetics theory, Harper & Row, New York (1970).

[12] FREDRICKSON, A.G., A mathematical theory of age structure in sexual populations: Random mating and monogamous marriage models, *Math. Biosci.* **20**:117–143 (1971).

[13] GURTIN, ME. AND C.R. MACCAMY, Non-Linear age dependent population dynamics, *Archive for Rational Mechanic and Analysis*, **54**(3):281–300 (1974).

[14] HADELER, K.P., Modeling AIDS in structured populations. *The 47th Session of the International Statistical Institute, Paris, August/September. Conf. Proc.*, **C1-2.1**:83-99 (1989).

[15] HADELER, K.P., Pair formation in age-structured populations. *Acta Applicandae Mathematicae*, **14**:91–102 (1989).

[16] HADELER, K.P, Pair formation with maturation period, *J. Math. Biol,* **32**:1–15 (1993).

[17] HADELER, K.P., Periodic solutions of homogeneous equations, *J. Diff. Equations,* **95**:183–202 (1992).

[18] HADELER, K.P. AND K. NGOMA, Homogeneous models for sexually-transmitted diseases. *Rocky Mountain Journal of Mathematics*, **20**:967–986 (1990).

[19] HADELER, K.P., WALDSTÄTTER, R., AND WÖRZ-BUSEKROS A., Models for pair-formation in bisexual populations. *Journal of Math. Biol.*,**26**:635–649 (1988).

[20] Hoppensteadt, F., Mathematical Theories of Populations: Demographics, Genetics and Epidemics *SIAM Regional Conference Series in Applied Math.*, num. **20**, Philadelphia (1975).

[21] Hsu Schmitz, S-F, Some theories, estimation methods and applications of marriage functions in demography and epidemiology, *PhD Cornell University dissertation* (1993).

[22] Hsu Schmitz, S-F. and C. Castillo-Chavez, Completion of mixing matrices for nonclosed social networks, In: *Proceedings to the First World Congress of Nonlinear Analysis*, Tampa, Florida, August 19–26 (1992).

[23] Hsu Schmitz, S-F. and Castillo-Chavez, C., Parameter estimation in non-closed social networks related to the dynamics of sexually-transmitted diseases. In: E.H. Kaplan and M.L. Brandeau (eds.), *Modeling the AIDS Epidemic: Planning, Policy, and Prediction*, 533–559. Raven Press, New York (1994).

[24] Iannelli, M. and Martcheva, M., Homogeneous dynamical systems and the age-structured SIR model with proportionate mixing incidence (submitted).

[25] Kendall, D.G., Stochastic processes and population growth, *Roy. Statist. Soc. Ser.* **B2**:230–264 (1949).

[26] Keyfitz, N., The mathematics of sex and marriage, *Proceedings of the Sixth Berkeley Symposium on Mathematical Statistics and Probability*, Vol. IV: Biology and Health, 89–108 (1949).

[27] Lubkin, S., S-F. Hsu Schmitz, and Castillo-Chavez, C., A framework for modeling inheritance of social traits, *In: Proceedings to the First World Congress of Nonlinear Analysis, Tampa, Florida,* August 19–26 (1992).

[28] Luo, X. and C. Castillo-Chavez, Limit behavior of pair-formation for a large dissolution rate. *Journal of Mathematical Systems, Estimation, and Control,* **3**(2):247–264 (1993).

[29] Malthus, T.R., An esssay on the principle of population, *J. Johnson in St. Pauls's Churchyard, London* (1978).

[30] Martcheva, M., An age-structured two-sex population model, *Ph. D. Thesis, Mathematics Department, Purdue University* (1998).

[31] May, R.M., Simple mathematical models with very complicated dynamics, *Nature*, **261**:459–469 (1977).

[32] May, R.M., Stability and complexity in model ecosystems, *Princeton University Press, Princeton.* (1974).

[33] May, R.M., Theoretical ecology principles and applications, *Blackwell Scientific Publications, Oxford* (1981).

[34] McFarland, D., Comparison of alternative marriage models. In (Greville, T. N. E., ed.), *Population Dynamics, Academic Press, New York London*: 89–106 (1972).

[35] Nicholson, A.J., Compensatory reactions of populations to stresses, and their evolutionary significance, *Aust. J. Zool.* **2**:1–65 (1954).

[36] Parlett, B., Can there be a marriage function? In (Greville, T.N.E., ed.), Population Dynamics, *Academic Press, New York London*: 107–135 (1992).

[37] Pollard, J.H., Mathematical models for the growth of human populations, *Chapter 7: The two sex problem, Cambridge University Press* (1973).

[38] Verhulst, P.F., Recherches mathématiques sur la loi d'accroissement de la population, *Mém Acad Roy, Brussels,* **20**(1) (1847).

[39] Waldstätter, R., Models for pair formation with applications to demography and epidemiology, PhD thesis, *University of Tübingen* (1990).

CENTER MANIFOLDS AND NORMAL FORMS IN EPIDEMIC MODELS*

CHRISTOPHER M. KRIBS-ZALETA†

Abstract. Stability analysis of endemic equilibria in epidemic models may be complicated. We apply techniques of center manifolds and normal forms to determine stability through bifurcation analysis. Although the technique is not new, the application and resulting insights are. Some examples lead to a discussion of backward bifurcations and multiple endemic equilibria for $R_0 < 1$. In particular, it is observed that backward bifurcations are sufficient but not necessary to cause endemic stationary states to occur when $R_0 < 1$.

In memory of Jerome Eisenfeld

1. Introduction. As further study is done in population modeling, there is a tendency for the models under study to become increasingly complicated. Modeling usually involves a compromise of sorts, incorporating as many details as possible without making the model too complex to analyze. Even so, the majority of the systems presented in recent literature are complicated enough that only a partial analysis is given. In epidemic models, typically one gives a complete stability analysis for the disease-free equilibrium, which procedure is simplified by the fact that all infective variables are set to zero there. Endemic equilibria do not offer this feature, and consequently their stability is often analyzed more by means of numerical examples and intuition than by traditional methods such as considering the characteristic equation.

At the same time, study of more complicated epidemic models has shown behaviors that diverge from the classical threshold behavior, in which the disease dies out if and only if a certain scalar quantity, called the disease's basic reproductive number or ratio (denoted R_0), is below one, and persists otherwise. In particular, the existence of multiple endemic equilibria has been observed in some cases where the basic reproductive number is less than one ([1], [7], [8], [9], [11], among others). Such behavior has serious biological as well as mathematical consequences; in particular, it may be possible for a disease to persist under conditions which would otherwise preclude an invasion.

This latter phenomenon has recently been associated ([4], [5], [7], [8], [13]) with the so-called "backward bifurcation", a transcritical bifurcation at the threshold point $R_0 = 1$ whose direction can affect the number of endemic equilibria existing on either side of the threshold. For the reader

*This research was partially supported by an REP grant from the University of Texas at Arlington during the summer of 1998.

†Department of Mathematics, University of Texas at Arlington, Arlington, TX 76019-0408.

unfamiliar with the term, a bifurcation is a point where a system's equilibria appear, disappear, and/or change stability.

Specifically, the picture of the bifurcation at $R_0 = 1$ has been understood as follows. In "forward" bifurcations, which occur in the earliest and simplest models, the disease-free equilibrium is globally stable for $R_0 < 1$, and the size of the endemic state grows from zero as R_0 passes 1 (see Figure 1a), so that for R_0 only slightly greater than 1, a small endemic persists. In "backward" bifurcations, however, a disease can persist for $R_0 < 1$ if a sufficient quantity of infectives are introduced into the population, because endemic equilibria exist there (see Figure 1b). Furthermore, as R_0 passes 1, the disease suddenly establishes a large endemic state, which can only be eradicated by reducing R_0 well below 1, to the point where the endemic states disappear. Consequently, deeper study of bifurcations appears warranted.

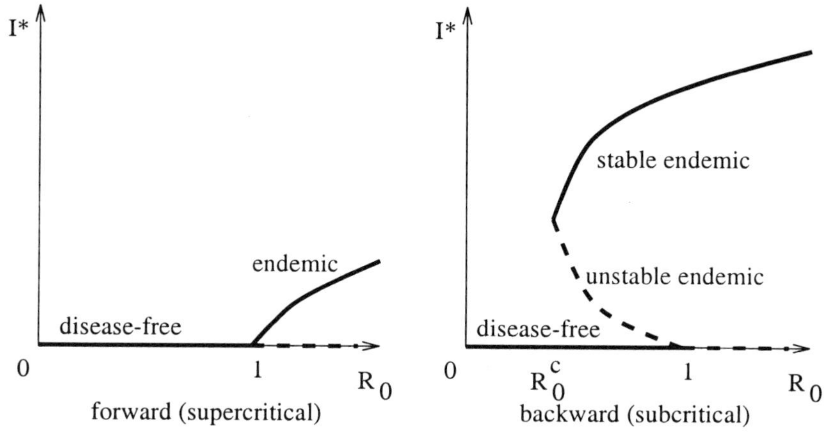

FIG. 1. *Bifurcation diagrams for simple (a) forward and (b) backward bifurcations at* $R_0 = 1$.

This paper presents a technique which addresses both of the above concerns. It provides an alternative way to analyze the stability of a system's equilibria by categorizing the dynamics at bifurcation points. The technique involves constructs called center manifolds and normal forms. This technique itself is not new: The finite-dimensional center manifold theorem can be traced back as far as the 1960's ([10], [14]), while the use of normal forms stems from the doctoral thesis of Poincaré [15]. More recently, Chow and Hale [2], Guckenheimer and Holmes [6] and Wiggins [16], among others, have discussed it in analyzing nonlinear dynamical systems. However, to the author's best knowledge, this approach has not been applied to population models, and as will be shown below, it yields some interesting insights with important consequences, regarding both the mathematics and the epidemiology of the systems of interest.

The idea is a simple one in theory, although the calculations can become involved. Since it is the complexity of the system which complicates analysis, one isolates only those dimensions of the system on which the interesting dynamics occur. Since, at a bifurcation, the number of eigenvalues of the system whose real part crosses zero is usually less than the dimension of the system — and is frequently only one — this isolation effectively reduces the dimension of the system. In the (simplest) case of a bifurcation of codimension one, when only one eigenvalue crosses the imaginary axis, the result is a one-dimensional system.

This subspace of the original state space is called a *center manifold*, i.e., a manifold tangent to the eigenvectors of the zero-crossing eigenvalues at the bifurcation point. Furthermore, since it is the dominant eigenvalue which is crossing $Re(\lambda) = 0$, all the other eigenvalues have negative real part. Consequently, the center manifold is an attractor in the state space. For this reason, it is sufficient to consider the dynamics on the center manifold for purposes of stability analysis.

Once one has reduced the dimension of the system as much as possible, one can compare the dynamics on the center manifold with known canonical (normal) forms, whose behavior is completely known. The normal forms are typically polynomial, with terms separated by order. One therefore performs a Taylor expansion on the vector field representing the dynamics on the center manifold, of as high an order as necessary to match terms with a normal form. A match then yields information about local asymptotic stability of equilibria.

The next section describes the procedure outlined above, and Section 3 provides several examples. Section 4 draws some conclusions from the insights yielded by the examples, and indicates directions for further study.

2. The procedure. We shall now detail the steps involved in applying center manifolds and normal forms to an epidemic model (or other dynamical system). The procedure below follows Wiggins [16].

We shall use an apostrophe to denote the derivative of a vector with respect to the independent variable t: $x' \equiv \frac{dx}{dt}$, and a capital D to denote the derivative of a vector with respect to state variables. Also, we shall use the notation $s(A)$ to denote the *spectral bound* of a matrix A, that is, the real part of its dominant eigenvalue. Bifurcations occur at a point where $s(A)$ crosses 0, for a system represented by the matrix A (in a way we shall describe more precisely below). To simplify the procedure, we shall assume the original vector field to be at least $\mathbf{C}^5$.

To determine the center manifold, we use a linear transformation to separate the dimension(s) of our system which correspond(s) to purely imaginary eigenvalues from those which correspond to eigenvalues with negative real part. (Recall that it is the dominant eigenvalue of the system whose real part crosses zero at a bifurcation, so there are no eigenvalues with positive real part.) The following steps are involved:

1. Suppose we begin with a system $W' = G(W, \rho)$. At the bifurcation point we must identify the equilibrium value W^* and parameter value ρ^*. We first translate the system to put the bifurcation point at the origin, letting $\tilde{W} \equiv W - W^*$ and $p \equiv \rho - \rho^*$ to give us the system $\tilde{W}' = \tilde{G}(\tilde{W}, p)$ with bifurcation point $\tilde{W}^* = 0$, $p = 0$. Now, in preparation for the linear transformation, we separate the linear and nonlinear terms in $\tilde{G}(\tilde{W})$, writing $\tilde{W}' = M\tilde{W} + Kp + F(\tilde{W}, p)$, where $M = d\tilde{G}/d\tilde{W}(0)$ is a constant matrix, $K = \frac{d}{dp}\tilde{G}(0)$ is a constant vector, and $F(\tilde{W}, p) = \mathcal{O}(\tilde{W} \cdot \tilde{W}, p^2)$.

2. We now form our transformation matrix T by augmenting the eigenvectors of M, placing the eigenvectors corresponding to purely imaginary eigenvalues first (since they indicate locally the dimensions along which the center manifold extends) — in other words, T puts M into Jordan canonical form. Our transformation, putting our systems in terms of this eigenvector basis, will be $\tilde{W} = TX$, so that $X \equiv T^{-1}\tilde{W}$ and $X' = T^{-1}\tilde{W}' = (T^{-1}MT)X + T^{-1}Kp + T^{-1}F(TX)$, where $T^{-1}MT$ is now block diagonal.

We can separate X into two vectors x and y, x corresponding to the purely imaginary eigenvalues of M and y to those with negative real part. In the (common) case $K = 0$, we can now write the system as

$$\begin{aligned} &x' = Ax + f(x,y,p), \quad f(0,0,0) = 0, \quad Df(0,0,0) = 0, \quad s(A) = 0,\\ (2.1)\quad &y' = By + g(x,y,p), \quad g(0,0,0) = 0, \quad Dg(0,0,0) = 0, \quad s(B) < 0,\\ &p' = 0. \end{aligned}$$

2a. If $K \neq 0$, then we must deal with the vector $T^{-1}K$ in the above equation for X'. We separate $T^{-1}K$ into two vectors Λ_x and Λ_y of lower dimension corresponding to x and y, and rewrite the system as

$$\begin{pmatrix} x \\ p \\ y \end{pmatrix}' = \begin{pmatrix} A & \Lambda_x & 0 \\ 0 & 0 & 0 \\ 0 & \Lambda_y & B \end{pmatrix} \begin{pmatrix} x \\ p \\ y \end{pmatrix} + \begin{pmatrix} f \\ 0 \\ g \end{pmatrix}$$

Now we must make another linear transformation $X = \tilde{T}\tilde{X}$ to put this new matrix into Jordan canonical form. Note that if $A = 0$, the matrix will not have a full set of eigenvectors, but we can fill in using generalized eigenvectors (i.e., vectors v such that $(P - \lambda I)^n v = 0$ for some $n > 1$, instead of $(P - \lambda I)v = 0$). This additional transformation puts the system into the form of (2.1) if we consider $\tilde{X} = [\tilde{x} \;\; \tilde{y}]^T$ where $\tilde{x}$ includes x and p, and $\tilde{y}$ includes y. Note that when $K \neq 0$ we are obliged to incorporate p into the matrix part of the system in a way that we are not when $K = 0$.

3. We now find a polynomial approximation $y = h(x,p)$ to the center manifold, by taking the derivative of both sides of the equation $y = h(x,p)$ with respect to t:

$$y' = D_x h(x,p)\, x'$$
$$B\, h(x,p) + g(x, h(x,p), p) = D_x h(x,p)\,[Ax + f(x, h(x,p), p)]$$
$$D_x h(x,p)\,[Ax + f(x, h(x,p), p)] - B\, h(x,p) - g(x, h(x,p), p) = 0$$

We can now substitute for $h(x,p)$ a general polynomial of the desired order, e.g., $a_2x^2 + a_1xp + a_0p^2 + \mathcal{O}(3)$, and solve for the coefficients a_i.

4. Finally, we write the differential equation(s) for the dynamics on the center manifold by substituting $h(x,p)$ for y in $f(x,y,p)$. Now we have the system $x' = Ax + f(x, h(x,p), p)$, $p' = 0$.

5. After we have reduced the system to the center manifold at the bifurcation of interest, we Taylor-expand $f(x, h(x,p), p)$ if necessary, so that we can compare it with the known normal forms.

It is important to note that terms of higher order than those specified in the normal forms on which comparison is based do not affect the behavior of a system near a bifurcation point ([16], Chapter 3). Therefore, one need only match polynomial expansions with known normal forms as far as terms are given in the latter.

Normal forms corresponding to the simplest types of bifurcation, including those encountered in the examples to follow, are cataloged in Table 1. The normal form for the Hopf bifurcation can be written in two ways:

Cartesian:

$$x' = \mu(p)x - \nu(p)y + (a(p)x - b(p)y)\,(x^2+y^2)$$
$$y' = \nu(p)x + \mu(p)y + (b(p)x + a(p)y)\,(x^2+y^2)$$

where $\mu(0) = 0$, $\nu(0) = \omega \neq 0$.

Polar:

$$r' = \tfrac{d\mu}{dp}(0)\, pr + a(0)r^3$$
$$\theta' = \nu(0) + \tfrac{d\nu}{dp}(0)\, p + b(0)r^2$$

3. Some examples. We shall now look at some applications of this technique to epidemic models which have already been studied in the context of backward bifurcations and multiple endemic equilibria.

3.1. The basic one-dimensional model. We shall first look at the simplest epidemic model, whose behavior is already completely known, just to see how to apply the technique. We consider the equation $I' = \beta SI - \frac{1}{\tau}I$, where $N = S + I$ is a constant. We can rewrite the equation in terms of a new variable $x \equiv I/N$ as $x' = \beta N\left[\left(1 - \frac{1}{\beta N\tau}\right)x - x^2\right]$.

Knowing that the usual threshold phenomenon manifests as a bifurcation at $R_0 \equiv \beta N\tau = 1$, we define our bifurcation parameter $p \equiv R_0 - 1$, so that the model becomes $x' = \beta N\left[(1 - \frac{1}{p+1})x - x^2\right]$. Since the model is already one-dimensional, we do not have to worry about reducing it to its center manifold (steps 1-4), so we are ready to put it in normal form. We note that there are two equilibria: $x^* = 0$ and $x^* = (1 - \frac{1}{p+1})$, the latter of which is only meaningful (positive) for $p > 0$. We can search for bifurcations of these equilibria by solving $|J - \lambda I| = 0$ for purely imaginary λ, where J is the system's Jacobian matrix, the linearization about a given

TABLE 1

The simplest bifurcations and their normal forms.

Bifurcation type	Normal form	Equivalent description with $x' = f(x,p)$, $f(0,0) = 0$	Bifurcation diagram
Saddle-node (also called turning point)	$x' = p \pm x^2$	$\frac{\partial f}{\partial x}(0,0) = 0$, $\frac{\partial f}{\partial p}(0,0) \neq 0$, $\frac{\partial^2 f}{\partial x^2}(0,0) \neq 0$	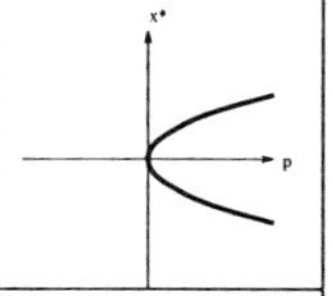
Transcritical	$x' = px \pm x^2$	$\frac{\partial f}{\partial x}(0,0) = 0$, $\frac{\partial f}{\partial p}(0,0) = 0$, $\frac{\partial^2 f}{\partial x\,\partial p}(0,0) \neq 0$, $\frac{\partial^2 f}{\partial x^2}(0,0) \neq 0$	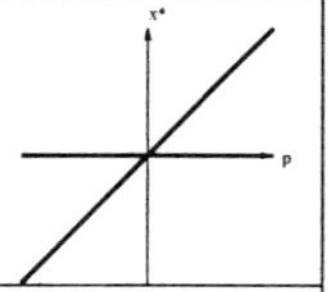
Pitchfork	$x' = px \pm x^3$	$\frac{\partial f}{\partial x}(0,0) = 0$, $\frac{\partial f}{\partial p}(0,0) = 0$, $\frac{\partial^2 f}{\partial x\,\partial p}(0,0) \neq 0$, $\frac{\partial^2 f}{\partial x^2}(0,0) = 0$, $\frac{\partial^3 f}{\partial x^3}(0,0) \neq 0$	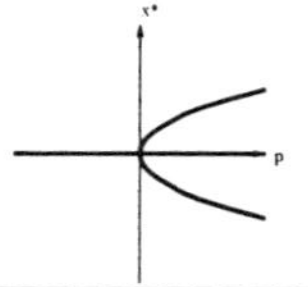
Hopf (Poincaré-Andronov-Hopf)	(see note in text)	$D_x f(0,0)$ has precisely two purely imaginary eigenvalues $\pm i\omega$	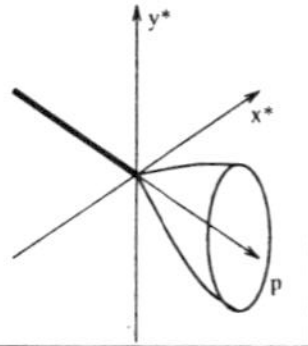

equilibrium. In this simple case, however, we will find that there is only one bifurcation: the one we expect, where the equilibria cross, at $p = 0$.

We can verify that this is a transcritical bifurcation (cf. Table 1) either by expanding $\frac{1}{p+1} = \Sigma_{n=0}^{\infty}(-p)^n = 1 - p + p^2 - \ldots$ for p small, or by showing that the expression for x' obeys the necessary equations and inequalities in the table. If we choose the former option, we find that $x' = \beta N x(p-x) + \mathcal{O}(x^3)$, which further tells us (see the diagram in Table 1) that this transcritical bifurcation is forward (or supercritical) in p, and thus in R_0. In other words, this model never manifests a backward bifurcation.

3.2. A simple two-dimensional model. Dushoff, Huang and Castillo-Chavez [4] present a criterion for determining the direction of the bifurcation at $R_0 = 1$, essentially by examining the sign of the quadratic coefficient of the normal form at that point. In the same paper, they present a $2n$-dimensional model which can exhibit backward bifurcations. When $n = 1$, this model looks like

$$\begin{aligned} I' &= c\lambda I \frac{T-I}{T} - \mu(\sigma+1)I \\ T' &= \Lambda - \mu T - \mu\sigma I \end{aligned}$$

for positive constants c (contact rate), λ (proportion of potentially infectious contacts which infect), μ (mortality rate), σ (disease-related increase in mortality), and Λ (birth rate).

Analysis of the model's characteristic equation finds $R_0 = \frac{c\lambda}{\mu(\sigma+1)}$, with a disease-free equilibrium $(I^*, T^*) = (0, \Lambda/\mu)$ which is globally stable for $R_0 < 1$ and an endemic equilibrium $\frac{\Lambda}{\mu}\left(\frac{R_0-1}{R_0+\sigma(R_0-1)}, \frac{R_0}{R_0+\sigma(R_0-1)}\right)$ which exists, and is locally stable, for $R_0 > 1$. From this analysis we can see that there should be no backward bifurcation at $R_0 = 1$ for the $n = 1$ model. Applying the technique of center manifolds and normal forms agrees with this result, as follows:

1. Consider the bifurcation of the disease-free equilibrium at $R_0 = 1$. We define $\tilde{T} \equiv T - \frac{\Lambda}{\mu}$ and $p \equiv R_0 - 1$, and expand the $\frac{1}{T}$ in the equation for I' using $\dfrac{1}{1+\frac{\mu}{\Lambda}\tilde{T}} = \sum_{n=0}^{\infty}\left(-\frac{\mu}{\Lambda}\tilde{T}\right)^n$. This yields

$$\begin{aligned} \begin{pmatrix} I \\ \tilde{T} \end{pmatrix}' &= \begin{pmatrix} 0 & 0 \\ -\mu\sigma & -\mu \end{pmatrix}\begin{pmatrix} I \\ \tilde{T} \end{pmatrix} + \begin{pmatrix} \mu(\sigma+1)pI - c\lambda\left(\frac{\mu}{\Lambda}\right)I^2 + c\lambda\left(\frac{\mu}{\Lambda}\right)^2 I^2\tilde{T} + \mathcal{O}(I^2\tilde{T}^2) \\ 0 \end{pmatrix} \\ p' &= 0 \end{aligned}$$

2. Based on the eigenvectors of the square matrix above, we make the linear transformation $x \equiv I$, $y \equiv \sigma I + \tilde{T}$ ($I = x$, $\tilde{T} = -\sigma x + y$) and obtain

$$\begin{aligned} x' &= 0x + \left[\mu(\sigma+1)px - c\lambda\left(\frac{\mu}{\Lambda}\right)x^2 + c\lambda\left(\frac{\mu}{\Lambda}\right)^2 x^2(-\sigma x + y) + \mathcal{O}(x^2(x+y)^2)\right] \\ y' &= -\mu y + \left[\mu\sigma(\sigma+1)px - c\lambda\sigma\left(\frac{\mu}{\Lambda}\right)x^2 + c\lambda\sigma\left(\frac{\mu}{\Lambda}\right)^2 x^2(-\sigma x + y) + \mathcal{O}(x^2(x+y)^2)\right] \\ p' &= 0 \end{aligned}$$

3. We next find that the center manifold is $y = -\frac{c\lambda\sigma}{\Lambda}x^2 + \sigma(\sigma+1)px + \mathcal{O}(3)$.

4, 5. On the center manifold, the dynamics are $x' = x[\mu(\sigma+1)p - c\lambda\left(\frac{\mu}{\Lambda}\right)x] + \mathcal{O}(3)$, or $x' = \mu(\sigma+1)x\left[p - (p+1)\left(\frac{\mu}{\Lambda}\right)x\right] + \mathcal{O}(3)$. In either case, we can see that the bifurcation in x is always transcritical, and forward in terms of p, i.e., the bifurcation in I is always forward in terms of R_0.

Hence we must have $n \geq 2$ in order for the model to exhibit a backward bifurcation; in fact, [4] gives an example of one with $n = 2$.

3.3. A vaccination model with a backward bifurcation. In [13], Kribs-Zaleta and Velasco-Hernández present a simple vaccination model which exhibits a backward bifurcation under certain conditions. The model can be written

$$I' = (N - I - (1-\sigma)V)\beta\frac{I}{N} - (\mu + c)I$$
$$V' = \phi(N - I - V) - \beta\sigma V\frac{I}{N} - (\mu + \theta)V$$

where I and V are the numbers of infectives and vaccinated individuals, respectively, the total population N is taken constant, and the parameters are the contact rate β, recovery rate c, natural mortality (and birth) rate μ, vaccination rate ϕ, rate θ at which the vaccine wears off, and factor σ by which the vaccine reduces infections ($\sigma = 0$ for a completely effective vaccine; $\sigma = 1$ for a useless one).

Traditional analysis of this model yields $R_0 = \frac{\beta}{\mu+c} \cdot \frac{\mu+\theta+\sigma\phi}{\mu+\theta+\phi}$, with the disease-free equilibrium $I^* = 0$, $V^* = \phi N/(\mu+\theta+\phi)$ locally asymptotically stable for $R_0 < 1$ and unstable for $R_0 > 1$. When $R_0 > 1$, there is a unique endemic equilibrium, as is usual, but when $R_0 < 1$, a pair of endemic equilibria can exist, iff

(a) $\beta > \mu + c + (\mu + \theta + \sigma\phi)/\sigma$ and

(b) $\beta > \mu + c - (\mu + \theta + \sigma\phi)/\sigma + (2/\sigma)\sqrt{(\mu + c)(1-\sigma)\sigma\phi}$.

Otherwise there are none.

Intuition suggests that when this pair exists, one is an attractor, and the other an unstable saddle point. The characteristic equation, however, is intractable at these equilibria. Now we need to turn to center manifolds and normal forms.

It is shown in [13] that this system exhibits two bifurcations: the expected one at $R_0 = 1$ and another with $R_0 < 1$ which exists when the inequality in (a) above is met, and the inequality in (b) is made an equality. Let us first consider the bifurcation at $R_0 = 1$, with $I^* = 0$, $V^* = \phi N/(\mu + \theta + \phi)$.

1. We define $\tilde{V} \equiv V - \frac{\phi N}{\mu+\theta+\phi}$ and $p \equiv R_0 - 1$, and obtain

$$\begin{aligned} \begin{pmatrix} I \\ \tilde{V} \end{pmatrix}' &= \begin{pmatrix} 0 & 0 \\ -\phi\left(1+\frac{\beta\sigma}{\mu+\theta+\phi}\right) & -(\mu+\theta+\phi) \end{pmatrix} \begin{pmatrix} I \\ \tilde{V} \end{pmatrix} + \begin{pmatrix} -\frac{\beta}{N}I^2 - (1-\sigma)\frac{\beta}{N}I\tilde{V} + (\mu+c)pI \\ -\frac{\beta\sigma}{N}I\tilde{V} \end{pmatrix}, \\ p' &= 0. \end{aligned}$$

2. Using the eigenvectors of the matrix above, we make the transformation

$$\begin{aligned} x &= -\frac{\phi(\mu+\theta+\phi+\beta\sigma)}{(\mu+\theta+\phi)^2} I & \qquad I &= -\frac{(\mu+\theta+\phi)^2}{\phi(\mu+\theta+\phi+\beta\sigma)} x \\ y &= \frac{\phi(\mu+\theta+\phi+\beta\sigma)}{(\mu+\theta+\phi)^2} I + \tilde{V} & \qquad \tilde{V} &= x + y \end{aligned}$$

and obtain

$$\begin{aligned} x' &= 0x + \frac{\beta}{N}\left[\frac{(\mu+\theta+\phi)^2}{\phi(\mu+\theta+\phi+\beta\sigma)} - (1-\sigma)\right] x^2 \\ &\quad -(1-\sigma)\frac{\beta}{N} xy + (\mu+c)px \\ y' &= -(\mu+\theta+\phi)y + (1-\sigma)\frac{\beta}{N}\left[1 - \frac{(\mu+\theta+\phi)^2}{\phi(\mu+\theta+\phi+\beta\sigma)}\right] x^2 \\ &\quad + \frac{\beta}{N}\left[(1-\sigma) + \sigma\frac{(\mu+\theta+\phi)^2}{\phi(\mu+\theta+\phi+\beta\sigma)}\right] xy - (\mu+c)px \\ p' &= 0 \end{aligned}$$

3. We find the center manifold

$$y = \frac{\beta}{N}(1-\sigma)\left[\frac{\phi(\mu+\theta+\phi+\beta\sigma) - (\mu+\theta+\phi)^2}{\phi(\mu+\theta+\phi+\beta\sigma)(\mu+\theta+\phi)}\right] x^2 - \frac{\mu+c}{\mu+\theta+\phi} xp + O(3).$$

4. On the manifold,

$$x' = (\mu+c)px - \frac{\beta}{N}\left[(1-\sigma) - \frac{(\mu+\theta+\phi)^2}{\phi(\mu+\theta+\phi+\beta\sigma)}\right] x^2 + \frac{\beta}{N}(1-\sigma)\frac{\mu+c}{\mu+\theta+\phi} x^2 p + O(x^3)$$

5. Comparing this with the normal forms in Table 1, we see that the bifurcation is transcritical iff $h \equiv \left[(1-\sigma) - \frac{(\mu+\theta+\phi)^2}{\phi(\mu+\theta+\phi+\beta\sigma)}\right] \neq 0$, and forward in x (and thus backward in I) iff $h > 0$. (A linear transformation can remove the x^2p term, so we consider the first two.)

Furthermore, this form gives local stability information about the endemic equilibrium: it is stable if the bifurcation is forward in I, and unstable if the bifurcation is backward in I (cf. Figure 1 (a) and (b) at $R_0 = 1$). This single condition may appear to conflict with the multiple conditions given above, but those are for the existence of endemic equilibria, and as can be seen in Figure 1(b), it is possible to have a backward bifurcation without endemic equilibria (if $R_0 < R_0^c$). Substituting $R_0 < 1$ (solved for $\mu + c$) into condition (a) above yields the inequality $h > 0$.

We now consider the other bifurcation this model can exhibit, when $R_0 < 1$, inequality (a) holds, and (b) is an equality. Note that this bifurcation only exists when the other bifurcation is backward in I and R_0, since it was pointed out above that $R_0 < 1$ and (a) together imply $h > 0$.

Here for ease of notation we define the quantity $B \equiv \sigma[\beta - (\mu + c)] - (\mu + \theta + \sigma\phi)$. Condition (a) is equivalent to $B > 0$, and from (b) we get the equation $B^2 + 4\beta\sigma(\mu + \theta + \sigma\phi)\left(1 - \frac{1}{R_0}\right) = 0$.

1. At the bifurcation point we define $p^2 \equiv B^2 + 4\beta\sigma(\mu+\theta+\sigma\phi)\left(1 - \frac{1}{R_0}\right)$, motivated by the equation above and the quadratic endemic equilibrium condition (cf. Section 2.2 of [13]). Now we have $I^* = \frac{(B+p)N}{2\beta\sigma}$ and $V^* = \frac{\phi N}{\beta\sigma}\cdot\frac{2\beta\sigma-(B+p)}{2(\mu+\theta+\phi)+B+p}$. We therefore define $\tilde{I} \equiv I - I^*\big|_{p=0}$ and $\tilde{V} \equiv V - V^*\big|_{p=0}$. This gives us

$$
\begin{aligned}
\begin{pmatrix} \tilde{I} \\ \tilde{V} \end{pmatrix}' &= \begin{pmatrix} -\frac{B}{2\sigma} & -(1-\sigma)\frac{B}{2\sigma} \\ -\frac{2\phi(\mu+\theta+\phi+\beta\sigma)}{B+2(\mu+\theta+\phi)} & -\left[\frac{B}{2} + (\mu+\theta+\phi)\right] \end{pmatrix} \begin{pmatrix} \tilde{I} \\ \tilde{V} \end{pmatrix} + \begin{pmatrix} \frac{BN}{4\beta\sigma^2[B+2(\mu+\theta+\phi)]} \\ 0 \end{pmatrix} p \\
&\quad + \begin{pmatrix} -\frac{\beta}{N}\tilde{I}^2 - (1-\sigma)\frac{\beta}{N}\tilde{I}\tilde{V} + \frac{1-[B+2(\mu+\theta+\phi)]}{2\sigma[B+2(\mu+\theta+\phi)]}\tilde{I}p - \frac{1-\sigma}{2\sigma}\tilde{V}p + kp^2 + \mathcal{O}(3) \\ -\frac{\beta\sigma}{N}\tilde{I}\tilde{V} + \frac{2\phi(\mu+\theta+\phi+\beta\sigma)}{[B+2(\mu+\theta+\phi)]^2}\tilde{I}p - \frac{1}{2}\tilde{V}p + \mathcal{O}(3) \end{pmatrix}, \\
p' &= 0,
\end{aligned}
$$

where $k = \left(\frac{(\mu+\theta+\phi)N}{2\beta\sigma^2[B+2(\mu+\theta+\phi)]^2} - \frac{(1-\sigma)\phi(\mu+\theta+\phi+\beta\sigma)BN}{\beta\sigma^2[B+2(\mu+\theta+\phi)]^3}\right)$.

2. We now use the eigenvectors of the matrix above to make the transformation

$$
x \equiv \frac{-\frac{\sigma}{1-\sigma}[B + 2(\mu+\theta+\phi)]\tilde{I} + B\tilde{V}}{B + \sigma[B + 2(\mu+\theta+\phi)]}, \quad y \equiv \frac{\frac{1}{1-\sigma}\tilde{I} + \tilde{V}}{B + \sigma[B + 2(\mu+\theta+\phi)]},
$$

$\tilde{I} = -(1-\sigma)x + (1-\sigma)By$, $\tilde{V} = x + \sigma[B + 2(\mu+\theta+\phi)]y$. We obtain the system

$$
\begin{aligned}
\begin{pmatrix} x \\ y \end{pmatrix}' &= \begin{pmatrix} 0 & 0 \\ 0 & -\frac{B+\sigma[B+2(\mu+\theta+\phi)]}{2\sigma} \end{pmatrix} \begin{pmatrix} x \\ y \end{pmatrix} \\
&\quad + \frac{BN}{4\beta\sigma^2(1-\sigma)(B+\sigma[B+2(\mu+\theta+\phi)])} \begin{pmatrix} -\sigma \\ \frac{1}{[B+2(\mu+\theta+\phi)]} \end{pmatrix} p + \mathcal{O}(2), \\
p' &= 0.
\end{aligned}
$$

2a. Here, the linear term in p obliges us to make the extra step detailed in the previous section. We first rewrite the system, using the abbreviation $Q \equiv [B + 2(\mu+\theta+\phi)]$:

$$
\begin{pmatrix} x \\ p \\ y \end{pmatrix}' = \begin{pmatrix} 0 & -\frac{BN}{4\beta\sigma(1-\sigma)(B+\sigma Q)} & 0 \\ 0 & 0 & 0 \\ 0 & \frac{BN}{4\beta\sigma^2(1-\sigma)Q(B+\sigma Q)} & -\frac{B+\sigma Q}{2\sigma} \end{pmatrix} \begin{pmatrix} x \\ p \\ y \end{pmatrix} + \mathcal{O}(2)
$$

Next we make the following linear transformation, based on the matrix's two eigenvectors and first generalized eigenvector (for $\lambda = 0$):

$$\tilde{x} \equiv x, \qquad x = \tilde{x}$$

$$\tilde{p} \equiv \frac{2\sigma}{B+\sigma Q} p, \qquad p = \frac{B+\sigma Q}{2\sigma}\tilde{p}$$

$$\tilde{y} \equiv y - \frac{BN}{2\beta\sigma(1-\sigma)Q(B+\sigma Q)^2} p, \qquad y = \frac{BN}{4\beta\sigma^2(1-\sigma)Q(B+\sigma Q)}\tilde{p} + \tilde{y}$$

This gives the system

$$\begin{pmatrix} \tilde{x} \\ \tilde{p} \\ \tilde{y} \end{pmatrix}' = \begin{pmatrix} 0 & -\frac{BN}{8\beta\sigma^2(1-\sigma)} & 0 \\ 0 & 0 & 0 \\ 0 & 0 & -\frac{B+\sigma Q}{2\sigma} \end{pmatrix} \begin{pmatrix} \tilde{x} \\ \tilde{p} \\ \tilde{y} \end{pmatrix} + \mathcal{O}(2)$$

3. We now find the center manifold in terms of x and $\tilde{p}$; it is $\tilde{y} = -\frac{\beta}{N}\frac{2\sigma^2(1-\sigma)}{(B+\sigma Q)^2}x^2 + bx\tilde{p} + c\tilde{p}^2 + \mathcal{O}(3)$, where b and c are constants defined in terms of the model parameters.

4. On the center manifold,

$$\begin{aligned} x' &= -\frac{BN}{4\beta\sigma(1-\sigma)(B+\sigma[B+2(\mu+\theta+\phi)])}p \\ &\quad + \frac{\beta}{N}\sigma(1-\sigma)\frac{B}{B+\sigma[B+2(\mu+\theta+\phi)]}x^2 \\ &\quad + O(xp) + O(p^2) + O(3). \end{aligned}$$

5. Comparing this form with those given in Table 1, we see that it is a saddle-node bifurcation.

This fact gives us information on the local stability of the two endemic equilibria which meet at this bifurcation, and (since we know in this case that there are no other bifurcations) confirms that the bifurcation diagram in Figure 1 holds for this system. We can classify its behavior as follows:

(i) if $R_0 < 1$ and conditions (a) and (b) above hold, then there are two endemic equilibria, one of which is locally stable and competes with the locally stable disease-free equilibrium;

(ii) otherwise, if $R_0 < 1$, the disease-free equilibrium is a global attractor;

(iii) if $R_0 > 1$, the unique endemic equilibrium is the global attractor. Note that the conditions which permit endemic equilibria when $R_0 < 1$ involve parameter values in an intermediate range: β, σ and ϕ neither too high nor too low. A more detailed discussion of these results are given in [13], and some conclusions are drawn in the final section of this paper.

Also given in [13] is an extension of this system which includes the model of Hadeler and Castillo-Chavez ([7], system (4)) by adding a term $+c\gamma I$ to the equation for V' above, where γ represents some proportion of recovering infectives who pass directly into the vaccinated class upon recovery. Bifurcation analysis for this more general model yields results identical to those obtained above, with analogous conditions (a') and (b'):

(a') $\beta > \mu + c + (\mu + \theta + \sigma\phi + (1-\sigma)c\gamma)/\sigma$,

(b') $\beta > \mu + c - (\mu + \theta + \sigma\phi - (1-\sigma)c\gamma)/\sigma + \frac{2}{\sigma}\sqrt{(\mu + c)(1-\sigma)\sigma\phi - c\gamma(1-\sigma)(\mu+\theta+\sigma\phi)}$,

and a backward bifurcation occurring when

$$h' \equiv \left[(1-\sigma) - \frac{(\mu+\theta+\phi)^2}{\phi(\mu+\theta+\phi+\beta\sigma) - c\gamma(\mu+\theta+\phi)}\right] > 0.$$

3.4. A core group model with recruitment. Kribs-Zaleta [11], [12] presents models for a heterosexually transmitted disease in which one gender is divided into core (very active) and noncore (less active) groups, with a nonlinear recruitment term into the core, dependent on the prevalence of disease in the core, and a linear back-recruitment, or defection, term for core members returning to the noncore. This type of multi-group movement, like that between the susceptible and vaccinated compartments in the model above, can cause multiple endemic equilibria to exist.

The simplest of the models given which exhibits multiple endemic equilibria (called the three-dimensional Case I model in the references) can be written as the following system of ODEs:

$$\begin{aligned} I_2'(t) &= c_2\beta_{23}\frac{I_3(t)}{T_3(t)}\left[T_2 - I_2(t)\right] - \frac{1}{\tau}I_2(t) \\ I_3'(t) &= c_2\beta_{32}\frac{T_3(t) - I_3(t)}{T_3(t)}I_2(t) - \frac{1}{\tau}I_3(t) \\ T_3'(t) &= r_0 e^{-bI_3(t)/T_3(t)}\left[T_f - T_3(t)\right] - \mu\left[T_3(t) - I_3(t)\right] \end{aligned} \tag{3.1}$$

where the subscript 2 denotes the male population, the subscript 3 denotes the female core, and parameters are: c_2 for male activity/contact rate (female core activity/contact rate is written as a function of c_2 and the core size $T_3(t)$, while the female noncore is assumed inactive), infection probabilities β_{23} (female to male) and β_{32} (male to female), average recovery rate $1/\tau$ written in terms of average infection duration τ, base recruitment rate r_0, back-recruitment rate μ, and dimensionless parameter b measuring how much the disease incidence in the core discourages recruitment into the core.

Note that the variability of the total female core causes a singularity at $T_3 = 0$, and indeed it is for small values of T_3 that the unusual behavior occurs. As usual for this type of epidemic model, there is always a disease-free equilibrium, in which $I_2^* = I_3^* = 0$, and $T_3^* = T_{3DF} \equiv \frac{r_0}{\mu + r_0}T_f$;

its (local) stability is determined by $R_0 = c_2\tau\sqrt{\beta_{23}\beta_{32}\frac{\mu + r_0}{r_0}\frac{T_2}{T_f}}$. The following rather technical result from [11] and [12] specifies the number of endemic equilibria.

Theorem. For the model (3.1), with R_0 as given above, the number of endemic equilibria is determined by the following conditions:

(C1) $b > b_{min} \equiv \frac{\beta_{23}(c_2\tau)}{1+\beta_{23}(c_2\tau)}(3 + 2\sqrt{2})\left(\frac{\beta_{32}(c_2\tau)T_2}{T_f} + 1\right)$;

(C2) $\mu_s(T_+) < \mu < \mu_s(T_-)$, where $\mu_s(T_+)$ and $\mu_s(T_-)$ are functions of all system parameters but μ, given in [11], [12];

(C3) $b < b_{split} \equiv \dfrac{[2 + \beta_{23}(c_2\tau)]T_f - \beta_{23}\beta_{32}(c_2\tau)^2 T_2}{T_f - \beta_{23}\beta_{32}(c_2\tau)^2 T_2}$;

(C4) $\left(\sqrt{2} - \beta_{23}(c_2\tau)\right) T_f < \beta_{23}\beta_{32}(c_2\tau)^2 T_2\,(1 + \sqrt{2})$;

(C5) $T_f < \beta_{23}\beta_{32}(c_2\tau)^2 T_2$, (or, equivalently, $R_0 > \sqrt{\frac{\mu+r_0}{r_0}}$).

If $R_0 < 1$, there are 2 endemic equilibria iff conditions (C1) and (C2), and either (C4) or $b > b_{split}$ (the reverse of (C3)), hold. Otherwise there are none. If $R_0 > 1$, then there are 3 endemic equilibria iff conditions (C1) and (C2), and either both (C3) and (C4), or (C5) alone, hold. Otherwise there is only one.

As in the previous example, the possible existence of endemic equilibria for $R_0 < 1$ gives reason to believe a backward bifurcation may be present. An important difference, however, from the previous example is that multiple endemic equilibria may also occur for $R_0 > 1$. We proceed with an analysis of the bifurcation at $R_0 = 1$ which will shed some light on this result.

1. We begin by defining $\tilde{T}_3 \equiv T_3 - T_{3DF}$ (not to be confused with the quantity $\tilde{T}_3$ used in [11], [12]) and expanding the $1/T_3$ and exponential terms, in order to rewrite the system as

$$\begin{pmatrix} I_2 \\ I_3 \\ \tilde{T}_3 \end{pmatrix}' = \begin{pmatrix} -\frac{1}{\tau} & c_2\beta_{23}\frac{T_2}{T_{3DF}} & 0 \\ c_2\beta_{32} & -\frac{1}{\tau} & 0 \\ 0 & \mu(1-b) & -(\mu + r_0) \end{pmatrix} \begin{pmatrix} I_2 \\ I_3 \\ \tilde{T}_3 \end{pmatrix}$$
$$+ \begin{pmatrix} -\frac{c_2\beta_{23}}{T_{3DF}} I_2 I_3 - \frac{c_2\beta_{23}T_2}{T_{3DF}^2} I_3\tilde{T}_3 + \mathcal{O}(3) \\ -c_2\beta_{32}\frac{1}{T_{3DF}} I_2 I_3 + \mathcal{O}(3) \\ \frac{\mu b^2}{2T_{3DF}} I_3^2 + \frac{(\mu+r_0)b}{T_{3DF}} I_3\tilde{T}_3 + \mathcal{O}(3) \end{pmatrix}$$

2. Now we define the bifurcation parameter $p \equiv R_0 - 1$ and implement the linear transformation

$$\begin{pmatrix} x \\ y_1 \\ y_2 \end{pmatrix} =$$

$$\begin{pmatrix} \frac{1}{2(p+1)(p+(\mu+r_0)\tau)} & \frac{1}{2\beta_{32}c_2\tau(p+(\mu+r_0)\tau)} & 0 \\ \frac{1}{2(p+1)(p+2-(\mu+r_0)\tau)} & -\frac{1}{2\beta_{32}c_2\tau(p+2-(\mu+r_0)\tau)} & 0 \\ -\frac{\mu\tau(1-b)\beta_{32}c_2\tau}{(p+(\mu+r_0)\tau)(p+2-(\mu+r_0)\tau)} & \frac{\mu\tau(1-b)((\mu+r_0)\tau-1)}{(p+(\mu+r_0)\tau)(p+2-(\mu+r_0)\tau)} & 1 \end{pmatrix} \begin{pmatrix} I_2 \\ I_3 \\ \tilde{T}_3 \end{pmatrix}$$

so that we can rewrite the system again, as

$$x' = 0x + \frac{1}{\tau}px + A_{200}x^2 + A_{110}xy_1 + A_{101}xy_2 + A_{020}y_1^2 + A_{011}y_1y_2 + \mathcal{O}(3)$$

$$y_1' = -\frac{2}{\tau}y_1 - \frac{1}{\tau}py_1 + B_{200}x^2 + B_{110}xy_1 + B_{101}xy_2 + B_{020}y_1^2 + B_{011}y_1y_2 + \mathcal{O}(3)$$

$$y_2' = -(\mu+r_0)y_2 + C_{200}x^2 + C_{110}xy_1 + C_{101}xy_2 + C_{020}y_1^2 + C_{011}y_1y_2 + \mathcal{O}(3).$$

where the A_{ijk}, B_{ijk} and C_{ijk} are given functions of system parameters. Note that in order to do all of this, we must have $(\mu + r_0)\tau \neq 2$, so that the eigenvalues corresponding to y_1 and y_2 are distinct. (The case $(\mu+r_0)\tau = 2$ would simply require a different transformation.)

3. We find that the center manifold is $y_1 = B_{200}\frac{\tau}{2}x^2 + \mathcal{O}(3)$, $y_2 = \frac{C_{200}}{\mu}x^2 + \mathcal{O}(3)$.

4. On the center manifold, we have $x' = \frac{1}{\tau}px + A_{200}x^2 + \mathcal{O}(3)$.

5. Comparing the above equation with those in the table, we see, as expected, that the bifurcation is transcritical iff $A_{200} \neq 0$, and backward in x and I_2 iff $A_{200} > 0$. Given that

$$A_{200} = -\frac{\mu + r_0}{2T_f\tau}(\beta_{32}c_2\tau)\frac{\mu}{r_0}\left[1 + \frac{\mu + r_0}{\mu}(1 + \beta_{23}c_2\tau) - b\right],$$

we can rewrite the criterion for a backward bifurcation by solving the term in square brackets for b: $b > b_{bif} \equiv 1 + \frac{\mu+r_0}{\mu}(1 + \beta_{23}c_2\tau)$.

Analysis of other bifurcation points of System (3.1) is complicated by the fact that one of the equilibrium conditions involves an exponential term. However, numerical examples can be used to verify the saddle-node bifurcation which typically accompanies the backward bifurcation in epidemic models (cf. Figure 1(b)).

If we now compare the condition $b > b_{bif}$ for a backward bifurcation with the existence conditions for two endemic equilibria, we will see that they are not equivalent. More precisely, it is possible to satisfy the latter conditions without having $b > b_{bif}$, which appears to contradict intuition. The explanation for this phenomenon also accounts for the possibility of having three endemic equilibria when $R_0 > 1$: namely, System (3.1) can exhibit a pair of saddle-node bifurcations in the absence of a backward bifurcation. The bifurcations create an extra pair of endemic equilibria in the region "between" them, which region may or may not extend into $R_0 < 1$. Figure 2 illustrates this possibility with a bifurcation diagram in terms of the activity rate c_2 (R_0 is a linear function of c_2) and the equilibrium value I_2^*, for which there is a forward transcritical bifurcation at $R_0 = 1$ but multiple endemic equilibria for both $R_0 < 1$ and $R_0 > 1$. Here we can see that the backwardness of the bifurcation at $R_0 = 1$ is not a necessary condition for the existence of endemic equilibria when $R_0 < 1$. One might call this a "forward-backward" bifurcation pair: a saddle-node bifurcation turns the equilibrium curve back across $R_0 = 1$ following the normal forward bifurcation.

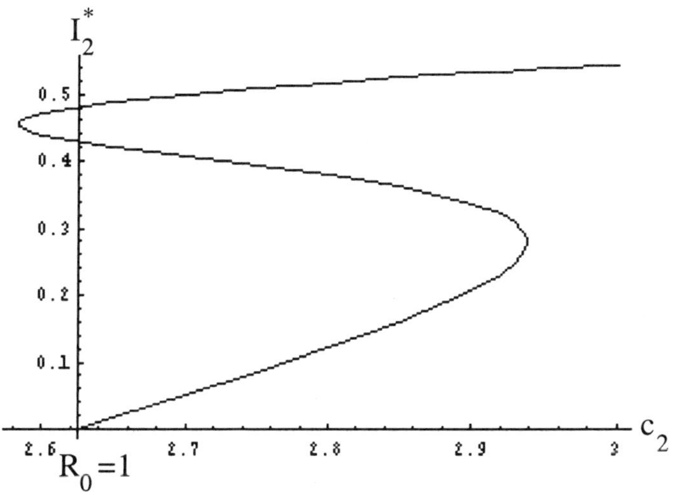

FIG. 2. *A bifurcation diagram showing a forward bifurcation at* $R_0 = 1$ *and multiple endemic equilibria for* $R_0 < 1$.

Proving that the backward bifurcation at $R_0 = 1$ and the extra pair of endemic equilibria for $R_0 > 1$ are mutually exclusive is hindered by the complicated expression for $\mu_s(T_-)$ (see [11], [12]), but a picture may serve to give an idea of what happens. Figure 3 graphs boundaries of the bifurcation and equilibrium criteria in terms of μ and b, for the case where (C4) holds but not (C5). (If (C4) does not hold, there can be no extra endemic equilibria for $b_{min} < b < b_{split}$. If (C5) holds, the region in the graph between b_{min} and b_{split} is extended to include the entire half-plane $b > b_{min}$. Note (C5) implies (C4).)

The conclusion, then, is that if $R_0 < 1$, a sufficiently large value of b will guarantee a locally stable endemic equilibrium which will compete with the disease-free equilibrium. If $R_0 > 1$, the possibility of multiple endemic equilibria depends on the parameters unrelated to recruitment and defection: If (C4) does not hold, there is only one endemic equilibrium. If (C4) but not (C5) holds, there is a range of μ for which three endemic equilibria exist iff $b_{min} < b < b_{split}$. If (C5) holds, for all values of b there is a range of μ in which three endemic equilibria exist.

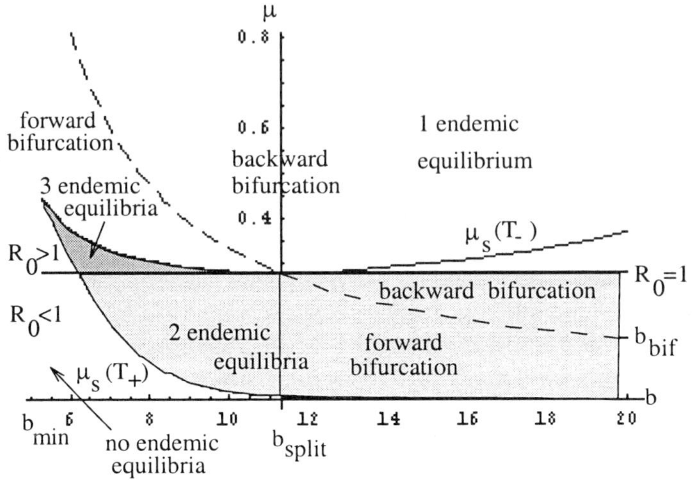

FIG. 3. *Number of endemic equilibria of model (3.1) in terms of* μ *and* b *given that condition (C4) holds and (C5) does not.*

4. Discussion. As evidenced in the above examples, the technique of center manifolds and normal forms provides an alternative way to obtain information analytically about the stability of equilibria and the behavior more generally of epidemic models. Approaches have been suggested before to determine the direction of the bifurcation at $R_0 = 1$ [4], [8], but the method of normal forms applies more generally to cases when this bifurcation may not be transcritical, and to other bifurcations of a system. Comparison of the criteria derived from this method with the conditions for existence of multiple endemic equilibria can also prove enlightening: for the models of [7] and [13], for example, we found the two essentially equivalent, implying that the backward bifurcation accounted for the equilibria, while for the model of [12] they were not, leading to the realization that multiple endemic equilibria can occur without a backward bifurcation. This last fact may have important ramifications in deciding precisely what question to ask: if we have been led to ask "What causes backward bifurcations?" by the fact that backward bifurcations can cause epidemiologically undesirable phenomena, we must now broaden our investigations to include other types of bifurcations which also affect model behavior.

As with other, more classical techniques, the complexity of the calculations required in this approach rises with the complexity of the model under study; one may obtain a criterion for backward bifurcation which is so complicated as to make biological interpretation difficult if not impossible. However, at the very least it remains within reach for some cases where more classical approaches do not.

We may now consider results from the examples above to try to explain what causes backward bifurcations. For the model of [13] generalized to include that of [7], the criterion is

$$\beta > \frac{(\mu+\theta+\phi)(\mu+\theta+\sigma\phi+c\gamma(1-\sigma))}{\sigma(1-\sigma)\phi}$$

Here we see that a backward bifurcation requires a high contact rate β, a mediocre vaccine efficiency σ (away from both 0 and 1), and an intermediate vaccination rate ϕ (away from both 0 and ∞), and, in the case where infection provides no immunity ($\gamma = 0$), the recovery rate is irrelevant. In [5] the infection rates must also be sufficiently high in order to have a backward bifurcation.

For the model of [12], the criterion $b > b_{bif}$ requires that disease prevalence in the core damp off recruitment sharply (via b), that the rate of defection μ out of the core be not too small compared to the base recruitment rate r_0 into the core, and, perhaps counterintuitively, that the rate of disease transmission into the male population $\beta_{23}c_2T$ not be too high.

For the AIDS model of Doyle [3], Hadeler and van den Driessche [8] obtained a criterion which states essentially that the mortality rate plus the rate of new infections must be less than the rate of transition from HIV-positive to AIDS. They also concluded that in general backward bifurcations are related to a large difference (asymmetry) between interacting groups, or multiple mechanisms for interactions between groups. Both the model of Doyle [3] and that of Kribs-Zaleta [12] incorporate an asymmetry in two-sex models, by defining one sex's activity rate in terms of the other's, thereby creating a potential for greatly disparate contact rates. In that of [12], for example, the core's activity rate is inversely proportional to its size, so that it may rise extremely high for a small core. In addition, the parameter b creates a disparity in the rates of migration between core and noncore. The model of [13] includes movement between a vaccinated compartment and the usual susceptible pool, a similar idea to that of a core and a noncore.

It is worth noting that in each case, the criterion cannot be met simply by exaggerating all the parameters that cause the asymmetry. In the first case, raising either of the rates ϕ and θ which control movement between the two compartments (S and V) orthogonal to infectedness, or making the vaccine effectiveness σ too extreme, will make it difficult for a backward bifurcation to occur. In the model of [12], raising the male activity level c_2 also raises the activity level of the female core, thereby accentuating the difference between core and noncore. One may speculate that it is for this reason that it makes a backward bifurcation less likely. Of course, it also makes an invasion more likely to succeed, but by raising R_0 rather than via a backward bifurcation. Likewise in the model of Doyle we see that raising the infection rate may make a backward bifurcation more difficult.

It is clear that further study of bifurcations causing additional endemic equilibria is warranted, and it is hoped that techniques like the one described in this paper will facilitate quantitative precision in determining their mathematical causes, in order to derive some qualitative generalizations about their biological causes.

REFERENCES

[1] C. Castillo-Chavez, K.L. Cooke, W. Huang, and J. Li, On the role of long incubation periods in the dynamics of AIDS. Part II: Multiple-group models, in *Mathematical and statistical approaches to AIDS epidemiology*, C. Castillo-Chavez, ed., Lecture Notes in Biomathematics 83, Springer-Verlag, New York, 1989, pp. 200–217.

[2] S.N. Chow and J.K. Hale, *Methods of bifurcation theory*, New York: Springer-Verlag, 1982.

[3] M.T. Doyle, A constrained mixing two-sex model for the spread of HIV, in *Mathematical population dynamics*, O. Arino, D. Axelrod, M. Kimmel, and M. Langlois, eds., Third International Conference proceedings, Vol. 1, Marcel Dekker, Winnipeg, 1995, pp. 209–228.

[4] J. Dushoff, W. Huang, and C. Castillo-Chavez, Backwards bifurcations and catastrophe in simple models of fatal diseases, *J. Math. Biol.* **36**: 227–248 (1998).

[5] D. Greenhalgh, O. Diekmann, and M.C.M. de Jong, Subcritical endemic steady states in mathematical models for animal infections with incomplete immunity, *Math. Biosci.* **165**(1): 1–25 (2000).

[6] J. Guckenheimer and P.J. Holmes, *Nonlinear oscillations, dynamical systems, and bifurcations of vector fields*, New York: Springer-Verlag, 1983.

[7] K.P. Hadeler and C. Castillo-Chavez, A core group model for disease transmission, *Math. Biosci.* **128**: 41–55 (1995).

[8] K.P. Hadeler and P. van den Driessche, Backward bifurcation in epidemic control, *Math. Biosci.* **146**: 15–35 (1997).

[9] W. Huang, K.L. Cooke, and C. Castillo-Chavez, Stability and bifurcation for a multiple-group model for the dynamics of HIV/AIDS transmission, *SIAM J. Appl. Math* **52**: 835–854 (1992).

[10] A. Kelley, The stable, center-stable, center, center-unstable, unstable manifolds, in *Transversal mappings and flows* (appendix), R. Abraham and J. Robbin, New York: Benjamin, 1967.

[11] C.M. Kribs, *Core recruitment effects in modeling a sexually transmitted disease*, Doctoral dissertation, University of Wisconsin, 1997.

[12] C. M. Kribs-Zaleta, Core recruitment effects in SIS models with constant total populations, *Math. Biosci.* **160**(2): 109–158 (1999).

[13] C.M. Kribs-Zaleta and J.X. Velasco-Hernández, A simple vaccination model with multiple endemic states, *Math. Biosci.* **164**(2): 183–201 (2000).

[14] V.A. Pliss, The reduction principle in the theory of stability of motion, *Soviet Math.* **5**: 247–250 (1964).

[15] H. Poincaré, Sur les propriétés des fonctions définies par les equations aux différences partielles, *Oeuvres*, Paris: Gauthier-Villars, pp. XCIX-CX, 1929.

[16] S. Wiggins, *Introduction to applied nonlinear dynamical systems and chaos*, New York: Springer-Verlag, 1990.

REMARKS ON MODELING HOST-VIRAL DYNAMICS AND TREATMENT

JORGE X. VELASCO-HERNÁNDEZ*, JOSÉ A. GARCÍA†, AND DENISE E. KIRSCHNER‡

1. Introduction. Mathematical modeling of host-pathogen interactions is playing an increasingly important role in our understanding of the pathogenesis of infectious diseases. Many of the results have shaped our understanding of disease processes both at the population and cellular levels. In this tutorial we give an introduction to modeling the interaction of the human immune system with viral pathogens. Our collective research experience is focused on HIV so we use that as our prime example to explore approaches to understanding host-pathogen interactions and the treatment of disease. We present basic principles on the interaction of the immune system in response to the diverse set of pathogens that challenge humans. We then present a brief review of models for host-pathogen interactions at the cellular level, a summary of modeling HIV disease progression and subsequent chemotherapy, and finally, we present a model for the treatment of AIDS using the novel approach of robust control theory.

2. Host-pathogen interactions. The immune response represents a complex defense system against invading pathogens. Its main features involve induction, specificity and memory. Most organisms posses a non-specific procedure for protection against pathogens: an innate response composed of physical and chemical barriers. Higher organisms also maintain an adaptive response comprised by humoral and cellular components that are pathogen specific (see [1]).

The most popular paradigm in immunology is that the key role of the immune response is to distinguish between self and non-self. This involves immune cells known as lymphocytes, that during their development, are elimintated if they recognize self [2]. Thus, immune cells that participate in the immune response recognize non-self molecules and can initiate an immune response cascade.

A second paradigm postulates that adaptive immune cells only respond if the antigen elicits different types and levels of tissue damage, not based on the nature of the antigen molecule [3, 4]. This model considers the immune response as a defense system against pathogens.

When a foreign pathogen invades, an immune response is triggered. The innate elements attempt to suppress the invader, and days later the

---

*Departamento de Matemáticas, UAM Iztapalapa, México.

†Departamento de Investigación, Universidad La Salle, México.

‡Department of Microbiology and Immunology, University of Michigan, Ann Arbor, MI 48109-0620, USA.

adaptive immune components are developed. As the response progresses, the pathogen attempts to survive by various evasion mechanisms. Thus, a series of complex interactions between the host and the parasite are established.

2.1. Immune response to viral pathogens. Unlike bacteria, viruses must infect host cells to survive and replicate, and thus by definition, are intracellular microbes. Once virus binds to the host cell, the virus introduces its genetic material into the cell nucleus, and it remains there until the cell is activated and the viral genetic material is replicated. This process eventually kills the host cell. New virions are produced that are able to infect other cells.

When the invading virus circulates through the blood its receptor could be blocked by neutralizing antibodies. However, once a virus has already infected a cell, specific antibodies cannot reach it, and thus a cellular immune response is needed in order to suppress infection. Infected cells also are recognized by natural killer cells and then killed through the action of perforin and other molecules secreted by the NK cell. Both CTLs and NK cells are activated by TH1 cells through the action of cytokines.

Perhaps the main immune evasion mechanism of viruses is mutation. As the body is preparing to fight the virus by developing specific responses, the virus changes some of its antigenic proteins, via mutation, so that it is no longer recognized. Retroviruses (like the human immunodeficiency virus (HIV)) have a high spontaneous rate of mutation due to the enzyme called reverse transcriptase that does not possess a repair domain (exonuclease activity) which DNA polymerases usually have. This facilitates the mutation process. A second evasion mechanism comes by virtue of the intracellular lifestyle of viruses. Residing within host cells offers them protection from the immune response. Viruses have even developed ways to downregulate expression of host proteins on cells that signal infection.

2.2. Modeling host-viral interactions. Models of host-viral infections, namely HIV-host models, have a successful recent history. Many of the key results that have shaped our understanding of the T-cell and viral dynamics in HIV disease have come from mathematical modeling approaches [5–7]. Many others have given insight into HIV-immune dynamics as well as progression [8–26]. There is also a first attempt on modeling the interaction of cytokines and the HIV-infected immune system. This work examined the role of IL-2 immunotherapy in HIV-1 infection ([27]). Other viruses that have captured recent attention through modeling are Hepatitis B and C viruses [28, 29]. Most viral-host models are developed using continuous and deterministic methods, and thus have been formulated using ordinary or partial differential equations. A few of these models e.g. [30–34] are discrete and stochastic. The choice of modeling method is based on several considerations; e.g., the time frame of a study, the population sizes, and the types of questions posed.

3. The human immunodeficiency virus. HIV has been recognized as the etiologic agent of the acquired immunodeficiency syndrome -AIDS ([35]. The United Nations estimates that there have been 8.4 million AIDS cases since the start of the global pandemic in the 1980s, with an estimated 30 million persons HIV-positive. Only 1.5 million cumulative cases have been officially reported by countries. An estimated 5 million adults and 1.5 million children have already died from AIDS. The impact of this emerging infectious disease is clear. Despite the impressive amount of research on this pathogen and the related areas of study, there are as yet no effective vaccines or treatment strategies that prevent the ultimate progression to AIDS and death. This is sentinel in realizing that many of the pathogenic mechanisms leading to disease progression are still unknown.

HIV is a retrovirus containing two single strands of RNA. It is an enveloped virus that carries its own reverse transcriptase for transcribing the viral RNA. HIV is transmitted via three primary routes: sexually, vertically (mother to child) and intravenously. Once infection takes place, the interaction of HIV and the immune system begins with $CD4^+$ cells. The CD4 receptor appears mostly on helper T cells and some macrophages, and binds with the protein (ligand) gp120 (on the surface of the virus) initiating cellular infection. This is a necessary, but insufficient step – a co-receptor is also vital for proper cellular infection, and the virus uses a cytokine receptor on the surface of the host cell near the CD4 receptor to finish the lock-and-key entry process. It has been shown that individuals lacking the co-receptor have a natural immunity to infection by HIV [36], although it is not known how this receptor mutation arose. It has been observed that initial infection with HIV usually occurs in macrophages, as the predominately-transmitted strain of HIV is tropic for the cytokine co-receptor on macrophages [37, 38]. These important phagocytes and antigen presenting cells serve as a cloak for virus that can now be carried through the blood and lymph to all parts of the body (including crossing the blood-brain barrier). As infection progresses, HIV expands its co-receptor usage repertoire, and can infect both T cells and macrophages. There is much evidence to support the observation that this infection process occurs more efficiently in activated cells, and that even when a resting cell binds virus, the viral DNA may never be inserted into the host genome [39, 40].

Once inside the host cell, the viral DNA can be inserted into the host-cell's genome only upon cellular activation, and new viral particles are created and released. For HIV, viral production per infected cell is estimated to be on the order of 500 virions per infected cell [41, 42]. It has been observed that these infected cells (whether resting or active) are at an increased risk for cell death via apoptosis or other pathways [43]. This enhanced cell death is also seen in bystander cells (cells not producing HIV) [44]. Infected cells are also cleared via a CTL response, or may die due to lysis from infection.

As the infection develops, immune cells are depleted and a disruption in the immune system is established so that the host becomes susceptible to opportunistic infections and pathologies, like *Pneumocystis carinii* pneumonia (PNP), Kaposi's sarcoma, candidiasis, tuberculosis, etc. AIDS is diagnosed when the count in $CD4^+$ T cells is less than $200/mm^3$ and/or the seropositive patient has one or more AIDS defining illnesses.

3.1. Modeling the mechanisms of HIV disease. Any theory or model of HIV disease progression needs to reconcile the following aspects of the disease process: (1) net loss of $CD4^+$ lymphocytes is gradual and takes, on the average, 10 years; (2) $CD4^+$ T cell numbers decrease in the blood earlier than in lymph nodes, and in the early symptomatic stages when $CD4^+$ lymphocytes are declining in the blood, their numbers are often increasing in the lymph nodes (lymphadenopathy); (3) there is some compartmentalization of HIV-infected cells to lymphatic tissues with the preponderance of cells producing virus residing there, as well as a large percentage of virus present on follicular dendritic cells; (4) the number of productively infected cells at any given time is very low, with approximately 10^7 productively infected cells present in the whole body out of a total of 10^{12} lymphocytes ($1{:}10^5$ ratio); and (5) $CD4^+$ lymphocytes that die, tend to die in lymph nodes, not in the peripheral blood, and those that are dying are mostly bystander cells. The factors determining the dynamics of the T-cell populations during HIV infection can be classified into 3 main areas: a change in cell productions, a change in cell migration patterns, and a change in cell life-spans (i.e. increased cell death). Each of these dynamics is modulated by cytokines as well as other influences. Two hallmarks of immunopathogenesis in the progression of HIV to AIDS are the loss of $CD4^+$ T cell function in response to antigens and the critical reduction of $CD4^+$ T cell numbers. It is probable that these two phenomena are related. Other data point to a reduction in $CD8^+$ T cell anti-HIV activity associated with disease progression, and recent evidence indicates that CD8 T cells can be infected directly by HIV [45].

3.1.1. HIV-1 disease progression. As mentioned above, models of HIV-immune dynamics have gained much attention since the mid 1980s. The first three works done in this area were by Cooper [46], Dolezal and Hraba [47] and Perelson [48]. For recent reviews of HIV-immune models, see [49, 50]. The Perelson et al. [25] model included populations of uninfected $CD4^+$ T cells, latently infected $CD4^+$ T cells, actively infected $CD4^+$ T cells, and free HIV virus. This model provided a reasonable first approximation to the clinical progression of the disease, although the T-cell populations never declined to very low levels. (Note that this model is used in Section 4 of this tutorial.) This model was modified to include macrophages as a possible site of virus replication [21]; the result was a slower disease progression and a lower T-cell count, but the collapse of immunity (the "crash to AIDS") was always very abrupt. With both of these models chemotherapy was explored using a treatment that was assumed to reduce viral production.

To improve the mechanistic basis for HIV models, we included anatomical compartments other than the peripheral blood compartment in which viral loads and T-cell counts are typically measure. We first included the thymus as there is much evidence that the thymus is infected with HIV and that this may impair production of naive $CD4^+$ T cells [51]. The compartment for the lymph system was included as there is evidence that lymph nodes become saturated early with infected T-cells and thus provides a constant supply of virus to the peripheral blood compartment throughout the infection [42, 52]. Our results have given the most accurate simulations yet of the disease progression – including the slow decrease in $CD4^+$ T cells, the quasi-constant viral load in peripheral blood until very late in the progression, and the long delay to the onset of AIDS [53].

3.1.2. Progression models of HIV. Any model of HIV disease progression should incorporate clinically determined dynamic information about the HIV-infected immune system. The essential elements are as follows. After an initial period of acute viremia in the first few weeks after seroconversion, $CD4^+$ T-cell counts decline gradually from approximately 600 to $800/mm^3$ to almost $0/mm^3$ over approximately 10 years (normal $CD4^+$ T-cell counts are 800 to $1200/mm^3$). Data from [54] is shown in Figure 1. The decline of $CD4^+$ T cells is more rapid early in the infection [55]. Infected $CD4^+$ T cells constitute 4% or less of the $CD4^+$ T-cell population [56]. The half-life of an infected $CD4^+$ T cell is approximately 2 days [5–7, 57]. After the initial viremia, plasma virus increases from below 10^4/ml to 10^7/ml or more during the variable course of infection with a sharper increase toward the end of the symptomatic phase [54]. The lifespan of a virus outside the cell is about 7.2 hrs [5–7].

To model the longest stage of HIV infection, the asymptomatic phase, we developed a model [19, 18] consisting of ordinary differential equations for the variables $T(t)$ (the $CD4^+$ T-cell population uninfected by virus at time t), $T^s(t)$ (the $CD4^+$ T-cell population infected by drug-sensitive virus (wild-type) at time t), $T^r(t)$ (the $CD4^+$ T-cell population infected by drug-resistant virus (mutant) at time t), $V_s(t)$ (the drug-sensitive virus population at time t), and $V_r(t)$ (the drug-resistant virus population at time t). All these virus populations reside in the circulating blood, in which the values of uninfected $CD4^+$ T cells and virus can be clinically measured. The equations are presented below (reprinted from [17]).

$$(1) \qquad \frac{dT(t)}{dt} = s(t) + p(t)T(t) - \mu_T T(t) - \mathbf{P_1} k_s T(t)V_s(t) - k_r T(t)V_r(t),$$

$$(2) \qquad \frac{dT^s(t)}{dt} = k_s T(t)V_s(t) - \mu_{T_i^s} T^s(t) - p_i^s(t)T^s(t),$$

$$(3) \qquad \frac{dT^r(t)}{dt} = k_r T(t)V_r(t) - \mu_{T_i^r} T^r(t) - p_i^r(t)T^r(t),$$

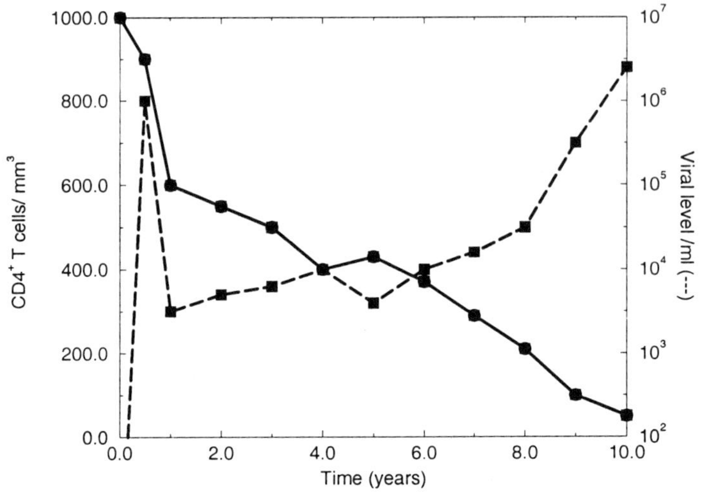

FIG. 1. *Data graph taken directly from [54]. Shown are averaged CD4+ T-cell counts and viral loads from a large number of untreated patients.*

$$\frac{dV_s(t)}{dt} = q \cdot p_n^s(t)T^s(t) + (1-q) \cdot p_n^r(t)T^r(t) - k_T T(t)V_s(t) + \mathbf{P_2} g_s(t), \tag{4}$$

$$\frac{dV_r(t)}{dt} = q \cdot p_n^r(t)T^r(t) + (1-q) \cdot p_n^s(t)T^s(t) - k_T T(t)V_r(t) + g_r(t). \tag{5}$$

Initial conditions are $T(0) = T_0$, $T^s(0) = 0$, $T^r(0) = 0$, $V_s(0) = V_{so}$, $V_r(0) = 0$. The model is explained as follows. The first two terms of Eqn. (1) represent the source of new T cells. This incorporates T cells from the bone marrow, thymus and general production. It is time dependent to represent the evidence that the source of new cells from the thymus, $s(t)$, is reduced during HIV infection [58]. The equation also includes a term to represent proliferative production (whether direct or indirect) due to the presence of antigen, $p(t)T(t)$. This production changes over the course of infection, which is accounted for in the time-dependent rate, $p(t)$. This general form allows for inclusion of different functional forms representing cell expansion. We choose to use Michaleis-Menten kinetics of the form $\frac{pV(t)}{V(t)+C}$. The other proliferation terms, $p_i^j(t)$ follow this same form. The next term is a natural death term, since cells have a finite lifespan; the average of which is $\frac{1}{\mu_T}$. The last two terms represent the infection of $CD4^+$ T cells by both resistant and sensitive strains of virus. These terms are mass-action type terms with constant rates of infectivity k_s, k_r. We assume the law of mass action applies here based on the large numbers of cells and virus involved. P_1 represents the effects of treatment on viral infectivity in the plasma. Equations (2) and (3) describe changes in the infected population of $CD4^+$ T cells, T^s and T^r, respectively. (We assume

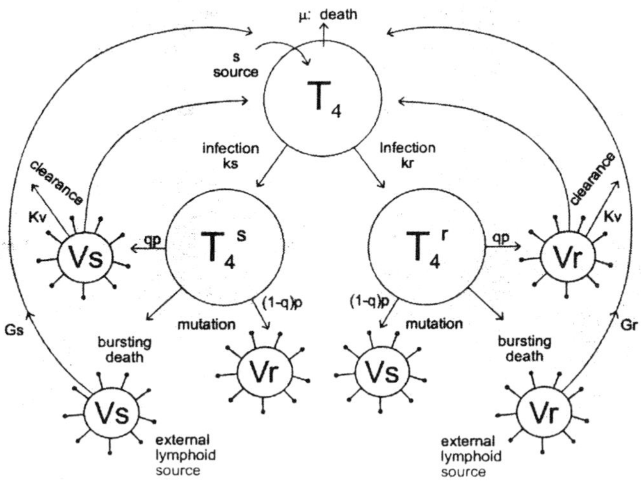

FIG. 2. *Model of HIV-immune system dynamics. The uninfected CD4$^+$ T-cell population has a source rate of s, and a death rate of μ. Cells are infected by either wild-type or resistant mutant virus, at rate k. These infected cells can produce either wild-type or mutant viral strains (which is dependent on the presence of drug for biased selection at rates q and p). Both infected cells and virus are cleared by immune response and death. There is an external source of virus (both types) from the lymph system.*

that, each T cell is dominated by, and hence producing, only one strain of the virus, either V_s or V_r.) The first gain terms for each carries over from the loss terms in Eqn. (1). Then, infected cells are lost by such processes as natural death, viral killing, apoptosis or homing to LS.

In Equations (4) and (5), the first terms are the source for the virus population. Newly produced virion come from production by infected CD4$^+$ T cells (from Eqs. (2) and (3)), in which new virion are produced at rates $p_n^s(t)$ and $p_n^r(t)$, respectively. We assume that upon each replication there is a probability of $(1-q)$ that a significant mutation will take place; and, that the proportion q remain faithful to the original strain. We account for the mutation effects directly in the production term, although mutation occurs during the transcription stage which is not directly accounted for in the model.

The next two terms in Equations (4) and (5), $-k_T T(t)V(t)$ represent anti-HIV cytotoxic responses. As we track only CD4$^+$ T cells in our model, and it is known that CD8$^+$ T cells can directly kill infected cells, we wish to account for this cytotoxic response. Quantitative evidence supports that CD8$^+$ T cells are present in numbers twice that of CD4$^+$ T cells during HIV infection (the opposite ratio exists in uninfected individuals). Thus we use twice the number of CD4$^+$ T cells to represent CD8$^+$ T cells. We then use them in mass action form to represent direct interaction for killing to occur.

As there is much evidence to support the major production of virus taking place in the lymphoid system (LS), we account for this phenomenon as a major contributor of virions, other than the small amount produced in the blood [52]. The input rates of lymphoid system virus are $g_s(t)$ and $g_r(t)$, for the sensitive and resistant viral strains, respectively. They are time dependent, as this will vary over the course of infection. We again use the Michaelis-Menten kinetics here as with the proliferation terms. P_2 represents the effects of treatment on viral infectivity in the LS. The model (1)–(5) describes the interaction of the immune system with HIV.

A typical untreated disease course (i.e. $P_1 = P_2 = 1$) based upon CD4$^+$ T-cell counts and viral load is simulated from the model in Figure 3. The initial virus level is determined by the model's parameters. This assumption is consistent with recent clinical findings that disease prognosis is correlated to a set-point of virus level established in each patient soon after the initial viremia, and viral levels and replication rates remain relatively stable after the set-point [59–62]. In the model, different set-points are obtained by varying key parameter values, such as viral burst size. This system is the only model to date that accurately captures clinic data [18]. This is now corroborated in published work from the Swiss HIV cohort study, where our model is used and gives consistent simulation of the clinical data during the long-term infection with HIV-1 [63].

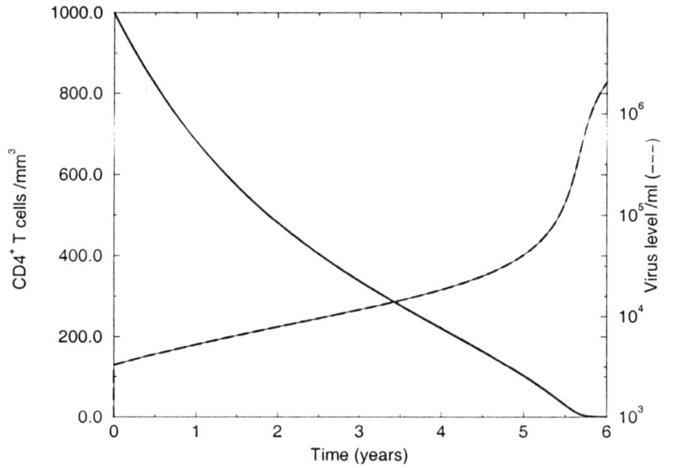

FIG. 3. *A simulation of HIV dynamics for the model with initial T-cell count at* 1000 $/mm^3$ *and initial viral load at* $10^4/ml$. *The curves correspond to data as shown in Figure 1. The set-point of the virus is in the middle range [61] and corresponds to a typical disease progression of about 6 years in this simulation.*

3.2. Antiretroviral therapy of HIV infection. Clearly there is a necessity for both prevention and treatment of HIV infection. There are no vaccines as yet available, but there are several drugs now employed to lower viral loads and raise $CD4^+$ T-cell counts. These antiviral drugs fall into two main categories: inhibitors of reverse transcriptase and inhibitors of protease. The role of reverse transcriptase inhibitors is to interfere with the transcription of the RNA to DNA thus, halting cellular infection; the role of protease inhibitors is to interfere with post-translational viral particle assembly. Unfortunately, these drugs are not cures for the infection, but only serve as maintenance programs to temporarily prevent further progress of the virus. Despite this drawback, there is much clinical evidence to support the use of combinations of these chemotherapies in HIV infected individuals. Aside from the possibility of prolonging life in an HIV positive individual, it may make them less infectious to their sexual partners [64], as well as reduce rates of mother to fetus transmission [65]. Controversy exists among clinicians, however, as to whom should be treated, when they should be treated, what treatment scheme should be used, and if it fails, what should be done in replacement therapy.

HAART (highly active antiretroviral therapy) is a cocktail of different antiretroviral drugs. The effectiveness of HAART in terms of slowing progression to AIDS is high for a large percentage of cases although it presents several problems in terms of drug resistance and compliance.

Most chemotherapies reduce viral production in a dose dependent manner to the expense of multiple side effects as well as ineffectiveness of the treatment after a certain time due to the capability of the virus to mutate and become resistant [66].

3.2.1. Treatment models. Recent clinical trials have had some success in using combined drug therapy [67, 59]. Ongoing trials with combinations of drugs have shown sharp declines of viral counts to undetectable levels within several weeks of treatment; these levels are sustained for 1 year or more [59, 68, 60]. At the same time, $CD4^+$ T-cell counts rise markedly before gradually leveling off [59, 68, 60]. This apparent remission of HIV infection offers hope for potential chronic control [57]. The long-term implications of patients on this therapy, however, are not yet fully understood. Mathematical models provide a means to understand the HIV infected immune system as a dynamic process. Models formulated as differential equations for the dynamic interactions of $CD4^+$ lymphocytes and virus populations thus can be useful in identifying essential characteristics of HIV pathogenesis and chemotherapy.

3.2.2. Relevance of HIV-1 progression models to treatment and resistance. In the absence of any chemotherapy, it can be assumed that the sensitive strain (wildtype) of virus is dominant; but in the presence of treatment, selection is for resistant strains (mutant). Because of the development of resistance and side effects during single drug chemotherapy, the time frame for which the drug can be administered is finite [69, 70]. This phenomenon can be modelled by treating, for example, for a 52 week window during the course of infection. Simulations of viral dynamics can be made using the total CD4$^+$ T-cell population over time together with HIV levels as indicators of drug effectiveness. To include monotherapy in the model, it is necessary to mathematically mimic the effects of a drug which is a reverse transcriptase inhibitor. Such drugs reduce viral infectivity, since they do not allow the viral DNA to be inserted into the host genome. Since multiple virions may infect a cell, such drugs may inhibit one virus, but allow another to get through or around the drug barrier. One can therefore model treatment by inhibiting the infectivity of the virus. This would affect both the viral infectivity of T cells, and also reduce the number of infectious virus flowing into the blood from the LS virus compartment. One can achieve this by multiplying the parameters k_s and g_s in the model by functions which are "off" outside the treatment period (thus having no effect) and "on" during the treatment period (thus reducing viral infectivity). Treatment functions which achieve this are of a piecewise continuous form with the value 1 outside the treatment period, and P_1 within the treatment period. P_1 is the treatment effectiveness, $0 < P_1 < 1$. If $P_1 = 1$, treatment is 0% effective; if $P_1 = 0$, treatment is 100% effective. A similar function, with treatment parameter P_2, is also applied to the external LS, however with less effect (i.e. $P_1 < P_2$, since it is proportionate reduction) as we assume the drug effectiveness is less there [52]. Drugs such as AZT reduce viral activity in a dose dependent manner. The efficacy of the chemotherapy may differ from patient to patient; therefore, P_i for $i \in \{1, 2\}$ represents the varying effectiveness of the drug in halting viral activity in a given patient.

Models of treatment by Kirschner and Webb (e.g. [19, 18]) have distinguished qualitatively two distinct outcomes as indicated by clinical trials. The first is resistance. Examples of resistance for three-drug combined therapy are reported for completed clinical trials by Collier et al. [71]. In these trials, there was on average an increase of CD4$^+$ T-cell counts by approximately 30% (peaking at approximately 8 weeks and returning to baseline at approximately 40 weeks) and a decrease of plasma virus by approximately 70% (peaking at approximately 4 weeks and recovering to half baseline at approximately 40 weeks). The second treatment outcome is *remission*. Examples of remission are indicated in preliminary reports of ongoing clinical trials [59, 60, 39, 72]. In these trials, two things were observed: 1) plasma virus decreased sharply to undetectable levels in 2 to 4 weeks, and these levels are sustained for periods of 1 year or more, and 2) CD4$^+$ T-cell counts increased steadily by 100/mm^3 or more before gradually leveling off to below normal levels (this below normal recovery is believed to be due to an impaired production of new CD4$^+$ T cells from the thymus and other sources [54, 73]; this assumption is incorporated into the model).

Multi-drug treatment can be incorporated into the existing model as the reduction of two separate rates. The reduction of these rates provides treatment control variables corresponding to the intensity and velocity of HAART drug action. The variables are the rate at which virus infects uninfected CD4$^+$ T cells and the rate of virus influx into the plasma from the lymph system. Reduction of this second rate is the most important for treatment outcome, since it is believed that as much as 98% of the virus in the circulating blood is contributed by the external lymphoid compartment [59, 60]. In the simulations, the dynamics in the lymphoid compartment are modeled as a viral source term rather than mechanistically, since limited data are available for the host-pathogen dynamics in this compartment [52, 42]. When treatment begins, the model assumes that a proportion of drug-sensitive virus mutates to drug-resistant virus. This proportion is also a treatment control variable corresponding to the combination of drugs used or the presence of genetic diversity at different disease stages [16]. Figure 4 shows the different outcomes of the treatment model simulations.

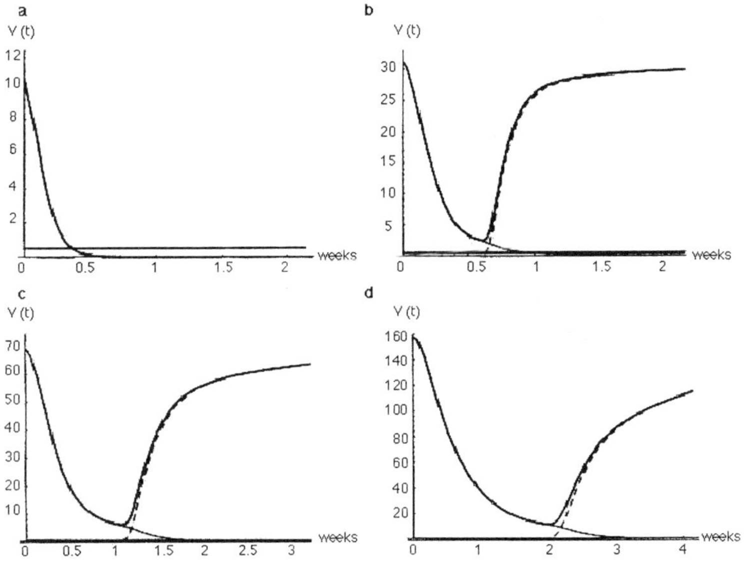

FIG. 4. *Treatment simulations for four starting viral levels. The simulations have a common viral set-point of disease progression, and the treatment starting values are from Figure 3. Initiation of treatment with the lowest starting viral load achieves remission (a), while the other three develop resistance.*

The model distinguishes primarily between resistance and remission in the assumption of a threshold condition for the virus population in the plasma (and thus for the virus population in the lymphoid compartment). The threshold condition is incorporated into the rate that controls the contribution of drug-resistant virus from the external lymphoid compartment to the plasma. When treatment drives the plasma virus level below the threshold, the drug-resistant virus population does not emerge, and the drug-sensitive virus population falls to undetectable levels. This threshold cannot be reached simply by gradually lowering the drug-sensitive virus population. Two additional factors must be considered: 1) when the virus population is above threshold, the high mutational capacity and short lifespan of the virus results in rapid production of drug-resistant variants; and 2) as the virus population approaches the threshold, Darwinian competition gives competitive advantage to the resistant viral strain as the sensitive viral strain diminishes in fitness and in numbers.

To reach the threshold, the virus population must be brought down extremely fast before mutation and selection pressure allow resistant virus to propagate in the drug-altered environment. In the simulations (see Figure 4, (reprinted from [17])), this rapid fall to the threshold can be achieved if treatment inhibits the rate of viral influx from the external lymphoid compartment term sufficiently fast. The threshold value depends on the drugs used and the capacity of the virus to mutate against these drugs. In some patients, plasma levels were reduced to undetectable levels, yet remission did not occur [5, 6]. In these cases, there may have been an extremely low threshold specific to the drugs used or a disproportionately lower suppression of virus in the lymphoid compartment than in the plasma.

Although computer models of HIV therapy are no substitute for clinical trials, they can bring into focus essential elements of the dynamic processes involved. The treatment simulations presented here identify the following qualitative dynamic elements involved in resistance and remission: 1) remission can occur if the viral production in the lymphoid tissues is suppressed below a threshold level; 2) drug action must be strong enough and fast enough to drive the virus population to the threshold before resistant virus appears and propagates; 3) combination therapy or early treatment lowers the capacity of the virus to mutate to resistant strains and thus forestalls their emergence until the threshold is reached. In the next section we present a different approach to modeling of chemotherapy in HIV.

4. A chemotherapy feedback control model. The question of whether or not treatment should be given in a constant or dynamic way remains open. Some scientists believe that it is too difficult to taylor treatment regimes for individual patients. Others believe that in life-threatening diseases such as HIV, we should treat each patient with all available options. To this end, Kirschner et al. [66] used optimal control methods to explore the issue of a dynamic treatment regime. They addressed this problem concentrating on when and how treatment should be initiated for patients who are in the early stages of infection where uninfected cell counts are high. Their optimal control approach has an objective function based on benefit, measured as the number of uninfected cell counts less the systemic cost of chemotherapy. Using a previously studied simple model of HIV-T cell dynamics ([25] given in (6–9) below), the authors concluded that a dynamically scheduled treatment protocol can maintain the uninfected cell counts in normal levels while reducing the side effects of chemotherapy.

Optimal control based solutions lack robustness against modeling errors and imperfect measurements, and depend strongly on the model used to compute the treatment scheduling. Host HIV dynamics are poorly understood. Therefore, misconstructed model dynamics and uncertainty in parameters may lead to faulty conclusions, such as failure of treatment due to unnecessary high doses or high virus counts due to low doses. We now present a different approach to HIV chemotherapy modeling using robust control summarizing the results from [74].

An alternative to optimal control strategies is the method of feedback control. The aim of this section is to summarize recent results that explore the use of robust control theory to design treatment scheduling for the treatment of HIV infected patients. Alvarez-Ramirez et al. [74] considers the percentage effect of the chemotherapy on viral production as the target variable seeking to regulate the viral production via a feedback function where the percent of effect of chemotherapy is computed from actual measurements of viral and cells counts.

4.1. The HIV-immune system model. To illustrate the possibilities of the application of feedback control, the authors in [74] make use of an early model for HIV dynamics from Perelson et al. [25] (given in (6–9) below), which was also used for the optimal control strategies applied to treatment as described above [66].

In the model, T denotes the numbers of uninfected CD4$^+$ T cells per mm^3, T_1 and T_2 denote respectively the numbers of both latently infected (cells that contains virus but do not release them) and actively infected CD4$^+$ T cells (virus releasing cells) per mm^3. The number of free infectious virus particles per ml is V. Definitions and numerical information for the parameters can be found in Table 2 of Kirschner et al. [66].

$$\frac{dT(t)}{dt} = \frac{s}{1+V(t)} - \mu_T T(t) + rT(t)(1-f(t)) - k_1 T(t)V(t), \tag{6}$$

$$\frac{dT_1(t)}{dt} = k_1 T(t)V(t) - \mu_T T_1(t) - k_2 T_1(t), \tag{7}$$

$$\frac{dT_2(t)}{dt} = k_2 T_1(t) - \mu_b T_2(t), \tag{8}$$

$$\frac{dV(t)}{dt} = N\mu_b T_2(t) - k_1 V(t)T(t) - \mu_V V(t), \tag{9}$$

where $f(t) = (T(t) + T_1(t) + T_2(t))/T_{\max}$.

The model is briefly explained as follows (for a more complete description see [25]). The first term of Equation (6) represents the source of new CD4$^+$ T cells from the thymus. As in the first model (see Eqn. 1) this term is a function of viral load to represent the reduction in the number of newly produced T cells during HIV infection [58]. The next term is a natural death term, followed by a term representing the stimulation of CD4$^+$ T to proliferate in the presence of virus. The last term represents the infection of CD4$^+$ T cells by virus and is determined by the rate of encounters of CD4$^+$ T cells with virus. This is based on the law of mass action. In Equation (7), latently infected CD4$^+$ T cells are assumed to have the same death rate μ_T as uninfected T cells, although other factors can augment their death rate [66]. Equation (8) models the rate of change of actively infected CD4$^+$ T cells. The first term represents the rate at which latently infected cells become actively infected cells. Actively infected cells produce virus and die at per capita rate μ_b. Equation (9) models the rate of change of free virus population. The model assumes that when an actively CD4$^+$ T cell becomes activated through exposure to antigen, replication of the virus is initiated and N virus are produced before the host cell dies. The middle term in the viral equation represents the idea that, as we are tracking only free viral particles in $V(t)$, The term $-\mu_V V$ accounts for viral loss and/or removal from the body. In the absence of virus, the T cell population has a unique steady state known as the *uninfected steady state* such that $T_0 > 0$. Reasonable initial conditions for the differential equations system are $T(0) = T_0$, $T_1(0) = T_1^0$, $T_2(0) = T_2^0$ and $V(0) = V_0$. In particular, if the initial innoculum is free virus and not infected cells, then $T_1(0) = T_2(0) = 0$.

The system (6)–(9) has a second steady state [25]. The uninfected steady state represents a healthy individual, while the second steady state corresponds to a successful invasion of HIV (*infected steady state*), in which uninfected T cells have a low, positive concentration. It has been shown in [25] that if the parameter N is below a critical value N_c, the uninfected steady state is stable and the infected steady state is unstable. If $N < N_c$, the uninfected steady state is globally asymptotically stable. At $N = N_c$ a transcritical bifurcation occurs. Once $N > N_c$ stability is reversed, and the infected state is locally stable. Model (6)–(9) can be used to study the effects of chemotherapy [66, 25] by representing the effect of drug treatment as a reduction of the viral production rate as shown in [66]. Obviously, if chemotherapy reduces the number of virus production below the value N, then the immune system could recover and lead to the uninfected steady state. Thus, a treatment scheduling design is required to avoid proliferation of free infectious virus particles.

4.2. The feedback treatment model. The control variable represents the percentage of effect the chemotherapy has on viral production. The authors in [74, 66, 25] mimic the effects of HAART, by assuming that chemotherapy reduces viral load; thus in Equation (9), the control $u(t)$ multiplies the number of free virus produced by $T_2(t)$ cells:

$$\frac{dV(t)}{dt} = u(t)N\mu_b T_2(t) - k_1 V(t)T(t) - \mu_V V(t). \tag{10}$$

We require the control to satisfy the restriction $0 \leq u(t) \leq 1$ where $u(t) = 1$ is the maximal use of chemotherapy. For design purposes, it is assumed that $N > N_c$, so the model does not evolve in the region of stability of the uninfected state (i.e. the individual has active HIV infection). Kirschner et al. [66] defined a control objective functional that maximizes chemotherapy benefits based on the uninfected T-cell counts. Alvarez-Ramirez et al [74] use a different control objective: the regulation of the free infectious virus particles about a low reference value by scheduling the chemotherapy dosage. This follows since a reduction of free infectious virus leads to a reduction of (latently and active) infected cells and, consequently, to an increase in uninfected cells. A feature of this approach is that the virus reference value is a design variable that can be prescribed in terms of the degree of infection and patient characteristics. As pointed out in [66], public health policies are being designed to determine the time and degree of infection of each particular case and therefore health officials may want to treat under asymptomatic or symptomatic infection scenarios depending on viral load.

If V_r denotes the virus reference value, then it is assumed that the dynamic behavior of the free infectious virus particles is:

$$\frac{dV}{dt} = -\tau_c^{-1}(V(t) - V_r), \tag{11}$$

where $\tau_c > 0$ is a closed loop time constant. Notice that the dynamics of the above equation are asymptotically stable around the reference value V_r with τ_c as the convergence time. The feedback control law is based on a matching scheme. Provided $N\mu_b T_2 \neq 0$ for all positive t, exact model matching between (10) and (11) is achieved by the following feedback function:

$$u(t) = \big(k_1 V(t)T(t) + \mu_V V(t) - \frac{dV(t)}{dt}\big)/N\mu_b T_2(t). \tag{12}$$

The above function corresponds to feedback treatment since it is a function of the actual values of actively infected cell concentration $T_2(t)$ and of free infectious virus particles $V(t)$. Under the above control (12), the controlled dynamics are given by system (6–8) plus Equation (11). It can be proved that feedback control $u(t)$ given above can regulate the immune system-HIV dynamics to either steady state.

A major drawback of the feedback control function (12) is that perfect knowledge of the parameters and dynamics are required for its implementation. It is in this sense that the feedback function (12) is called *an ideal scheduling treatment.* The model above is only an approximation of the real immune system-HIV dynamics and in fact, it does not account for some key aspects of the dynamics. In particular, parameter estimation from actual clinical data parameters is inexact as well as time varying, and even some model parameters are unobtainable from clinical data. For instance, only rough estimates of the number of free virus produced by $T_2(t)$ cells are presently available. As in the case of optimal control based approaches [66], the design of treatment scheduling under these uncertainties may lead to undesired results (e.g. premature ineffectiveness of treatment due to unnecessary high doses or high virus counts due to low doses). The aim of this section is to use control theory tools to design a robust treatment scheduling in the face of model uncertainties.

The following assumptions are made for control design purposes:

- Free infectious virus particles and actively infected cell concentrations are available from (periodic) measurements. This is a reasonable assumption, since cell and virus counts can be obtained with present clinical techniques.
- Estimates of N, μ_b, μ_V are known denoted by $\hat{N}$, $\hat{\mu}_b$, $\hat{\mu}_V$ respectively. Clinical data are becoming more accessible, making it possible to get estimates for them.

We write the viral dynamics, $V(t)$, as

$$V'(t) = -\mu_V V(t) + \eta(V(t), T_2(t), u(t)) + \hat{\beta} u(t),$$

where $\hat{\beta} = \hat{N}\hat{\mu}_b$ and

$$\eta(V(t), T_2(t), u(t)) = -(\mu_V - \hat{\mu}_V)V(t) - k_1 V(t)T(t) + (N\mu_b - \hat{\beta})T_2(t)u(t)$$

is the model error function. The aim is to estimate $\eta(V(t), T_2(t), u(t))$ and to design a feedback function to approximate the optimal scheduling treatment function (12).

To estimate the model error $\eta(t)$, we introduce the observer

$$\hat{\eta}'(t) = \omega_e(\eta(t) - \hat{\eta}(t)),$$

where $\hat{\eta}(t)$ is the estimate of $\eta(t)$ and $\omega_e > 0$ is the estimation frequency, which is an adjustable parameter. If $e = \eta - \hat{\eta}$ is the estimation error then $e' = -\omega_e e + \eta'$. If the model error dynamics are bounded the idea is to pick a sufficiently large estimation frequency value and push the estimate modeling error towards the real modeling error. The implementation of this idea can be consulted in [74]. We now proceed to some numerical examples.

4.2.1. Numerical simulations. In this section we study the controlled immune system HIV dynamics numerically to illustrate our treatment scheduling design as well as to provide evidence that our feedback control design is likely to work in more general situations. We assumed the following scenarios:

- Free virus and actively infected cell concentrations are measured every P days. Moreover, such measurement is delayed P days. This means that the sample for measurement is taken every P days and the actual measurement is available at the next sampling instant.
- An upperbound for the parameter N is $\hat{N} = 1800$ virus counts/cell [25]. Note that the estimated value $\hat{N} = 1800$ virus counts/cell has about 80% error with respect to the real value.

- We use the estimate $\hat{\mu}_b = 0.3/d$, such that the death rate of the $T_2(t)$ cell population is overestimated about 25%.
- Chemotherapy begins D days after the onset of infection. The estimated parameter becomes $\hat{\beta} = 240$ virion counts cell^{-1}d^{-1}.

Initial conditions are: $T(0) = 1000$ cells mm^{-3}, $T_1(0) = T_2(0) = 0$ cell mm^{-3}, and $V(0) = 0.001$ particles mm^{-3}. The control parameters are: $\tau_c = 7$ and $\omega_e = 0.05$ d^{-1}; therefore, the desired reference value can ideally be achieved in about a week, and the cutoff period of the modeling error estimation about two weeks. Thus, system parameter changes can be detected in at most two weeks.

For comparison purposes the dynamical behavior of the uninfected cells and virus populations in absence of treatment are presented in Figure 5. Notice that for this set of parameters, the stage where the uninfected cell concentration decreases rapidly starts 2–2.5 years after the onset of infection. In the first year, the virus and infected cell concentration are very small. This can be a drawback for treatment scheduling based on feedback control because the modeling error estimator may be insensitive to excessively small values of virus concentrations. Based on the numerical simulation displayed in Figure 5, we propose to use our feedback control scheme for treatment scheduling about 400 days after the onset of infection.

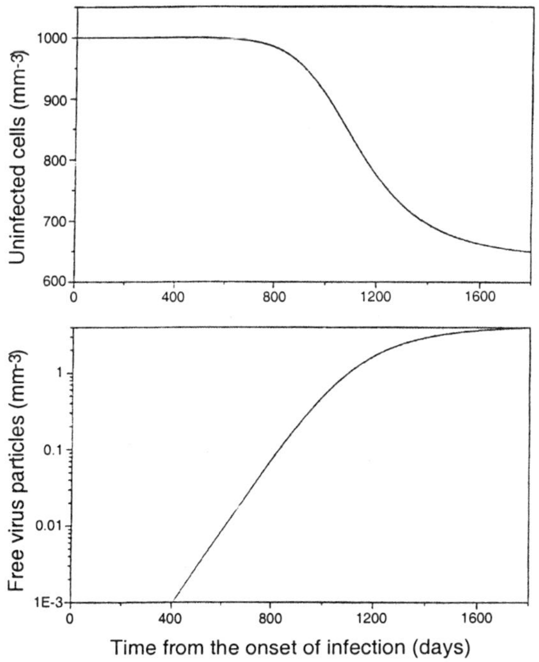

FIG. 5. *Time series plot of the solution to the model in Equations (6–9) showing the virus and uninfected T-cell populations.*

Let the reference $V_r = 0.05$ particles mm^{-3}, correspond to a steady state with about a 10% decrease in the normal uninfected T-cell population. Figure 6 presents the dynamics of the immune system-HIV interactions under chemotherapy computed from the proposed feedback control for three different values of the sampling period P; namely, 7, 15 and 30 days, and $D = 1000$, corresponding to the beginning of the catastrophic stage of fast, uninfected T cell decrease. Examining the results, two things are evident. First, the reference value V_r is achieved in about 250 days. After this time, the treatment achieves a stationary value. Second, the smaller the sampling period, the better the performance of the chemotherapy administration. This point highlights the importance of monitoring frequently the evolution of T cell populations in HIV infected patients.

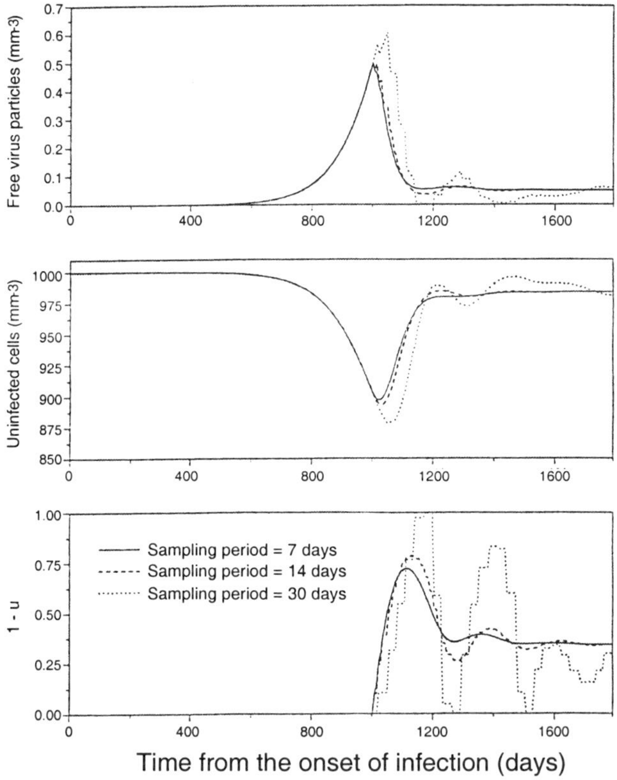

FIG. 6. *Dynamics of the immune-HIV interaction for different reference values of the sampling period, P at 7, 15 and 30 days.*

We also did studies where we varied the treatment initiation times, D at times 1500, 1000 and 2000 days. These results reveal that early treatment leads to moderate treatment scheduling. On the other hand, late treatment induces the highest dose possible for long periods, which may lead to premature resistance (data not shown).

Finally, we studied the performance of the feedback-control based treatment under the instantaneous development of viral resistance to chemotherapy (data not shown). To this end, we assumed a successive 15% sudden change at day 1500 of the parameter $\hat{N}$; the number of free virus produced by $T_2(t)$ cells. Although the parameter $\hat{N}$ can not verified from clinical data, the modeling error estimator is able to detect these changes. In this case after a sudden change in $\hat{N}$, the control feedback has to rectify the steady state value of chemotherapy, which increases as N also increases. These results suggest that the steady state value of the control, say u, can be used to monitor mutations and resistance of the virus to drugs. In this way, large values of u may indicate adaptation of the virus to chemotherapies.

It should be stressed that the numerical results presented above do not imply that the feedback control approach to HIV chemotherapy proposed in this work is a finished methodology. Instead, our objective has shown the strength of using control theory tools within a cross disciplinary framework to attack problems in medicine.

Acknowledgements. JXVH acknowledges support from a CONACYT (1998) grant and finished his part of this work while on sabbatical leave at the Seccion de Metodologia y Teoria de la Ciencia CINVESTAV-IPN. DEK acknowledges support from NIH grant # R01 HL62119.

REFERENCES

[1] R. Medzhitov and C.A. Jr. Janeway. Innate immunity: impact on the adaptive immune response. *Curr. Opin. Immunol*, 9:4–9, 1997.

[2] F.M. Burnet. *The clonal selection theory of acquired immunity.* Cambridge University Press, UK, 1959.

[3] P. Matzinger. Tolerance, danger and the extended family. *Ann. Rev. Immunol*, 12:991–1045, 1994.

[4] J.P. Ridge, E.J. Fuchs, and P. Matzinger. Neonatal tolerance revisited: turning on newborn T cells with dendritic cells. *Science*, 271:1723–1726, 1996.

[5] D.D. Ho, A.U. Neumann, A.S. Perelson, and et al. Rapid turnover of plasma virions and CD4 lymphocytes in HIV-1 infection. *Nature*, 373:123–126, 1995.

[6] X. Wei, S.K. Ghosh, M.E. Taylor, V.A. Johnson, and et al. Viral dynamics in HIV-1 infection. *Nature*, 373:117–122, 1995.

[7] A.S. Perelson, A.U. Neumann, M. Markowitz, and et al. HIV-1 dynamics in vivo: Virion clearance rate infected cell life span and viral generation time. *Science*, 271:1582–1586, 1996.

[8] R.W. Anderson, M.S. Ascher, and H.W. Sheppard. Direct HIV cytopathicity cannot account for CD4 decline in AIDS in the presence of homeostasis: A worst-case dynamical analysis. *J. AIDS and Human Retrov.*, 17:245–252, 1998.

[9] R.W. Anderson. How adaptive antibodies facilitate the evolution of natural antibodies. *Immun. Cell Biol.*, 74:286–291, 1996.

[10] Z Agur. A new method for reducing cytotoxicity of the anti-AIDS drug AZT. *Biomedical Modeling and Simulation ed. D.S. Levine. J.C. Baltzer A.G. Scientific Publishing Co.* **IMACS**, 1:59–61, 1989.

[11] M.A. Nowak, R.M. May, and R.M. Anderson. The evolutionary dynamics of HIV-1 quasispecies and the development of immunodeficiency disease. *AIDS*, 4:1095–1103, 1990.
[12] M.A. Nowak and R.M. May. Mathematical biology of HIV infections: Antigenic variation and diversity threshold. *Math. Biosciences*, 106:1–21, 1991.
[13] M.A. Nowak and R.M. May. Coexistence and competition in HIV infection. *J. Theoret. Biol.*, 159:329–342, 1992.
[14] M.A. Nowak and C.R.M. Bangham. Population dynamics of immune responses to persistent viruses. *Science*, 272:74–79, 1996.
[15] A. McLean and M. Nowak. Interactions between HIV and other pathogens. *J. Theoret. Biol.*, 155:69–86, 1991.
[16] A. McLean and M. Nowak. Competition between AZT sensitive and AZT resistant strains of HIV. *AIDS*, 6:71–79, 1992.
[17] D Kirschner and G.F. Webb. A model for treatment strategy in the chemotherapy of AIDS. *Bulletin of Mathematical Biology*, 58(2):367–390, 1996.
[18] D Kirschner and G.F. Webb. Qualitative differences in HIV chemotherapy between resistance and remission outcomes. *Emerging Infectious Diseases*, 3(3):273–283, 1997.
[19] D. Kirschner and G.F. Webb. Understanding drug resistance in the monotherapy treatment of HIV infection. *Bulletin of Mathematical Biology*, 59(4):763–785, 1997.
[20] D Kirschner and G.F. Webb. A mathematical model of combined drug therapy of HIV infection. *Journal of Theoretical Medicine*, 1, 1997.
[21] D Kirschner and A Perelson. A model for the immune system response to HIV: AZT treatment studies. *Mathematical Population Dynamics*, 1:296–310, 1995.
[22] R.M. Anderson and R.M. May. Complex dynamical behaviour in the interaction between HIV and the immune system. *Cell-to-cell signalling: experiments to theoretical models*, pages 335–349, 1989.
[23] N. Stilianakis, K. Dietz, and D. Schenzle. Analysis of a model for the pathogenesis of aids. *Math. Biosci.*, 145:27–46, 1997.
[24] R.J. DeBoer and A Perelson. Target cell limited and immune control models of HIV infection: A comparison. *J. theoret. Biol.*, 190:201–214, 1998.
[25] A. Perelson, D. Kirschner, and R. De Boer. The dynamics of HIV infection of CD4+ T-cells. *Journal of Mathematical Biosciences*, 114:81–125, 1993.
[26] A. Perelson and P. Nelson. Mathematical analysis of HIV-1 dynamics in vivo. *SIAM Review*, 41:45–76, 1999.
[27] D. Kirschner and G.F. Webb. Immunotherapy of HIV-1 infection. *J. Biol. Systems*, 6:71–83, 1997.
[28] A.U. Neumann, N.P. Lam, H. Dahari, M. Davidian, T.E. Wiley, B.P. Mika, A.S. Perelson, and T.J. Layden. Differences in viral dynamics between genotypes 1 and 2 of hepatitis C virus. *Journal of Infectious Diseases*, 182:28–35, 2000.
[29] A.U. Neumann, N.P. Lam, H. Dahari, D.R. Gretch, T.E. Wiley, T.J. Layden, and A.S. Perelson. Hepatitis C viral dynamics in vivo and the antiviral efficacy of IFN-α therapy. *Science*, 282:103–107, 1998.
[30] S.J. Merrill. AIDS: Background and the dynamics of the decline of immunocompetence. *Theoretical Immunology, Part Two: A.S. Perelson ed.*, pages 59–75, 1987.
[31] S.J. Merrill. Modeling the interaction of HIV with cells of the immune response. *Mathematical and Statistical Approaches to AIDS Epidemiology: C. Castillo-Chavez ed.*, 83:371–385, 1989.
[32] W.Y. Tan. Estimation of HIV infection and incubation in space state models. *Math. Biosci.*, 167:31–50, 2000.
[33] W.Y. Tan. Some state space models of HIV pathogens under treatment by antiviral drugs in HIV infected individuals. *Math. Biosci.*, 156:69–94, 1999.

[34] W.Y. TAN. Stochastic models of the dynamics of cd4 + T cells infected by HIV and some monte carlo studies. *Math. Biosci.*, 147:173–205, 1998.

[35] F. BARR-SINOUSSI AND ET AL. Isolation of a T-cell lymphotropic virus from a patient at risk for the acquired immunodeficiency syndrome (AIDS). *Science*, 220:868–871, 1983.

[36] M.P. D'SOUZA AND V.A. HARDEN. Chemokines and HIV-1 second receptors: Confluence of two fields generates optimism in AIDS research. *Nature Medicine*, 2:1293–1300, 1996.

[37] M.T.L. ROOS, J.M.A. LANGE, R.E.Y. DEGOEDE, AND ET AL. Viral phenotype and immune response in primary HIV-1 infection. *J Infect Dis*, 165:427–432, 1992.

[38] T. ZHU, H. MO, N. WANG, D.S. NAM, Y. CAO, AND ET AL. Genotypic and phenotypic characterizations of HIV-1 in patients with primary infection. *Science*, 261:1179–1181, 1993.

[39] G. PANTALEO, C. GRAZIOSI, J.F. DEMAREST, L. BUTINI, M. MONTRONI, C.H. FOX, AND ET AL. HIV infection is active and progressive in lymphoid during the clinically latent stage of disease. *Nature*, 362:355–358, 1996.

[40] T.W. CHUN, L. CARRUTH, D. FINZI, X. SHEN, AND ET AL. Quantification of latent reservoirs and total body viral load in HIV-1 infection. *Nature*, 387:183–187, 1997.

[41] W. CAVERT, D.W. NOTERMANS, K. STASKUS, AND ET AL. Kinetics of response in lymphoid tissues to antiretroviral therapy of HIV-1 infection. *Science*, 276:960–964, 1997.

[42] A.T. HAASE, K. HENRY, M. ZUPANCIC, AND ET AL. Quantitative image analysis of HIV-1 infection in lymphoid tissue. *Science*, 274:985–989, 1996.

[43] J. ESTAQUIER, . TANAKA, T. SUDA, S. NAGATA, P. GOLSTEIN, AND J.C. AMEISEN. Fas-mediated apoptosis of CD4+ and CD8+ T cells from human immunodeficiency virus-infected persons: differential in vitro preventive effect of cytokines and protease antagonists. *Blood*, 87:4959–4966, 1996.

[44] M. CLERICI, J.A. SARIN, A. SANDERZOFSKY, A.L. LANDAY, H.A. KESSLER, F. HASHEMI, C.W. HENDRIX, S.P. BLATT, J. RUSNAK, M.J. DOLAN, R.L. COFFMAN, P.A. HENKART, AND G.M. SHEARER. Antigen-stimulated apoptotic T-cell death in HIV infection is selective for CD4+ T cells, modulated by cytokines and effected by lymphotoxin. *AIDS*, 10:603–611, 1996.

[45] K. SAHA, K.J. ZHANG, A. GUPTA, R. DAVE, M. YIMEN, AND B. ZERHOUNI. Isolation of primary HIV-1 isoltates that target $CD8^+$ T cells using CD8 as a receptor. *Nature Medicine*, 7:65–73, 2001.

[46] L.N. COOPER. Theory of an immune system retovirus. *Proc. Natl. Acad. Sci.*, 83:9159–9163, 1986.

[47] J. DOLEZAL AND T. HRABA. Application of mathematical model of immunological tolerance to HIV infection. *Folia Biologica*, 34:336–340, 1988.

[48] A.S. PERELSON. Modeling the interaction of the immune system with HIV. *Mathematical and Statistical Approaches to AIDS Epidemiology: Lecture Notes in Biomathematics*, 83:350–370, 1989.

[49] A.S. PERELSON AND P.W. NELSON. Matematical analysis of HIV-1 dynamics in vivo. *SIAM Review*, 41:3–44, 1998.

[50] D. COVERT AND D. KIRSCHNER. Revisiting the early models of the host-pathogen interactions in HIV infection. *Comments on Theoretical Biology*, 5:383–411, 2000.

[51] D. KIRSCHNER, R. MEHR, AND A. PERELSON. The role of the thymus in pediatric HIV-1 infection. *J. AIDS and Hum. Retrov.*, 18:95–108, 1998.

[52] A. LAFEUILLADE, C. POGGI, N. PROFIZI, AND ET AL. Human immunodeficiency virus type 1 in lymph nodes compared with plasma. *J. Infec. Diseases*, 174:404–407, 1996.

[53] D. KIRSCHNER, G.F. WEBB, AND M. CLOYD. A model of HIV-1 disease progression based on virus-induced homing and and homing induced apoptosis of $cd4^+$ T cells. *J. AIDS and Human Retro.*, 24:352–362, 2000.

[54] E. PENNISI AND J. COHEN. Eradicating HIV from a patient: not just a dream? *Science*, 272:1884, 1996.
[55] A.N. PHILIPS, C.A. SABIN, A. MOCROFT, AND G. JANOSSY. Antiviral therapy. *Nature*, 375:195, 1995.
[56] J. EMBRETSON, M. ZUPANCIC, J.L. RIBAS, R.A. BURKE, P. RACZ, K. TENNER-RACZ, AND A.T. HAASE. Massive covert infection of helper T lymphocytes and macrophages by HIV during the incubation period of AIDS. *Nature*, 362:359–362, 1993.
[57] J.M. COFFIN. HIV population dynamics in vivo: implications for genetic variation, pathogenesis and therapy. *Science*, 267:483–489, 1995.
[58] D.C. DOUEK, R.D. MCFARLAND, P.H. KEISER, AND ET AL. Changes in thymic function with age and during the treatment of HIV infection -see comments. *Nature*, 396:690–695, 1998.
[59] D.D. RICHMAN. HIV therapeutics. *Science*, 272:1886–1887, 1996.
[60] C.J. CARPENTER, M.A. FISCHL, S.M. HAMMER, M.S. HIRSCH, D.M. JACOBSEN, D.A. KATZENSTEIN, AND ET AL. Antiretroviral therapy for HIV infection. *JAMA*, 276:146–154, 1996.
[61] D. HO. Viral counts in HIV infection. *Science*, 272:1124–1125, 1996.
[62] J.W. MELLORS, C.R. RINALDO, P. GUPTO, R.M. WHITE, J.A. TODD, AND L.A. KINGSELY. Prognosis in HIV-1 infection predicted by the quantity of virus in plasma. *Science*, 272:1167–1170, 1996.
[63] R.W. CONE, P. GOWLAND, M. OPRAVIL, P. GROB, B. LEDERGERBER, AND ET AL. Levels of HIV-infected peripheral blood cells remain stable throughout the natural history of HIV infection. *AIDS*, 12:2253–2260, 1998.
[64] D.J. ANDERSON, T.R. O'BRIEN, J.A. POLITCH, A. MARTINEZ, G.R. SEAGE, AND ET AL. Effects of disease stage and azt therapy on the detection of HIV-1 in semen. *JAMA*, 267:2769–2774, 1992.
[65] M. NOZYCE, M. HOBBERMAN, S. ARPADI, A. WIZNIA, G. LAMBERT, AND ET AL. A 12-month study of the effects of oral AZT on neurodevolopmental functioning in a cohort of vertically HIV-infected inner-city children. *AIDS*, 8:635–639, 1994.
[66] D. KIRSCHNER, S. LENHART, AND S. SERBIN. Optimizing chemotherapy of HIV infection: Scheduling, amounts and initiation of treatment. *Journal of Mathematical Biology*, 35:775–792, 1997.
[67] M. PIATAK, M.S. SAAG, L.C. YANG, S.J. CLARK, AND D. HO. High levels of HIV-1 in plasma during all stages of infection determined by competitive PCR. *Science*, 259:1749–1754, 1993.
[68] J. STEPHENSON. New anti-HIV drugs and treatment strategies buoy AIDS researchers. *JAMA*, 275:579–580, 1996.
[69] G.X. MCLEOD AND S.M. HAMMER. Zidovudine: 5 years later. *Annals of Internal Medicine*, 117:487–501, 1992.
[70] P.A. VOLBERDING AND ET AL. The duration of zidovudine benefit in persons with asymptomatic HIV infection. *JAMA*, 272:437–442, 1994.
[71] A.C. COLLIER, R.W. COOMBS, D.A. SCHOENFELD, R.L. BASSETT, J. TIMPONE, A. BARUCH, AND ET AL. Treatment of human immunodeficiency virus infection with saquinavir, zidovudine, and zalcitabine. *N. Engl. J. Med.*, 334:1011–1017, 1996.
[72] J. COHEN. Shooting for the moon with drugs. *Science*, 273:302, 1996.
[73] W.W. GRODY, S. FLIGIEL, AND F. NAEIM. Thymus involution in the acquired immunodeficiency syndrome. *Am. J. Clin. Pathol.*, 84:85–95, 1985.
[74] J. ALVAREZ-RAMIREZ, M. MERAZ, AND J.X. VELASCO-HERNANDEZ. A feedback control strategy for the chemotherapy of HIV. *International J. Of Bif. and Chaos*, 10:2207–2220, 2000.

A MULTIPLE COMPARTMENT MODEL FOR THE EVOLUTION OF HIV-1 AFTER HIGHLY ACTIVE ANTIRETROVIRAL THERAPY*

G. COCHO†, L. HUERTA‡, G. MARTINEZ-MEKLER§, AND C. VILLARREAL¶

Abstract. We present a brief discussion of some basic features of HIV dynamics. Within a multiple compartment framework, we model the dynamics of HIV subsequent to the application of a highly active antriretroviral therapy (HAART) considering blood and lymphatic system compartments. We show that T-cell and HIV decay rates after HAART correspond to time dependent effective coefficients which include transfer between the compartments, stressing that a main component in the evolution of viral concentration is redistribution. In our analysis the viremia decay rate appears to be mainly determined by the effective lymph node-viral decay rate rather than by the decay constant of infected T CD4 cells. We also show that in a two type T cell model with a transition from type 1 to type 2, the more active cells with a shorter life are the porgenitors of the less active ones.

Key words. HIV-1 dynamics, compartment models, viral redistribution, infected T-Cell decay.

1. Introduction. The precise pathogenic mechanisms underlying the acquired immunodeficiency syndrome (AIDS) have remained elusive. After the initial infection by the human immunodeficiency virus (HIV), the gradual progression of the disease involves multiple complex processes with overlapping phases until the fatal outcome of AIDS [1]. Since the appearance of AIDS in 1981, an enormous amount of clinical studies have been carried out, together with very accurate characterizations of the molecular structure of HIV. However, central questions such as how does HIV kill or what is the origin and effects of the severe depletion of T-CD4 lymphocytes in blood plasma (BP), remain unanswered [2]. One of the main challenges is to clarify how a virus with an impressive turnover rate of 10^{10} virions per day [3–5] induces a disease with a long asymptomatic period of approximately 10 years. Several of these aspects have been contemplated in a variety of mathematical models [6–11, 13]. Trying to gain further insight into these fundamental questions, in this work we propose a multiple compartment model for the dynamics of HIV subsequent to the application of a highly active antiretroviral therapy (HAART) [14]. The therapy is based on the administration of potent drugs that inhibit viral repro-

*Financial support from DGAPA-UNAM project IN-116198 is gratefully acknowledged.

†Instituto de Física, Universidad Nacional Autónoma de México, Apdo. Postal 20-364, 01000 México, D.F., México. E-mail cocho@fenix.ifisicacu.unam.mx.

‡Instituto de Investigaciones Biomédicas, UNAM, Circuito Exterior, Ciudad Universitaria, 04510 México, D.F., México.

§Centro de Ciencias Físicas, UNAM, Apdo. Postal 48-3, 62210 Cuernavaca, Morelos, México. E-mail: mekler@fis.unam.mx.

¶Instituto de Física, UNAM.

duction. These drugs act either by blocking the integration of viral RNA into the host CD4 cells, therefore stopping its duplication process, or by inhibiting the production of enzymes that favour proper cleavage of viral polyproteins inside a cell. This last mechanism conduces to the creation of defective non-infectious viral particles [13].

At the initial stage of HIV-1 infection (for details of HIV pathogenesis see Refs. [15, 16]), the viral concentration in blood plasma (BP) reaches very high levels. After several weeks, this acute period recedes and the viremia decreases drastically. This stage is the onset of a long asymptomatic period in which the lymph nodes (LN) become the major viral reservoir. HIV is mainly found in these nodes in the form of virus-antibody immune complexes attached to the follicular dendritic cell (FDC) network [17]. In addition, HIV-1 RNA is detected in mononuclear cells (MNCs) such as CD4+ T lymphocytes, monocytes or macrophages, lying in the lymphoid tissue [18]. Quantitative image analysis and in situ hybridization have been combined to show [14, 18] that during this asymptomatic period the number of viral RNA copies in the FDC pool exceeds the number of those in BP by factors of 10^2 to 10^4, and the number of virions in MNC's in the LN by a factor of ~ 50 (see Table 1).

TABLE 1

Characteristic values of T-cell and viral populations during presymptomatic and late stages of HIV infection: a) T_B, number of non-infected CD4 T-cells per mm^3 in BP; b) T_L^*, total load of infected CD4 T-cells; c) N, number of HIV-RNA particles produced per infected cell; d) V_L, total load of HIV-RNA particles produced by MNC's cells in LN; e) V_F, total load of HIV-RNA particles attached to FDC's in LN; g) V_B, total load of HIV-RNA particles in BP. Total loads have been calculated assuming 700 g of LN tissue and 5 l of blood (adapted from Ref. [16]).

Infection stage	T_B	T_L^*	N	V_L	V_F	V_B
Presymptomatic	402	4×10^7	74	3×10^9	10^{11}	9×10^8
Late	194	8×10^7	50	4×10^9	10^{11}	2×10^9

In vitro studies show that HIV-1 remains tightly bound to the FDCs for at least several days [14]. However, when HAART is applied HIV is rapidly eliminated, following closely the decline observed in the number of productively infected MNCs in BP and lymphoid tissue. This is an evidence of a pre-treatment state in which the binding and dissociation of virion-antibody complexes in FDCs is in equilibrium with the production and clearance of virus from peripheral circulation [14]. A mathematical analysis of the dissociation mechanism of HIV from FDC's has been recently carried out in Ref. [19].

In this work we propose a multiple compartment model that describes the evolution of HIV-1 after the application of HAART. In particular, we focus our attention on the experiments of Haase *et al.* [14, 18], where they studied the viral evolution of in three different compartments: peripheral blood plasma, LN-MNCs, and FDCs. We consider that before HAART treatment the virus exists in a quasi-steady state and transits among the three compartments with given rates k_{ij}, where the subindexes mean the transit form compartment i to compartment j. Later on, we discuss a simplified two-compartment approach which provides some further understanding of the immunological dynamics during HIV infection.

2. Basic dynamics. A method to analyze the dynamics of the cell populations of the immune system and its interaction with the HIV virus was introduced by Perelson, Ho, and collaborators, by studying their transient response to the application of an external stimulus [5, 13, 20, 21]. For this purpose they administered either reverse transcriptase or protease inhibitors to HIV-infected patients.

After the therapy, an exponential decline of the viral concentration in BP is observed. The simplest model showing this behavior is

$$\frac{dV}{dt} = P - cV, \tag{2.1}$$

where V is the number of virions per mm^3 of plasma, P the source of viral production, and c the clearance rate constant. The clinical condition of infected patients generally evolves slowly along the asymptomatic period; therefore, before the therapy is initiated the patients are found in a quasi-steady state defined in the model by $dV/dt = 0$. Thus, the initial concentration of HIV in BP is given by $V_0 = P/c$. After the drug therapy is initiated viral production ceases and P vanishes. Under these circumstances Eq. (2.1) leads to an exponential decay:

$$V(t) = V_0 e^{-ct}. \tag{2.2}$$

By examining the after-therapy viral decay in BP of 20 patients, Ho *et al.* [5] obtained a mean clearance rate of $c = 3$/day, implying an HIV half-life time $t_{1/2} = \ln 2/c = 0.23$ days. This value allows an estimation of the minimal viral production for each patient: $P = cV_0$, whose mean value is $P = 0.7 \times 10^9$ virions/day.

A better characterization of AIDS dynamics is obtained by explicitly introducing the therapy-induced changes in the population of productively infected CD4 T-cells. The basic equation set is then:

$$\frac{dT^*}{dt} = kVT - \delta T^* \tag{2.3}$$

$$\frac{dV}{dt} = N\delta T^* - cV. \tag{2.4}$$

In this model HIV infects target T CD4 cells with a rate constant k, causing them to become productively infected cells T^*. Each one of these dies at a rate δ and produces N new virions during its life-span (an additional equation for the evolution of T could be considered; however, the transient responses under drug therapy are determined by considering $k = 0$, in which case the evolution of T decouples from that of T^* or V). Proceeding as before, the quasi-steady state values of infected CD4 cells and HIV are determined by the vanishing of the respective derivatives, leading to the pre-treatment concentrations

$$T_0^* = \frac{kV_0T_0}{\delta}, \quad V_0 = \frac{N\delta T_0^*}{c}. \tag{2.5}$$

On the other hand, the vanishing of the infectivity induces an exponential decay of productively infected cells

$$T^*(t) = T_0 e^{-\delta t}, \tag{2.6}$$

and by using this result in the equation for the viral population, a more complex decay of HIV follows:

$$V(t) = \frac{V_0}{c-\delta}\left(ce^{-\delta t} - \delta e^{-ct}\right). \tag{2.7}$$

Given the symmetry of this last equation with respect to parameters c and δ, a mere measurement of $V(t)$ cannot provide a unique identification for them. Thus, measurements of the decay of infected CD4-cell population are also necessary. An alternative path was followed by Perelson *et al.* [20]by analyzing the response of patients under application of protease inhibitors. In that case they considered differential equations for the populations of infectious (V_I) and non-infectious viruses (V_{NI}). The equation for the total viral population $V = V_I + V_{NI}$ displays an asymmetric behavior in c and δ. In this new study, the average value for the clearance rate was $c = 3$ per day, as before, while the value of δ was 0.5 per day.

3. Multiple compartment model. With the above parameters we can estimate the viral population in BP using Eq. (2.5). We can rewrite the viral production in the form $cV_0 = N\delta(T_0^*/T_B)T_B$, where T_0^*/T_B, is the fraction of (productively) infected to non-infected CD4 cells in BP. From Ref. [11] this fraction is $\sim 10^{-4}$, and from Table 1 we get $T_B \sim 2 - 4 \times 10^2$ per mm^3. Now, according to Ref. [14, 18] the number of virions produced by each cell is $N \approx$ 100–200, hence, we obtain $cV_0 \approx$ 2–4 virions per mm^3 per day , or considering a blood volume of 5 liters, a total daily production of $\approx 10^7$ virions. This number is two orders of magnitude smaller than the value of P obtained above, and does not coincide with a direct calculation of cV_0 by using the data from Table 1 for the viremia. This is an indication that the main source of virus in BP should reside elsewhere. We therefore formulate in this section a three-compartment model in which HIV in equilibrium is shared amongst BP, MNC's in lymph nodes and FDC's. We first consider the infected T-cell dynamics, then we look into the HIV dynamics, and eventually we collapse the model to a 2 compartment version.

3.1. Infected T-cell dynamics. Haase *et al* [14]investigated the frequency distribution of viral RNA copies in MNC's before and after HAART. At baseline, the frequency decreases as the number of intracellular copies increases, with the maximum lying around 20 copies per cell (corresponding also to the minimum detection level). They observed that by day 2 most of the cells with more than 75 RNA copies had been eliminated from the distribution, and that this rapid drop in the frequency of MNC's was followed by a much slower decay of the rest of infected cells (see Table 2). They thus proposed that the population with high viral levels consists of cells in the late stages of the viral life cycle in infections initiated asynchronously in vivo. This population would turn over rapidly and would contribute to most of the viral production.

TABLE 2

Temporal evolution of the relative population $\tau^*(t) = T^*(t)/T^*(0)$ of infected CD4 cells after HAART administration to 10 patients at days 0, 2, and 22, according to Ref. [14].

Case	Baseline T^*	$\tau^*(0)$	$\tau^*(2)$	$\tau^*(22)$
1	4.6×10^5	1	0.565	0.196
2	9.7×10^5	1	0.046	–
3	2.5×10^5	1	0.480	0.480
4	4.0×10^4	1	0.625	0.033
5	5.0×10^5	1	0.005	0.002
6	1.0×10^5	1	0.700	0.075
7	1.4×10^5	1	0.107	0.026
8	2.0×10^5	1	0.100	–
9	6.5×10^4	1	0.231	0.063
10	1.5×10^5	1	0.800	0.027
Average	–	1	0.366	0.113

In order to incorporate the above observations in the modeling of the T-cell dynamics, we consider evolution equations for two different types of infected cells, with decay rate constants δ_1 and δ_2, and such that type-1 cells are transformed into type-2 cells at a rate μ_{12}:

$$\frac{dT_1^*}{dt} = M_1 - (\delta_1 + \mu_{12})T_1^*, \tag{3.1}$$

$$\frac{dT_2^*}{dt} = -\delta_2 T_2^* + \mu_{12} T_1^*. \tag{3.2}$$

Here, $M_1 = kVT$ is the source of infection. We observe that the transfer rate μ_{12} induces an effective decay constant $\overline{\delta}_1 = \delta_1 + \mu_{12}$. According to this model, before HAART treatment the baseline population of productively infected cells is

$$T_1^*(0) = \frac{M_1}{\bar{\delta}_1}, \tag{3.3}$$

$$T_2^*(0) = \frac{\mu_{12} T_1^*(0)}{\delta_2}, \tag{3.4}$$

while the after-HAART evolution, obtained by considering $M_1 = 0$ is

$$T_1^*(t) = T_1^*(0) e^{-\bar{\delta}_1 t}, \tag{3.5}$$

and

$$T_2^*(t) = \frac{T_2^*(0)}{\delta_2 - \bar{\delta}_1} \left[\delta_2 e^{-\bar{\delta}_1 t} - \bar{\delta}_1 e^{-\delta_2 t} \right]. \tag{3.6}$$

The parameters of the model can be determined by analyzing clinical data of HIV-infected patients before and after antiretroviral treatments. Haase and collaborators [14] have also identified two different decay regimes for infected MNC's. A fast one, with a decay rate $\delta_{fast} = 0.77$, and a slow one with $\delta_{slow} = 0.046$. In order to relate these rates with the decay rates of our model the following considerations come into hand. There are two possible identifications: either $T_1^*(0) = T_{slow}^*$ and $T_2^*(0) = T_{fast}^*$, or $T_2^*(0) = T_{slow}^*$ and $T_1^*(0) = T_{fast}^*$. If, as suggested in Ref. [14], we associate the slow component to the infected MNC's with 20 to 80 viral RNA copies, then the ratio $T_{slow}^*(0)/T_{fast}^*(0)$ is $\approx 3:1$. However, if we reexamine the same data, focusing our attention on the slow dynamics instead of on the fast one, we observe that in the after-treatment change of the viral frequency distribution, the histogram band from 20 to 40 viral RNA particles decays much slower than the other bands. Hence, an alternative choice is to place the separation between slow and fast at 40, in which case, the ratio is reversed: $T_{slow}^*(0)/T_{fast}^*(0) \approx 1:3$. This leaves us with the following four alternatives: two choices for the slow component regarding types 1 and 2, and two values for the ratio $T_{slow}^*(0)/T_{fast}^*(0)$. However, parameter constraints associated to Eq. (3.4) exclude some of these options. Consider the following two cases:

Case 1. Let the younger infected cells T_1^* be associated with a slow decay. Then, $\bar{\delta}_1 = 0.046$, $\delta_2 = 0.77$. Using the values of 3 and 1/3 for $T_2^*(0)/T_1^*(0)$, we then obtain for μ_{12}, via Eq. (3.4), the values 2.31 or 0.26 respectively. Given that the effective decay constant of the type-1 component is $\delta_1 + \mu_{12} = 0.046$, both values of μ_{12} imply a negative value for δ_1, which is impossible. This case is compatible with the proposal of Haase and Cols. [18], where they assume that the subpopulation T_2^* of infected T cells showing the faster turnover consists of cells in the late stages of viral life. Since quantitative analysis shows that these cells present the highest intracellular concentration of HIV RNA, they would constitute a pool contributing most of the daily viral production.

Case 2. Let the older infected cells T_2^* be associated with a slow decay. Then $\bar{\delta_1} = 0.77$, and $\delta_2 = 0.046$, leading to values of the transfer rate of $\mu_{12} = 0.14$ or $\mu_{12} = 0.015$. On this occasion $\delta_1 + \mu_{12} = 0.77$, implying a positive value of δ_1 for both values of the ratio $T_2^*(0)/T_1^*(0)$. In this case, there are no contradictions. With this choice, after HAART treatment, the younger infected T cells disappear more rapidly than the older ones.

We hence adopt case 2 for the comparison of the solutions of our model with clinical data. In Fig. 1 we plot $T^*(t) = m_1T_1^* + m_2T_2^*$, given by Eqs. (3.5) and (3.6), with $m_1 = 0.25$ and $m_1 = 0.75$. We also show data corresponding to days 2 and 22 of the therapy Ref. [18]. The better correspondence using $m_1 = 0.75$ indicates that the association of the slow decaying T-cells with a low (20–40) RNA HIV content, and the fast decaying type with those with higher (more than 40 virions) viral content is more appropriate.

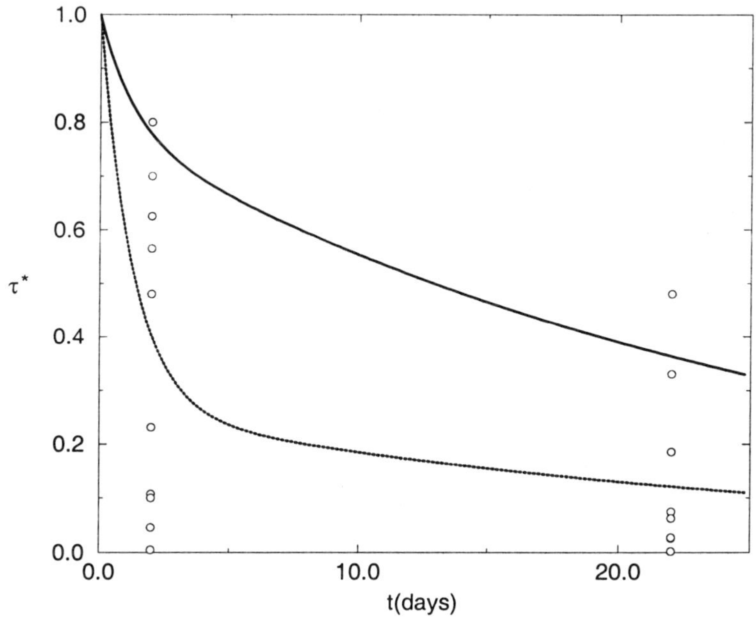

FIG. 1. *Evolution of the relative fraction $\tau^*(t) = T^*(t)/T^*(0)$ of productively infected T cells after HAART. Circles represent clinical data of HIV-infected patients corresponding to days 2 and 22 of HAART taken from Ref. [18]. For the continuous curve the infected-cell ratio is m_1 is 0.25 while for the dotted curve it is $m_1 = 0.75$.*

3.2. HIV dynamics. For the 3 compartment modeling of the HIV dynamics, we denote V_B the concentration of virus in blood plasma, V_L the virus in the lymph vessels and the MNC's in lymph nodes, and V_F the virus attached to the FDC's. We assume that each productively infected cell of type i and decay rate δ_i, produces N_i viral particles during its life span (this number should not be confused with the intracellular concentration of HIV at a given time). Thus, the sources of HIV production must have the form $S_i(t) = N_i\delta_i T_i^*$, and the total source is $S(t) = S_1(t) + S_2(t)$. The rate of change of the number of virus in blood plasma is then given by:

$$\frac{dV_B}{dt} = S_B(t) - c_B V_B - k_{BL} V_B + k_{LB} V_L, \tag{3.7}$$

where $S_B(t)$ is the source of virus in blood stream, and k_{BL} and k_{LB} are the viral transfer rates from blood plasma to lymph nodes and viceversa. The viral rate of change arising from the MNC's in LN is:

$$\frac{dV_L}{dt} = S_L(t) - c_L V_L + k_{BL} V_B - k_{LB} V_L + k_{FL} V_F - k_{LF} V_L, \tag{3.8}$$

with $S_L(t)$ the source of HIV associated to MNC's, k_{LF} and k_{FL} the transfer rates of virus from MNC's in lymph nodes to FDC's and viceversa. For V_F we have:

$$\frac{dV_F}{dt} = k_{LF} V_L - k_{FL} V_F - c_F V_F. \tag{3.9}$$

The stationary solutions of this set of differential equations give the relative amount of viral particles which are on a quasi-steady equilibrium stage before drug therapy. Thus, the amount of virus in blood plasma is:

$$V_B(0) = \frac{S_B(0) + k_{LB} V_L(0)}{\bar{c}_B}, \tag{3.10}$$

with $\bar{c}_B = c_B + k_{BL}$, while the amount of virus associated to MNC's in lymphoid tissue is

$$V_L(0) = \frac{S_L(0) + k_{BL} V_B(0) + k_{FL} V_F(0)}{\bar{c}_L}, \tag{3.11}$$

with $\bar{c}_L = c_L + k_{LB} + k_{LF}$, and the amount of virus attached to FDC's:

$$V_F(0) = \frac{k_{LF} V_L(0)}{\bar{c}_F}, \tag{3.12}$$

where $\bar{c}_F = c_F + k_{FL}$. Since only around 2% of the virus is present in BP [16], S_B is negligible compared to other viral sources. If we disregard it, then from Eq. (3.10) we get

$$\frac{V_B(0)}{V_L(0)} \approx \frac{k_{LB}}{\bar{c}_B} \sim 10^{-2}. \tag{3.13}$$

Similarly, from Eq. (3.12) we obtain the relative fraction

$$\frac{V_F(0)}{V_L(0)} = \frac{k_{LF}}{\bar{c}_F} \sim 10^2. \tag{3.14}$$

Note that these relationships pose strong restrictions on the possible values for the decay and transfer constants.

We have solved numerically this set of differential equations for the HIV evolution. Here we summarize some of our results reported in Ref. [22]. With the restrictions imposed by the parameter ratios discussed above, the number of virus decays in a parallel fashion in both compartments. During the first days of treatment there is a fast decay, approximately two orders of magnitude higher than the much slower decay that sets in during the following weeks. The inflection point dividing the fast/slow stages is shifted towards later times in the FDC compartment when compared with the BP compartment. This shift is consistent with the fits for viral decay in BP reported in Refs. [14, 21], as well as with those obtained from Table 3. Furthermore, our model shows consistency with data for HIV load up to 180 days, which is the maximum range reported in FDC samples in patients. We also find in Ref. [22] that the viral change in the three different compartments is mainly determined by the viral production of MNC's in lymph nodes.

TABLE 3

Temporal evolution of the relative population of LN HIV-RNA particles $v_N(t) = V_N(t)/V_N(0)$ after administration of HAART to 10 HIV-infected patients, at days 0, 2, 22, and 168, according to Ref. [14].

Case	Baseline V_N	$v_N(0)$	$v_N(2)$	$v_N(22)$	$v_N(168)$
1	3×10^8	1	0.197	0.200	1.3×10^{-3}
2	1.6×10^8	1	0.443	–	$< 0.6 \times 10^{-4}$
3	5.5×10^8	1	0.543	0.486	7.1×10^{-4}
4	2×10^7	1	0.950	0.100	7×10^{-4}
5	2×10^8	1	0.220	0.090	$< 0.5 \times 10^{-4}$
6	–	1	–	–	–
7	1.3×10^8	1	0.300	0.011	$< 0.8 \times 10^{-4}$
8	6.2×10^7	1	0.290	-	4.2×10^{-4}
9	2.5×10^7	1	0.440	0.120	$< 4.2 \times 10^{-4}$
10	1.3×10^8	1	1.231	0.131	2×10^{-3}
Average	–	1	0.512	0.163	–

3.3. Two compartments. A shortcoming of the above approach is that the distinction between the comparments is no clear cut, the boundaries cirumscribing the compartments within the lymphatic system are not sharply defined. Another drawback is that it often involves ratios of relevant parameters such as the transfer coefficients for which complete information is still lacking. We may circumvent this difficulty by considering a simplified model involving only two compartments. In this new formulation, the follicular and lymph compartments conform a single compartment. The virus lying there satisfies $V_N = V_F + V_L$, and may be transferred to and from the blood compartment. The population dynamics is now obtained by summing up Eqs. (3.8) and (3.9):

$$\frac{dV_N}{dt} = S_L(t) - \overline{c}_L V_L - \overline{c}_F V_F + k_{BL} V_B. \tag{3.15}$$

$$\frac{dV_B}{dt} = -\overline{c}_B V_B + k_{LB} V_L. \tag{3.16}$$

In the last equation we have discarded the HIV source in BP, since as we mentioned before, its contribution to the viremia is negligible. By summing now Eqs. (3.15) and (3.16), we obtain an equation for the total amount of virus:

$$\frac{dV}{dt} = -\overline{c}V + S, \tag{3.17}$$

with $S \equiv S_L$ and $\overline{c} \equiv (\overline{c}_L V_L/V + \overline{c}_F V_F/V + \overline{c}_B V_B/V)$. The decay parameter $\overline{c}$ will in general be a function of time. Here we adopt the simplifying assumption of only contemplating the constant values $\overline{c}^b$ and $\overline{c}^a$, which in general shall be different before and after the application of HAART.

We introduce the parameter $r \equiv \overline{c}^b/\overline{c}^a$, as a measure of the relative change in the viral clearance rate after treatment. As before, we take the viral evolution after HAART to be a superposition of exponentially decaying sources, which we write as follows:

$$S(t) = S(0) \sum_i s_i e^{-\overline{\delta}_i t}, \tag{3.18}$$

where the subindex i refers to the population of productively infected cells with effective decay rate $\overline{\delta}_i$, and the relative source weights s_i satisfy $\sum_i s_i = 1$. Under the action of this generalized source, the viral decay, which we express in terms of the relative fraction $v(t) = V(t)/V_0$, takes the form:

$$v(t) = e^{-\overline{c}^a t} + r \sum_i s_i \frac{\overline{c}^a}{\overline{c}^a - \overline{\delta}_i} \left(e^{-\overline{\delta}_i t} - e^{-\overline{c}^a t} \right). \tag{3.19}$$

We may similarly introduce, for the after-HAART evolution of infected T cells in BP, the parameter $r_B \equiv \overline{c}_B^b/\overline{c}_B^a$ and the fraction $v_B(t) \equiv V_B(t)/V_B(0)$. The solution of Eq. (3.16) may be then written in the form:

$$
\begin{aligned}
v_B(t) = & \left[1 - r_B \frac{\overline{c}_B^a}{\overline{c}_B^a - \overline{c}^a} - r_B r \sum_i s_i \frac{\overline{c}_B^a}{\overline{c}_B^a - \overline{\delta}_i}\right] e^{-\overline{c}_B^a t} \\
& + r_B \frac{\overline{c}_B^a}{\overline{c}_B^a - \overline{c}^a} e^{-\overline{c}^a t} + r_B r \sum_i s_i \frac{\overline{c}_B^a}{\overline{c}_B^a - \overline{\delta}_i} e^{-\overline{\delta}_i t}.
\end{aligned}
\tag{3.20}
$$

We should remark that for both $v(t)$ and $v_B(t)$, the ratios r and r_B control the slope of the curve at $t = 0$. If r and r_B are equal to one, then the slope is zero, whereas when they are smaller (bigger) than one, the slope is negative (positive).

Since the relative ratio $V_N/V \approx 1$ and $V_B \ll 1$, the HIV dynamics is basically determined by the LN pool, and we shall often make no distinction here after between $V(t)$ and $V_N(t)$. As we examine the data of Table 3 for the evolution of v_N ($\approx v$), we note that for most patients it decreases from $t = 0$ to 2 (quite drastically in some patients). This suggests that in most cases $r < 1$. On the other hand, in Eq. (3.20), if r is sufficiently small, the last term involving the exponential decay $e^{-\overline{\delta}_i t}$ is small, and the time evolution of $v_B(t)$ is mainly determined by the exponentials involving $\overline{c}_B^a$ and $\overline{c}^a$. Under these circumstances, when comparing with the experimental determinations of the viremia after HAART, a good fit with the data should be attained if $\overline{c}^a \approx 0.5$. Notice also, from Eqs. (3.19) and (3.20) that the slope for moderate (not large) values of t is given by $\overline{c}^a$ (i.e., mainly its $\overline{c}_F$ component), instead of $\overline{\delta}$, the decay rate of the T^* sources. We now procede for the 2 compartment case in analogy with the presentation of section 3.2 for the 3 compartment model. In the steady state before HAART, V_N and V_B are related by the equation $\overline{c}_B V_B(0) = k_{NB} V_N(0)$ where k_{NB} is the LN-BP transfer rate. If, according with our previous considerations, we take $\overline{c}_B \approx 3$ per day and $V_B(0)/V_N(0) \approx 10^{-2}$, then k_{NB} should be ≈ 0.03. On the other hand, if the interstitial plasma is taken into account (with a volume of $\sim$ 10 liters), and if we assume that the viral concentration and physiological conditions in the interstitial plasma are similar to those of BP, then k_{NB} rises up to ~ 0.09. Since $\overline{c}_N^b \equiv c_N^b + k_{NB}$, if we assume that c_N^b is small (about 0.01), we get $\overline{c}_N^b \approx 0.10$, which corresponds to a mean life of about one week. Taking into account that there are of the order of 10^{11} virions in the LN, the above value for c_N^b implies a daily production of 10^{10} virions. Now, since there are 5×10^7 productively infected MNC's in the whole body, each of these should produce ~ 200 virions per day. On the other hand, if we had only considered the BP compartment the daily production per cell would be ~ 60 virions. Both numbers are consistent with experimental findings.

In order to plot the viral decay given by Eq. (3.19) we need a criterium for the choice of the daily viral production by an infected cell of type i, which is given by $s_i = N_i \overline{\delta}_i T_i^*(0)$. For the 2 compartment model we only need to specify the ratio:

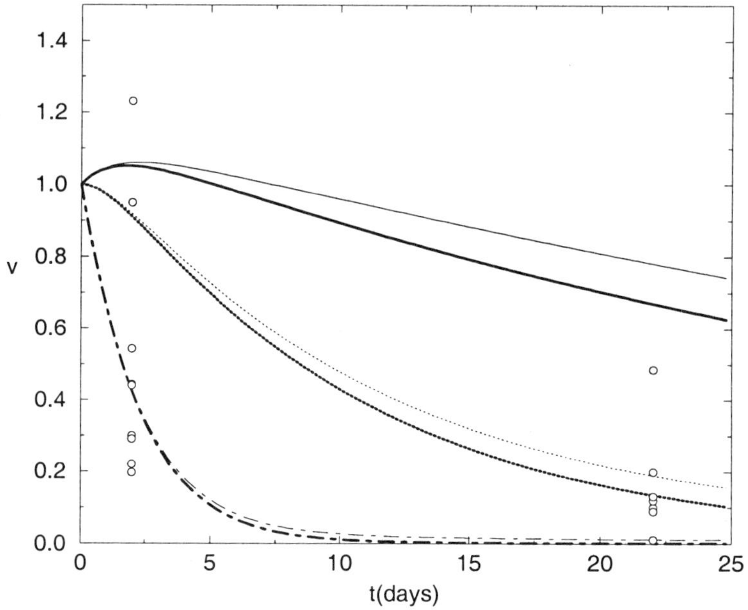

FIG. 2. *Evolution of the relative fraction $v(t) = V(t)/V(0)$ of viral RNA particles after HAART. We assume that type-1 and type-2 infected T-cells produce approximately the same number of virions along their life span: $N_1 = N_2$. Circles represent $v_N(t) = V_N(t)/V_n(0)$ clinical data of HIV-infected patients corresponding to days 2 and 22 of treatment. All graphs are plots of Eq. (3.19) using parameter values specified in the text. For the dash-dotted curves $\overline{c}^a = 0.5$ (suggested by the BP viral evolution after HAART), for the dotted lines, $\overline{c}^a = 0.1$, and for the continuous lines $\overline{c}^a = 0.025$. In all cases we consider $\overline{c}_b = 0.1$. The light lines correspond to an infected-cell ratio $m_1 = 0.25$ while bold lines to $m_1 = 0.75$. Agreement with clinical data at the second day of treatment is improved with $\overline{c}^a = 0.5$, regardless of the value of m_1.*

$$\frac{s_1}{s_2} = \frac{N_1}{N_2} \frac{\overline{\delta}_1 T_1^*(0)}{\overline{\delta}_2 T_2^*(0)}, \tag{3.21}$$

for which the only undetermined quantity is N_1/N_2. We consider two alternatives:

a) Both types of infected cells produce approximately the same number of virions along their life span: $N_1 = N_2$.

b) The viral production per unit time of each type of cell is approximately the same: $N_1\overline{\delta}_1 = N_2\overline{\delta}_2$.

In Figs. 2 and 3 we present the evolution of the viral load after HAART resulting from Eq. (3.19) using alternatives (a) and (b) respectively. The remaining parameters comply with our previous considerations. For each figure we show three pairs of graphs which are distinguished by considering three possible values for the effective HIV decay rate $\bar{c}^a$ with $\bar{c}^b \approx c_N^b \approx 0.10$ fixed, namely: $\bar{c}^a = 0.50 > \bar{c}^b$ as suggested by the viremia evolution after HAART, $\bar{c}^a = 0.10 = \bar{c}^b$ and, finally, $\bar{c}^a = 0.025 < \bar{c}^b$. In each pair the upper curve has a younger:older infected T-cell ratio $m_1 = 0.25$, while for the lower curve $m_1 = 0.75$. We also show the after-HAART clinical data. The correspondence with this data at the second day is improved when $\bar{c}^a = 0.5$. Notice that it does not depend significantly on the choice of m_1, showing that the viral evolution is practically insensitive (within our model) to the ratio N_1/N_2.

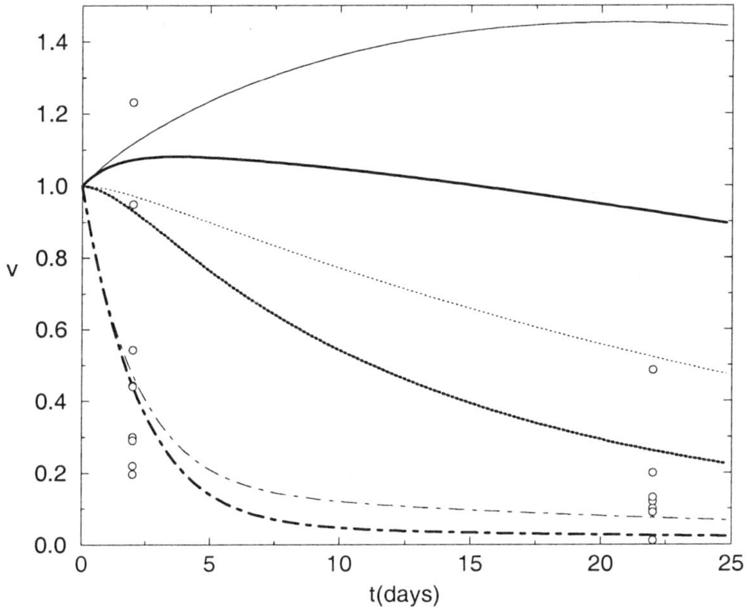

FIG. 3. *Evolution of the relative fraction $v(t) = V(t)/V(0)$ of viral RNA particles after HAART. We assume that the viral production per unit time of each type of type-1 and type-2 infected T-cells is approximately the same: $N_1\bar{\delta}_1 = N_2\bar{\delta}_2$. Circles represent $v_N(t) = V_N(t)/V_n(0)$ clinical data of HIV-infected patients corresponding to days 2 and 22 of treatment. All graphs are plots of Eq. (3.19) using parameter values specified in the text, for the dash-dotted curves $\bar{c}^a = 0.5$ (suggested by the BP viral evolution after HAART). For the dotted lines, $\bar{c}^a = 0.1$, and for the continuous lines $\bar{c}^a = 0.025$. In all cases we consider $\bar{c}_b = 0.1$. The light lines correspond to an infected-cell ratio $m_1 = 0.25$ while bold lines to $m_1 = 0.75$. Agreement with clinical data at the second day of treatment is improved with $\bar{c}^a = 0.5$, regardless of the value of m_1.*

4. Conclusion. Our model links viral dynamics in body compartments previously studied as dissociated. According to our results the viral load in plasma and FDC's is slaved by the viral production in lymph node MNC's. The decay rates involved in the T-cell and viral dynamics under HAART may be interpreted as *effective coefficients* which include transfer rates amongst different compartments during HIV-disease. Thus, a main component in the evolution of viral concentration in these compartments may be due to redistribution processes rather than to HIV clearance.

For this scheme to hold, the viral transfer rate from blood to lymph nodes k_{BL} must necessarily be much smaller than the converse transfer k_{LB}. This flow pattern is reminiscent of the T-cell dynamics through LN's [23]: CD4 T cells mainly arrive from blood vessels, cross a barrier represented by high endothelial venules (HEV), and migrate through the lymphoid tissue for a period of 12 hours. Afterwards, they leave the lymph by the efferent lymphatic vessels. This physiological mechanism suggests that the HIV could encounter some difficulty in crossing passively (as a free virion) from the blood stream to the LN's through the HEV, and might only be able to cross by means of infected T cells. HIV virions would then be produced mainly in LN, leaving through the efferent channels into the blood stream, where they would be cleared out without returning to the LN's. Consequently, the HIV transfer rate from blood to LN's would be very small, while the viral transfer from LN's to BP would, in comparison, be considerably bigger. On the other hand, it is well known [1, 15] that the architecture of the FDC network in the LN's gradually degenerates in the course of HIV infection. Thus, the viral transfer between the BP and LN compartments should be strongly influenced by the physiological state of HIV-infected individuals and change with time accordingly.

Another result of our approach is that we find internal consistency in the parameters of the infected-cell evolution model only by assuming that the more actively HIV-producing cells (with a higher decay rate) are the progenitors of the less active ones, contrarily to the proposition of Haase ad Cols. [14]. On the other hand, medical data presented in the same reference suggest a more or less continuous transition instead of the two state dynamics we have considered. It is hence appealing to model such a continuous dynamics in order to test further some of the conclusions of this work.

REFERENCES

[1] Fauci, A.S. Host factors and the pathogenesis of HIV-induced disease. *Nature*, 384:529–534, 1996.

[2] Dalgleish, A.G. The immune response to HIV: potential for immunotherapy? *Immunol Today*, 16:356–358.

[3] Coffin, J.M. HIV population dynamics in vivo: implications for genetic variation, pathogenesis, and therapy. *Science*, 267:483–489, 1995.

[4] Wei, X., Ghosh, S.K., Taylor, M.E., Johnson, V.A., Emini, E.A., Deutsch, P., Lifson, J.D., Bonhoeffer, S., Nowak, M.A., and Hahn, B.H. Viral dynamics in human immunodeficiency virus type 1 infection. *Nature*, 373:117–122, 1995.

[5] Ho, D.D., Neumann, A.U., Perelson, A.S., Chen, W., Leonard, J.M., and Markowitz, M. Rapid turnover of plasma virions in CD4 lymphocytes in HIV-1 infection. *Nature*, 377:123–126.

[6] Perelson, A.S. Modeling the Interactions of HIV with the Immune System. In Mathematical and Statistical Approaches to AIDS Epidemiology. Lecture Notes in Biomathematics, Vol. 83. Springer-Verlag, New York, 1989.

[7] Phillips, A.N. Reduction of HIV concentration during acute infection: Independence from a specific immune response. *Science*, 271:497–499.

[8] Nowak, M.A., Anderson, R.M., McLean, A.R., Wolfs, T.F.W., Goudsmit, J., and May, R.M.. Antigenic diversity threshold and the development of AIDS, *Science*, 254:963–969, 1991.

[9] Frost, S.D.W. and McLean, A.R. Germinal centre destruction as a major pathway of HIV pathogenesis, J. AIDS, 7:236–244, 1994.

[10] Nowak, M.A., Bonhoeffer, S., Shaw, G.M., Anderson, R.M., and May, R.M.. Antiviral drug treatment: Dynamics of resistance in free virus and infected cell populations, J. Theor. Biol., 184:205–219, 1997.

[11] Perelson, A.S., Kirschner, D.E., and DeBoer, R. Dynamics of HIV infection of $CD4^+$ T cells. *Math Biosciences*, 114:81–125 (1993).

[12] Clark, D.R., DeBoer, R.J., Wolthers, K.C., and Miedema, F. T Cell Dynamics in HIV Infection, *Adv Immunol*, 73:301–327, 1999.

[13] Perelson, A.S. and Nelson. Mathematical Analysis of HIV-1 Dynamics in Vivo. Preprint (1999).

[14] Cavert, W., Notermans, D.W., Staskus, K., Wietgrefe, W., Zupancic, M., Gebhard, K., Henry, K., Zhang, Z.Q., Mills, R., McDade, H., Goudsmit, J., Danner, S.A., and Haase, A.T. Kinetics of Response in Lymphoid Tissues to Antiretroviral Therapy of HIV-1 Infection. *Science*, 276:960–964, 1997.

[15] Pantaleo, G. and Fauci, A.S. New concepts in the immunopathogenesis of HIV infection. *Ann Rev Immunol*, 13:487–512, 1995.

[16] Haase, A.T. Population Biology of HIV-1 Infection: Viral and $CD4^+$ Demographics and Dynamics in Lymphatic Tissues. *Annual Review of Immunolgy*, 17:625–656, 1999.

[17] Pantaleo, G., Graziosi, C., Demarest, J.F., Cohen, O.J., Vacarezza, M., Gantt, K., Muro-Cacho, C., and Fauci, A.S. Role of lymphoid organs in the pathogenesis of human immunodeficiency virus infection. *Immunol Rev*, 140:106–130, 1994.

[18] Haase, A.T., Henry, K., Zupancic, M., Sedgewick, G., Faust, R.A., Melroe, H., Cavert, W., Gebhard, K., Staskus, K., Zhang, Z.Q., Dailey, P.J., Balfour Jr., H.H., Erice, A., and Perelson, A.S. Quantitative iamge analysis of HIV-1 infection in lymphoid tissue. *Science*, 274:985–989, 1996.

[19] Hlavacek, W.S., Wofsy, C., and Perelson, A.S.. Dissociation of HIV-1 from follicullar dendritic cells during HAART: Mathematical analysis. *PNAS*, 96:14681–14686, 1999.

[20] Perelson, A.S., Neumann, A.U., Markowitz, M., Leonard, J.M., and Ho, D.D. Virion clearance rate, infected cell life-span, and viral generation time. *Science*, 271:1582–1586, 1996.

[21] Perelson, A.S., Essunger, P., Cao, Y., Vesanen, M., Hurley, A., Saksela, K., Markowitz, M., and Ho, D.D. Decay characteristics of HIV-1-infected compartments during combination therapy. *Nature*, 387:188–191, 1997.

[22] Cocho, G., Huerta, L., Martinez-Mekler, G., and Villarreal, C. A mathematical model of HIV and lymphocyte evolution under antiretroviral therapy. Preprint IFUNAM (1999).

[23] Young, A.J. The Physiology of lymphocyte migration through the single lumph node *in vivo*. *Sem. in Immunol.* 11:73–83, 1999.

MODELING CANCER AS AN INFECTIOUS DISEASE: THE EPIDEMIOLOGY OF HELICOBACTER PYLORI

H.B. GERSHENGORN†* AND S.M. BLOWER†

Abstract. *Helicobacter pylori* is a bacterium that invades the human intestinal tract. Infection with *H. pylori* results in acute gastritis and has also been associated with chronic atrophic gastritis, peptic ulcers, gastric lymphoma, and intestinal gastric adenocarcinoma. Two important phenomena have been noted in *H. pylori* epidemiology. First, the prevalence of *H. pylori*-related diseases vary with geographic region; the prevalence of *H. pylori* infection in developing countries is significantly higher than in developed countries, and gastric adenocarcinoma is more common in parts of Asia and South America than elsewhere in the world. Second, in developed countries the prevalence of *H. pylori* infection and gastric cancer has decreased significantly over the past century. Here, we analyze the epidemiology of *H. pylori* by modeling cancer as an infectious disease. We use the theoretical framework that we develop: (1) to understand the geographic variation in the prevalence of *H. pylori* infection and disease in the United States, Japan, the Ivory Coast, and Peru, and (2) to explore the potential impact of increasing population size and improving general hygiene on decreasing the *H. pylori* epidemic in the United States over the past century.

1. Introduction.

Viruses are known to be responsible for certain human cancers. Infection with human papilloma virus is the cause of most cervical cancer, viral hepatitis increases risk for liver cancer in some patients, and Kaposi's sarcoma-associated herpesvirus (KSHV) can lead to the development of Kaposi's sarcoma [1]. Five years ago, the presence of the bacterium *Helicobacter pylori* was determined to be a risk factor for gastric adenocarcinoma by the International Agency for Research on Cancer [2]. A large number of mathematical models exist in the literature describing the transmission dynamics of infectious diseases throughout a population [3–7]. There are also many mathematical models that explore the dynamics of cancer growth within an individual [8–10]. Here, we unite these two previously disjoint fields of infectious disease and cancer modeling by developing and analyzing a mathematical model of the transmission dynamics of an *H. pylori* epidemic.

H. pylori are corkscrew-shaped, gram-negative bacteria that live primarily within the gastric mucosa of their host. The bacterium's constitutive production of urease allows it to protect itself from the harsh environment of the stomach until it is able to retreat beneath the mucousal lining [2]. While the mode of transmission is not yet completely understood, it is generally believed that the major transmission mode of *H. pylori* is either fecal-oral or oral-oral [2]. Acute infection with *H. pylori* results in gastritis

*Harvard Medical School, Boston, MA 02115.

†Department of Biomathematics, School of Medicine, University of California Los Angeles, 10833 Le Conte Avenue, Los Angeles, CA 90095-1766, USA. Corresponding Author; Email: sblower@biomath.medsch.ucla.edu; http:\\www.biomath.medsch.ucla.edu/faculty/sblower/.

[2], and once infected, the host remains so for life [2]. Chronic infection is associated with peptic (both duodenal and gastric) ulcer, gastric lymphoma (particularly mucosa-associated lymphoid tissue (MALT)), and also adenocarcinoma of the stomach [11].

Two interesting observations have been made concerning *H. pylori* epidemiology. First, significant geographic variation has been documented in the prevalence of *H. pylori*-related diseases and infection. Approximately 80% of individuals in developing countries are infected with *H. pylori*, whilst in developed countries no more than 50% are infected [12]. Furthermore, in certain countries in Asia and South America, gastric cancer rates are up to ten times higher than elsewhere in the world [13]. The second epidemiological observation is that, in developed countries, the prevalence of gastric cancer [14] and overall *H. pylori* infection [2] have steadily decreased over the past century (in developing countries, no decrease in prevalence has been observed). Better hygiene has been cited to rationalize the lower prevalence of *H. pylori* infection in developed countries [15]; while different diets [16, 17] and genetic diversity in bacterial strains [18] have been suggested as explanations to account for the disparate gastric cancer rates. Improvements in hygiene have been suggested to explain the decreasing prevalence of both *H. pylori* infection and gastric cancer [2]. These explanations, however, remain speculative.

Here, we first develop a mathematical model and then use it to investigate: (1) the geographic variation in the prevalence of both *H. pylori* infection and gastric cancer, and (2) the declining prevalence of *H. pylori* infection and gastric cancer in developed countries. We demonstrate that varying only two factors (the transmission rate and the rate of progression from infection to cancer) is sufficient to explain the observed geographic heterogeneity in both *H. pylori* infection and gastric cancer rates. We then explore the potential effects of improvements in hygiene and population growth on the *H. pylori* epidemic in developed countries. We conclude with a brief discussion of the future utility of our model for designing epidemic control strategies based upon antimicrobials and vaccines.

2. A mathematical model for an H. pylori epidemic. We developed a mathematical model based upon the current biomedical understanding of the transmission processes and the pathogenesis of *H. pylori*; a flow diagram of our model is shown in Figure 1. Our model reflects the following biological and medical facts that are known about *H. pylori* infection and *H. pylori* associated diseases. In the vast majority of cases, the human immune response to *H. pylori* infection is not sufficient to clear the bacteria; consequently, infection is life-long. Those infected with *H. pylori* initially experience acute gastritis; in the chronic stages of disease, infected individuals can progress to peptic ulcers, chronic atrophic gastritis, and/or intestinal gastric cancer. Although, *H. pylori* can affect a large percentage of a population, only a small percentage of carriers will develop peptic ulcers or gastric cancer. (The possible development of lymphoma due to *H. pylori* infection is not included in our model as evidence for the link between *H. pylori* infection and both ulcer disease and gastric adenocarcinoma is much stronger than that connecting the bacterium to lymphoma [2]).

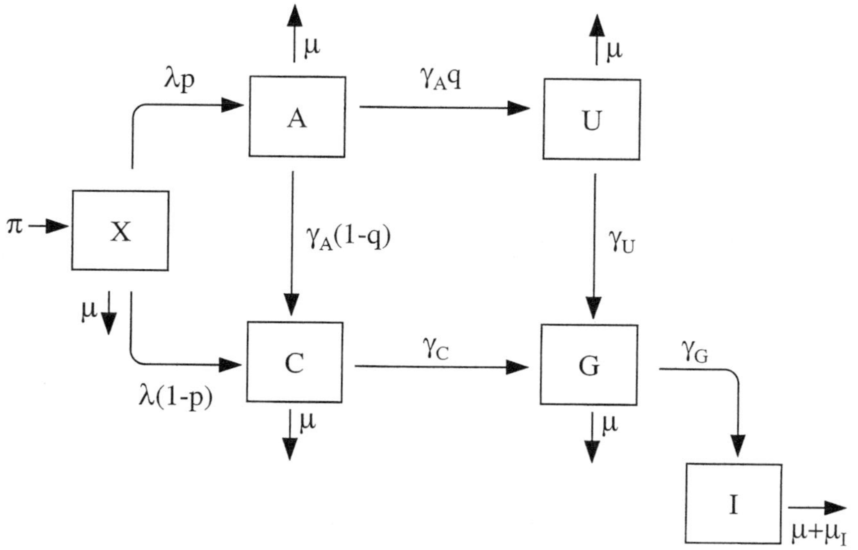

FIG. 1. *Flow diagram of the transmission dynamics of H. pylori infection and resultant diseases. The model specifies the rates of change over time of susceptible individuals (X) in the community and five subgroups of H. pylori-infected people: individuals with acute antral gastritis (A), individuals with acute corpus gastritis (C), individuals with peptic ulcers (U), individuals with chronic atrophic gastritis (G), and individuals with intestinal gastric adenocarcinoma (I). The transmission of H. pylori through the community is described completely by ten parameters: the transmissibility coefficient (β), the probability of developing acute antral (versus corpus) gastritis following initial infection (p), the probability of progressing from acute antral gastritis to peptic ulcers (versus corpus gastritis) (q), the progression rates from one stage of disease to the next (γ_A, γ_C, γ_U, and γ_G), the birthrate in the community (π), the rate of death from natural causes (μ), and the rate of death as a result of gastric cancer (μ_I).*

Our mathematical model specifies the rates of change (over time) of susceptible individuals (X) and individuals in five infection states: antral gastritis (A), corpus gastritis (C), peptic ulcer (U), chronic atrophic gastritis (G), and intestinal gastric adenocarcinoma (I). Six ordinary differential equations specify our model; see Equations 1 to 6. There is a background death rate (μ) in all states.

$$(1) \qquad \frac{dX}{dt} = \pi - (\lambda + \mu)X.$$

The number of susceptible individuals (X) increases over time as new susceptible individuals enter the community at a constant rate (π). The size of the group decreases as new susceptible individuals become infected with *H. pylori* (λX). Since *H. pylori* is thought to be transmitted through either a fecal-oral or an oral-oral route, transmission is modeled using a mass action process [19]; and the force of infection (λ) is determined by the absolute number of infectious individuals in the population at any given time t:

$$\lambda = \beta(C + A + U + \alpha G).$$

We assume that individuals with acute gastritis (A and C), ulcers (U), or chronic atrophic gastritis (G) are all infectious and can transmit *H. pylori*. However, those with chronic atrophic gastritis (G) are the least infectious (with relative weighting $\alpha < 1$) because of the atrophy associated with late stage disease. We assume that the atrophy effects are even more pronounced in individuals with gastric cancer (I); thus, we assume that they are unable to transmit *H. pylori* [20].

People who become infected with *H. pylori* almost inevitably experience acute gastritis [2]. Symptoms of gastritis can actually be manifestations of infection with *H. pylori* in the antrum (A), the corpus (C), or both (pangastritis) [21]. Gastritis in the antrum and the corpus affect the secretions of acid, gastrin, and pepsin in the intestinal tract differently [21]. Consequently, the prognosis for individuals with chronic *H. pylori* infection differs depending on the type of gastritis they experienced acutely. Therefore, we modeled separately people with antral (A) and corpus (C) gastritis. The progression through *H. pylori*-related diseases for individuals with pangastritis is similar to that for people suffering from antral gastritis alone [21]. Thus, the possibility of developing pangastritis was not considered separately.

$$\frac{dA}{dt} = p\lambda X - (\gamma_A + \mu)A. \tag{2}$$

The number of people with antral gastritis (A) increases as susceptible individuals become infected with *H. pylori* and develop (with probability p) antral inflammation. The size of this group decreases as some people with antral gastritis (A) progress to more chronic stages of disease (at a per capita rate γ_A).

$$\frac{dC}{dt} = (1 - p)\lambda X + (1 - q)\gamma_A A - (\gamma_C + \mu)C. \tag{3}$$

The number of people with corpus gastritis (C) increases as susceptible individuals become infected with *H. pylori* and experience corpal symptoms (with probability $(1-p)$) and people with antral gastritis (A) progress to the corpal form (C) (at a per capita rate γ_A and with probability $(1 - q)$) [20]. The size of this group decreases as people with corpus gastritis (C) progress to more chronic stages of disease (at a per capita rate γ_C). As a result of the specific secretory abnormalities associated with corpus gastritis, people with corpus gastritis (C) are protected against the development of peptic ulcers (U) [21]. In the progression to chronic disease, therefore, people with acute corpus gastritis (C) generally develop atrophic gastritis (G) [2].

$$\frac{dU}{dt} = q\gamma_A A - (\gamma_U + \mu)U. \tag{4}$$

The number of people with peptic ulcers (U) increases as those with antral gastritis (A) progress to more chronic disease (at a per capita rate γ_A and with probability q). Unlike with corpus gastritis, the intestinal tract secretory abnormalities associated with antral gastritis increase the risk of developing ulcers [21]. The size of the peptic ulcer group (U) decreases as some people with peptic ulcers progress to chronic atrophic gastritis (G) (at a per capita rate γ_U). Chronic atrophic gastritis (G) is not accompanied or followed by ulcers (U), because the limited acid secretion resulting from the disease is protective [2]. Yet, there is evidence that people currently experiencing chronic atrophic gastritis may have had ulcers in the past [21].

$$\frac{dG}{dt} = \gamma_C C + \gamma_U U - (\gamma_G + \mu)G. \tag{5}$$

The number of people experiencing chronic atrophic gastritis (G) increases as people with either corpus gastritis (C) or peptic ulcers (U) progress to later stages of disease. The size of this group decreases as some people with chronic atrophic gastritis (G) progress to intestinal gastric adenocarcinoma (I) (at a per capita rate γ_G). Increased cell proliferation and the formation of free radicals have been reported at sites chronically inflamed due to atrophic gastritis [22, 23]. Such effects provide an ideal environment for cancer growth.

$$\frac{dI}{dt} = \gamma_G G - (\mu_I + \mu)I. \tag{6}$$

The number of people with intestinal gastric adenocarcinoma (I), therefore, increases as people progress from chronic atrophic gastritis (G) to this end-stage disease. The size of this group decreases as people die as a result of the cancer (at a per capita rate μ_I).

3. Using the model to understand geographic differences in prevalence. *H. pylori* was first cultured only 17 years ago [24, 25], thus relatively little is known about the speed with which it is transmitted through a population or the rate of progression from one stage of infection to the next. Most of the available evidence points to fecal-oral as the route of transmission of *H. pylori* from one person to another. For this reason, and because rates of *H. pylori* have been seen to decrease over time, it has been postulated that hygiene plays a large role in determining the rate of transmission [2]. Consequently, it is thought that the more developed countries (e.g., the United States and Japan), with large-scale sanitation systems, have lower rates of transmission than the less developed countries (e.g., the Ivory Coast and Peru). In addition, the prevalence of gastric cancer is known to be highest in certain countries in Asia and South America. In these countries (e.g., Japan and Peru), diets high in salt, pickled foods, and nitrates [16, 17] are the norm. It has been suggested that these types of diets might speed up the rate of progression from earlier-stage *H. pylori* disease to its end-stage of intestinal gastric adenocarcinoma [17].

We used our model to investigate geographic differences in the prevalence of *H. pylori* infection and gastric cancer for four countries: the United States, Japan, the Ivory Coast, and Peru. The epidemics in these four countries were modeled using exactly the same parameter values (listed in Table 1), except for three parameters that were country-specific: the population size, the transmissibility coefficient of *H. pylori*, and the rate of progression from chronic atrophic gastritis to intestinal gastric adenocarcinoma. Currently, the exact value of the transmissibility coefficient of *H. pylori* and the rate of progression to cancer are unknown. Assumptions of poorer hygiene in the Ivory Coast and Peru suggested a higher transmissibility of *H. pylori* in these two countries. Assumptions about diets higher in salt, pickled foods, and/or β-carotene and the effects these would have on the intestinal environment indicated that progression rates (from chronic atrophic gastritis to intestinal gastric cancer) would be higher in Japan and Peru than in the United States or the Ivory Coast. To produce realistic values for the prevalence of both *H. pylori* infection and gastric cancer for the United States, we assumed that, on average, 8 out of every 300,000 people with chronic atrophic gastritis progress to cancer each year and that, on average, every person infected with *H. pylori* infects 2.6 other people during his/her lifetime. The parameter values used for the other three countries were selected relative to the choices made for the United States (Table 2). More importance should be placed on the relative weightings of these parameters (between the countries) than on their absolute values.

In each of the four countries, an epidemic was initiated by the introduction of one infected individual into a population of susceptible individuals (Figure 2). The epidemics were then simulated for 2,000 years. The population sizes in the four countries resulted in different time dynamics for the four epidemics. The long-term (equilibrium) prevalence of both *H. pylori* infection and intestinal gastric adenocarcinoma, though, were unaffected by the initial population sizes. By using the parameters in Tables 1 and 2, a realistic epidemic for each country was generated (see Table 3). It is clear that differences in only the transmissibility of the bacteria and the rate of progression of the host from chronic atrophic disease to gastric adenocarcinoma are sufficient to account for the disparate prevalences that are currently observed in the United States, Japan, the Ivory Coast, and Peru. It is important to note that we have not modeled the specific causal fac-

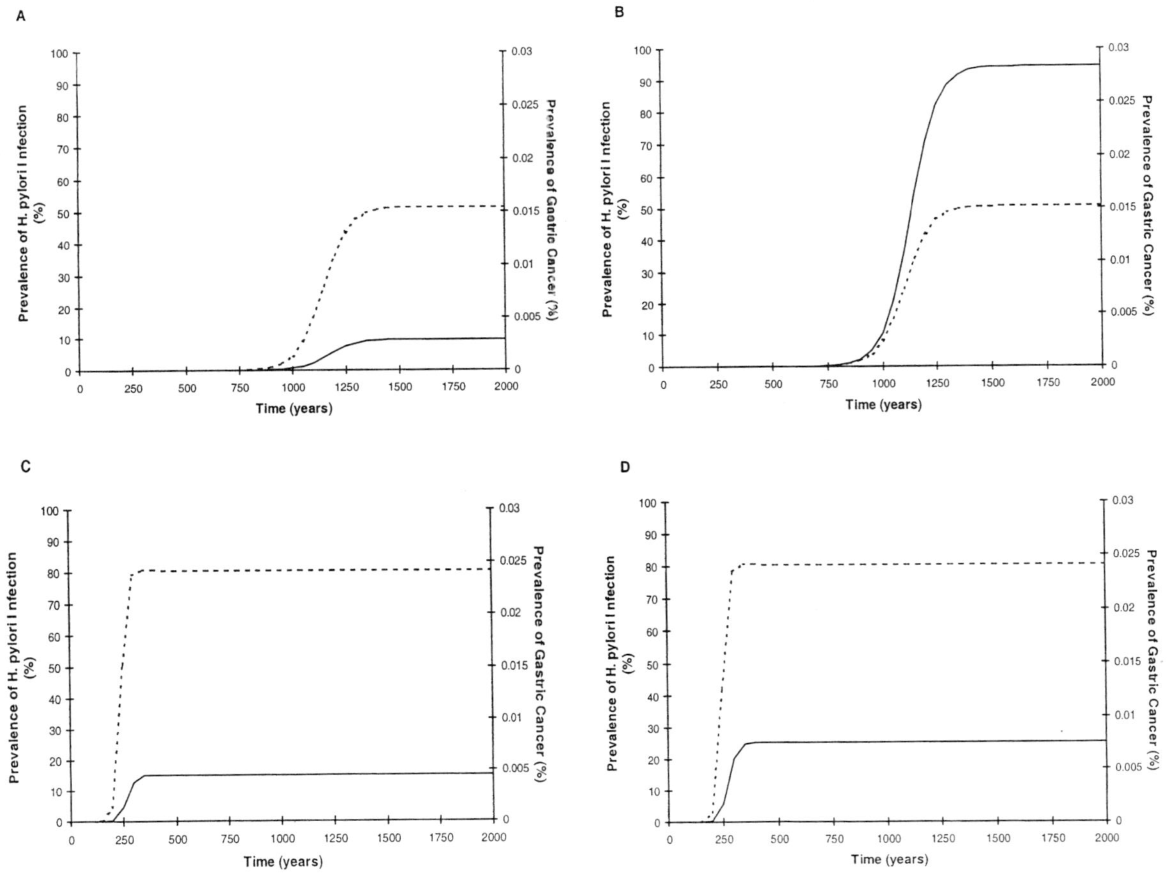

FIG. 2. *Simulated prevalences of H. pylori infection (dashed line) and intestinal gastric adenocarcinoma (solid line) in (**A**) the United States, (**B**) Japan, (**C**) the Ivory Coast, and (**D**) Peru. In each of the four countries, an epidemic was initiated by the introduction of 1 infected person into a population of susceptibles (the 1 infected person being split into 0.5 people with antral and 0.5 people with corpus gastritis).*

Table 1. Model Parameters

Symbol	Biogical Interpretation	Value	Notes
$1/\mu$	average life span	75 years	
$1/\mu_I$	average time to death, due to cancer, after diagnosis	3.1 years	corresponds with 80% death in 5 years [21, 26]
p	probability of developing antral (versus corpus) gastritis following acute infection	0.5	because acute infection often goes undiagnosed [2], this value is entirely unknown
q	probability of developing duodenal ulcers (versus corpus gastritis) following antral gastritis	0.25	because acute infection often goes undiagnosed [2], this value is entirely unknown
γ_A	average rate of progression from antral gastritis to later-stage disease	5 out of every 100 per year	agrees with reports that progression through the antral phase takes greater than 10 years [2]
γ_C	average rate of progression from corpus gastritis to later-stage disease	5 out of every 100 per year	
γ_U	average rate of progression from duodenal ulcers to chronic atrophic gastritis	5 out of every 100 per year	agrees with reports that progression takes 10-20 years [27]
α	relative transmissibility of *H. pylori* from people with chronic atrophic gastritis (versus those with acute antral and corpus gastritis or duodenal ulcers)	0.7	

Table 2. Differing Parameters for the United States, Japan, the Ivory Coast, and Peru

	Population Size (ref #) *(in millions)*	Number of Infections Caused in a Lifetime *(relative to the United States)*	Rate of Progression to Gastric Cancer *(relative to the United States)*
The United States	270.3	1	1
Japan	125.1	1	10
The Ivory Coast	15.5	2.5	1
Peru	24	2.5	1 2/3

Table 3. Prevalence of *H. pylori* Infection and Gastric Cancer: Observed (Real-World Data) & Predicted (Model)

	H. pylori Infection		Gastric Cancer	
	Observed	Predicted	Observed	Predicted
The United States	Up to 50%	51.57%	0.003%	0.0029%
Japan	Up to 50%	50.72%	0.028%	0.028%
The Ivory Coast	~80%	80.62%	0.004%	0.0045%
Peru	~80%	80.59%	0.007%	0.0075%

* *all "observed" data from [13] (values shown are those observed divided by 2, as H. pylori accounts for 50% of gastric cancer [28])*

tors that lead to differences in transmissibility or disease progression rates. Thus, our results indicate that it is possible that differences in hygiene and diet, or other differences such as genetic diversity in bacterial strains or host susceptibility, that lead to country-specific fairly small differences in transmissibility and disease progression rates are sufficient to explain the substantial geographic variation in *H. pylori* infection and gastric cancer rates.

4. Using the model to understand the declining prevalence of *H. pylori* infection and gastric cancer in developed countries. The incidence of *H. pylori* infection [2] and the prevalence of gastric adenocarcinoma [14] have been decreasing over the past century. Because *H. pylori* is likely transmitted from person to person in a fecal-oral manner, both the absolute size of the population as well as the general hygiene of the population under investigation will impact the epidemic spread of the bacteria (see Equation 2). Since 1900, the population of the United States has increased approximately five-fold [29]. In addition, hygiene has greatly improved in the United States during that time period. We used our model to explore the separate effects of population growth and improved hygiene on the diseases associated with *H. pylori* in the United States. We then analyzed the effects of the two factors in combination. Thus, we examined three cases: (i) population growth in the absence of improved hygiene, (ii) improved hygiene in the absence of population growth, and (iii) population growth coincident with improved hygiene. All but two of the parameter values used for these scenarios were identical to those used to simulate *H. pylori* transmission in the United States in the previous section. Only the population size (in the absence of disease) and the transmissibility coefficient (determined, at least in part, by hygiene) were varied. Over the past century, the population in the United States has grown in a near linear fashion from approximately 50 million to about 250 million (Figure 3, data from [29]). Thus, for case 1 and case 3, the population size (without disease) was set to increase (as a result of increasing recruitment into the population), linearly, from 50 million in the year 1900 to 250 million in 2000. For case 2, the disease-free population size was held constant at 150 million (the average value actually recorded over this 100 year time period).

Hygiene has improved substantially in the United States over the past century. Thus, we assumed (as *H. pylori* is transmitted in a fecal-oral manner) that this improvement in hygiene was translated into a decreased transmissibility coefficient (β) for the bacterium. Even if it were possible to quantify hygienic improvements, however, there is no obvious way to use this information to determine the amount by which *H. pylori* transmissibility coefficients have decreased over time. Thus to model the effect of hygiene on decreasing transmissibility we assumed that the average number of susceptible individuals that an infected person would infect in a year (transmissibility coefficient (β) * disease-free population size) was the same in 1900 as it would be in 2000. We set this average number of new infections per year at 0.035 (which corresponds to the value of 2.6 new cases per lifetime used previously for the United States); hence, we calculated that the transmissibility coefficient in 1900 (β_{1900}) was 7×10^{-10} whilst that in 2000 (β_{2000}) would be 1.4×10^{-10}. For cases 2 and 3 we assumed that the

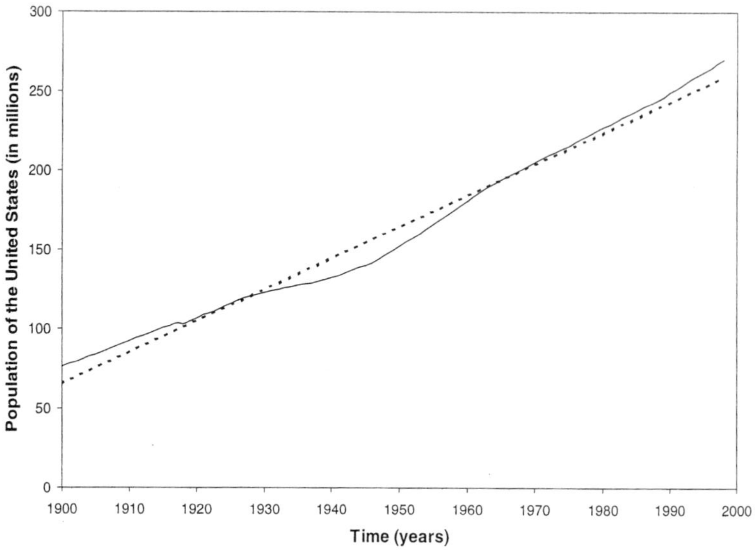

FIG. 3. *Population growth of the United States since 1900. The solid line representing the actual population growth [29] is shown to be well approximated by linear growth from about 50 million people in 1900 to about 250 million people in the year 2000.*

transmissibility coefficient decreased, linearly, from 7×10^{-10} (in 1900) to 1.4×10^{-10}(by 2000). For case 1, we held the transmissibility coefficient constant at 4.2×10^{-10} (the average of the two extreme values).

Figure 4 shows the three simulated epidemics describing the past 100 years of *H. pylori* infection in the United States. It is clear that population growth alone is not a sufficient explanation for the decreases in *H. pylori* and gastric cancer infection that have been observed in the United States (Figure 4A). In fact, after an initial decrease, the prevalence of gastric adenocarcinoma and *H. pylori* infection in the population increases under these conditions of only population growth (Figure 4a). An initial decrease in prevalence is observed because population growth increases the number of susceptible individuals (thus the percentage of people with *H. pylori* infection initially decreases), but eventually an increased pool of susceptible individuals results in increasing transmission rates and an increase in the absolute number of infected individuals. It may be seen that improvements in hygiene (in the absence of population growth) can lead to persistent decreases in the prevalence of both *H. pylori* infection and gastric cancer (Figure 4B). Over the past 70 years, however, the prevalence of gastric cancer has decreased to approximately 27% of its prevalence in 1930 [14]. In case 2 (Figure 4B), the prevalence of gastric cancer at the year 2000 is predicted to be 85% of its value in 1930. Improved hygiene alone, therefore,

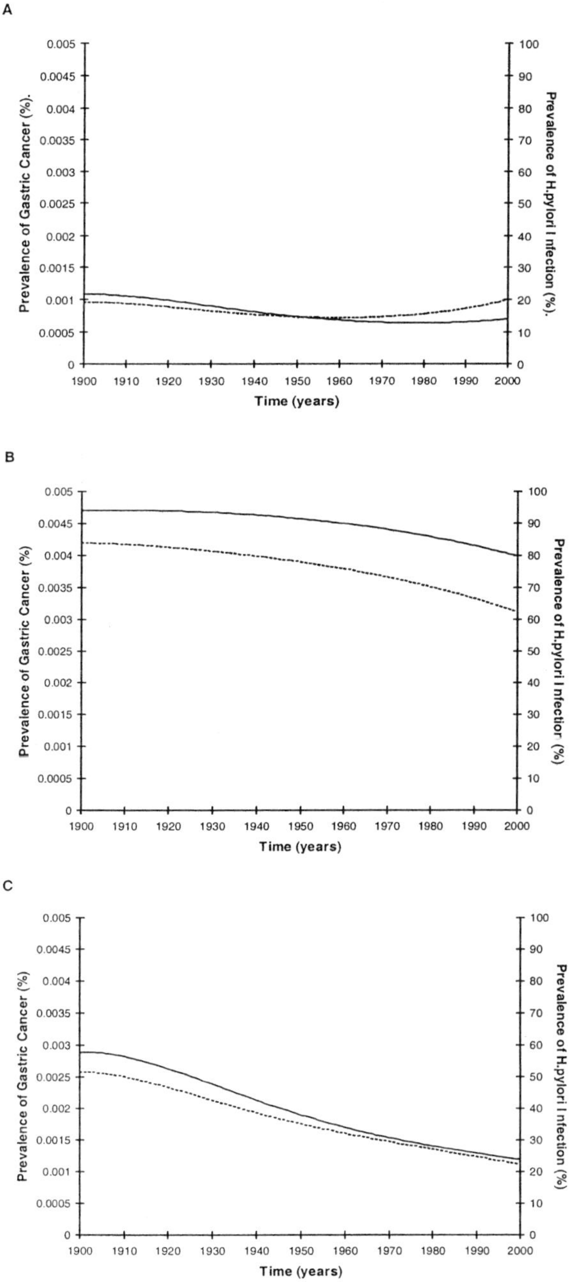

FIG. 4. *Simulated prevalences of H. pylori infection (dashed line) and intestinal gastric adenocarcinoma (solid line) in the United States from 1900–2000. Results under three different assumptions are shown: (**A**) population growth in the absence of improved hygiene, (**B**) improved hygiene with a constant population size, and (**C**) population growth coincident with improved hygiene.*

appears to be insufficient to explain the observed decline in gastric cancer rates. However, when both population growth and improved hygiene are considered together (case 3), then realistic trends in both the prevalence of *H. pylori* infection and gastric cancer are observed (Figure 4C). In this case, there is a persistent decrease in both *H. pylori* infection and gastric cancer rates. Moreover, the prevalence of gastric cancer that is predicted for the year 2000 is 50% of that reported for 1930. This predicted decrease in still less than what has been observed. To produce a more realistic decline in prevalence, we could have modeled the decrease in the transmissibility coefficient differently (i.e., having it attain lower values or having it decrease non-linearly). Even without these modifications, though, it is clear that this situation of both increased population size and decreased transmission rates is more effective in explaining the observed trends in *H. pylori* infection and gastric cancer rates than either factor alone.

5. Discussion. The mathematical model that we have developed to analyze the transmission dynamics of *H. pylori* infection can increase our understanding of the geographic differences in the prevalence of *H. pylori* infection and gastric cancer. We have also shown that our model can be used to explore the historical epidemiology of *H. pylori* in terms of the potential impact of population growth and improvements in hygiene on *H. pylori*-related disease. Due to the current state of the biomedical knowledge on the transmission dynamics and the pathogenesis of *H. pylori*, both the structure of our model and the parameter values that we have used in our analyses remain rather speculative. Our model is only the beginning of a theoretical framework for understanding *H. pylori* infection and gastric cancer. As more empirical studies are performed and as data accumulate, the specific biological mechanisms by which *H. pylori* acts as a risk factor for ulcers and gastric adenocarcinoma will be determined. At that point it will be possible to refine the model that we have presented here and to develop more detailed and complex models.

In addition once better estimates exist for the model's parameter values, then the model can be used to explain other epidemiological phenomenon that are currently only poorly understood. For example, recent evidence suggests that the prevalence of *H. pylori* infection in men is as much as 20–30% higher than it is in women [30]. Other studies have shown similar rates of *H. pylori* infection across gender, but higher rates of late stage disease (peptic ulcers and intestinal gastric adenocarcinoma) in men [30, 31]. Building gender differences into the model structure would enable these gender-specific disease-differences to be examined. Other phenomenology that could be investigated through the use of our model include: (i) people with peptic ulcers seem to be protected from the development of gastric cancer [11], (ii) some people's immune systems better protect them from progression to later stage disease than those of others, (iii) the 'clustering effect' [2]—close contacts of infected children (primarily their families) become quickly infected, and (iv) people are infected earlier in life in developing (most by age 10) than in developed (most not until adulthood) countries [2]. It would be relatively simple to incorporate heterogeneous protection from chronic disease, a clustering phenomenon, and/or age structure into the model to explore and hopefully explain these findings. Furthermore, our model could be expanded and used to investigate the recently identified effects of genetic diversity in both bacterial strains [32] and host susceptibility [33, 34].

Most importantly, our model could be used to design and to evaluate epidemic control strategies. Elimination of the diseases caused by *H. pylori* may be desirable, but elimination must be weighed against the loss of protection from gastroesophageal reflux disease (GERD) that is thought to be conferred upon people who are infected with the bacteria [35]. Antimicrobial therapy is effective in curing *H. pylori* infection [2]. Currently, however, the National Institutes of Health is recommending [31] it be given only to people with active ulcer disease (in 1995, less than 5% of people diagnosed with peptic ulcers received treatment for *H. pylori* infection [36]). The antimicrobial regimens used are a cocktail of three drugs. Despite this precaution, however, bacterial strains resistant to the drugs have been emerging [11]. As has been done previously using models for other infectious diseases (i.e., tuberculosis [37, 38], HIV/AIDS [39] or genital herpes [40]) our model for *H. pylori* infection could be used to weigh the costs (i.e., drug resistance) against the benefits (i.e., decreased transmission) of increasing antimicrobial therapy use. Despite potential positive effects of increasing antimicrobial treatments, however, there is the realistic concern that, especially in developing countries, it will never be possible to achieve the levels of treatment necessary for elimination [11]. Preventive vaccination has been suggested as the best, and perhaps the only realistic, way in which to eliminate *H. pylori* infection worldwide. Prophylactic vaccines are currently being tested in animals [2, 11]. The model framework that we have presented here would be very useful in evaluating the effectiveness of different vaccination strategies (mass vaccination, vaccination of high-risk individuals, etc.) to determine the optimal vaccination program. A combination of theoretical insights and genetic and virological advances may allow for gastric cancer to be made a killer of the past.

REFERENCES

[1] GANEM, D. Infectious Avenues to Cancer. *Science* **284**:1279 (1999).

[2] SMITH, K.L. AND PARSONNET J. *Helicobacter pylori*, in: *Bacterial infections of humans: epidemiology and control* (A.S. Evans and P.S. Brachman, eds.), pp. 337–353, Plenum Publishing Co., New York, 1998.

[3] BLOWER, S.M., MCLEAN, A.R., PORCO, T.C., SMALL, P.M., HOPEWELL, P.C., ET AL. The intrinsic transmission dynamics of tuberculosis epidemics. *Nature Medicine* **4**:815–821 (1995).

[4] EDMUNDS, W.J., MEDLEY, G.F., AND NOKES, D.J. The transmission dynamics and control of hepatitis B virus in The Gambia. *Statistics in Medicine* **15**:2215–2233 (1996).

[5] GAY, N.J. A model of long-term decline in the transmissibility of an infectious disease: implications for the incidence of hepatitis A. *International Journal of Epidemiology* **25**:854–861 (1996).

[6] LINDSAY, S.W. AND BIRLEY, M.H. Climate change and malaria transmission. *Annals of Tropical Medicine and Parasitology* **90**:573–588 (1996).

[7] MAY, R.M. AND ANDERSON, R.M. Transmission dynamics of HIV infection. *Nature* **326**:137–142 (1987).

[8] SOLYANIK, G.I., BEREZETSKAYA, N.M., BULKIEWICZ, R.I., AND KULIK, G.I. Different growth patterns of a cancer cell population as a function of its starting growth characteristics: analysis by mathematical modeling. *Cell Proliferation* **28**:263–78 (1995).

[9] PANETTA, J.C. A mathematical model of breast and ovarian cancer treated with paclitaxel. *Mathematical Biosciences* **146**:89–113 (1997).

[10] GATENBY, R.A. AND GAWLINSKI, E.T. A reaction-diffusion model of cancer invasion. *Cancer Research* **56**:5745–5753 (1996).

[11] COVACCI, A., TELFORD, J.L., DEL GIUDICE, G., PARSONNET, J., AND RAPPUOLI, R. Helicobacter pylori Virulence and Genetic Geography. *Science* **284**:1328–1333 (1999).

[12] PARKIN, D.M., PISANI, P., AND FERLAY, J. (1999). Global Cancer Statistics. *Ca: a Cancer Journal for Clinicians* **49**:33–64. Retrieved April 26, 1999 from the World Wide Web: http://www.ca-journal.org/frames/articles/articles_1999/49_033-064.html.

[13] http://www-dep.iarc.fr/dataava/globocan/globoJava.html.

[14] Bristol Hospital. Stomach cancer: can we prevent it? Retrieved June 22, 1999 from the World Wide Web: http://www.bristolhospital.org/stomach.html.

[15] PARSONNET, J. *Helicobacter pylori. Emerging Infectious Diseases* **12**:185–197 (1998).

[16] FUNG, M.C. (February 20, 1996). Outline summary of stomach cancer. Retrieved April 27, 1999 from the World Wide Web: http://oncolink.upenn.edu/disease/gastric/gastric_review.html.

[17] http://rex.nci.nih.gov/WTNK_PUBS/stomach/cause.htm.

[18] ALM, R.A., LING, L.-S.L., MOIR, D.T., KING, B.L., BROWN, E.D., ET AL. Genomic-sequence comparison of two unrelated isolates of the human gastric pathogen *Helicobacter pylori. Nature* **397**:176–180 (1999).

[19] ANDERSON, R.M. AND MAY, R.M. *Infectious diseases of humans: dynamics and control.* Oxford University Press, Oxford, 1991.

[20] PARSONNET, J. Personal communication. (1998).

[21] SIPPONEN, P. Natural history of gastritis and its relationship to peptic ulcer disease. *Digestion* **51**(suppl 1):70–75 (1992).

[22] DAVIES, G.R., SIMMONDS, N.J., STEVENS, T.R.J., ET AL. *Helicobacter pylori* stimulates antral mucosal reactive oxygen metabolite production *in vivo. Gut* **35**:179–185 (1994).

[23] LYNCH, D.A.F., MAPSTONE, N.P., CLARKE, A.M.T., ET AL. Cell proliferation in *Helicobacter pylori* associated gastritis and the effect of eradication therapy. *Gut* **36**:345–350 (1995).

[24] MARSHALL, B.J AND WARREN, J.R. Unidentified curved bacilli in the stomach of patients with gastritis and peptic ulceration. *Lancet* **1**:1311–1315 (1984).

[25] MARSHALL, B.J. History of the discovery of *C. pylori*, in: *Campylobacter pylori* in Gastritis and Peptic Ulcer Disease, Igaku-Shoin, New York, 1989.

[26] SIPPONEN, P., VARIS, K., FRAKI, O., KORRI, U.-M., SEPPALA, K., ET AL. Cumulative 10-year risk of symptomatic duodenal and gastric ulcer in patients with or without chronic gastritis: a clinical follow-up study of 454 outpatients. *Scandinavian Journal of Gastroenterology* **25**:966–973 (1990).

[27] MAAROOS H.-I., SALUPERE, V., UIBO, R., KEKKI, M., AND SIPPONEN, P. Seven-year follow-up of chronic gastritis in gastric ulcer patients. *Scandinavian Journal of Gastroenterology* **20**:198–204 (1985).

[28] The Helicobacter pylori Foundation. Diseases related to *H. pylori*. Retrieved April 26, 1999 from the World Wide Web: http://www.helico.com/newsite/disease.html.

[29] http://www.census.gov/population/estimates/nation/popclockest.txt. Retrieved June 10, 1999.

[30] REPLOGLE, M.L. GLASER, S.L., HIATT, R.A., AND PARSONNET, J. Biologic sex as a risk factor for Helicobacter pylori infection in healthy young adults. *American Journal of Epidemiology* **142**:856–863 (1995).

[31] NIH Consensus Development Panel on *Helicobacter pylori* in Peptic Ulcer Disease. NIH Consensus Statement **12**:1–22 (February 7–9, 1994).

[32] GERHARD, M. ET AL. Clinical relevance of the *Helicobacter pylori* gene for blood-group antigen-binding adhesion. *Proc. Natl. Acad. Sci.* **96**:12778–12783 (1999).

[33] EL-OMAR E. ET AL. Interleukin-1 polympoorphisms associated with increased risk of gastric cancer. *Nature* **404**:398–402 (2000).

[34] BLASER, M. Linking *Helicobacter pylori* to gastric cancer. *Nature Medicine* **6(4)**:376–377 (2000).

[35] WERDMULLER, B.F.M. AND LOFFELD, R.J.L.F. *Helicobacter pylori* infection has no role in the pathogenesis of reflux esophasgitis. *Dig. Dis. Sci.* **42**:103–105 (1997).

[36] MUNNANGI, S. AND SONNENBERG, A. Time trends of physician visits and treatment patterns of peptic ulcer disease in the United States. *Archives of Internal Medicine* **157**:1489–1494 (1997).

[37] BLOWER, S.M., SMALL, P.M., AND HOPEWELL, P.C. Control strategies for tuberculosis epidemics: new models for old problems. *Science* **273**:497–500 (1996).

[38] BLOWER, S.M. AND GERBERDING, J.L. Understanding, predicting, and controlling the emergence of drug-resistant tuberculosis: a theoretical framework. *Journal of Molecular Medicine* **76**:624–636 (1998).

[39] BLOWER, S.M., GERSHENGORN, H.B., AND GRANT, R.M. A Tale of Two Futures: HIV and Anti-Retroviral Therapy in San Francisco. *Science* **287**: 650–654 (2000).

[40] BLOWER, S.M., PORCO, T.C., AND DARBY, G. Predicting and preventing the emergence of antiviral drug resistance in HSV-2. *Nature Medicine* **4**:673–678 (1998).

FREQUENCY DEPENDENT RISK OF INFECTION AND THE SPREAD OF INFECTIOUS DISEASES

JUAN P. APARICIO*†, ANGEL F. CAPURRO*‡, AND CARLOS CASTILLO-CHAVEZ*§

Abstract. Disease evolution is not only intimately connected to changes in social dynamics but highly driven by them. Disease emergence and re-emergence is tightly linked to shifts on contact structures. Contact sub-structures and, consequently, local networks become epidemiologically active only when infectious individuals are present. In this article, we study the impact of networks on disease evolution. Our work is based on the idea that the "birth" of an infectious individual gives rise to a local epidemiologically active network or generalized household or an epidemiologically-active cluster, of individuals who are likely to have intimate contacts with the source case. Each source case is also a potential source of secondary infections, in the general population, via casual contacts and this is also considered in this paper. Hence, our focus is on the development and analysis of models of disease dynamics in networks that include local dynamics. Our work is applicable to slow diseases which are transmitted via casual and via (local) intimate contacts.

Key words. epidemic models, social networks, tuberculosis, dynamical systems.

1. Introduction. A useful classification of contacts can only be given in the context of a particular disease. Here, we study the transmission dynamics of communicable diseases like tuberculosis that, in general, have long periods of latency followed by short periods of infectiousness, recovery without permanent immunity, and/or death. The "birth" of an infectious individual gives rise to a local network or an epidemiologically active generalized household or active cluster. This local network is composed of individuals who are extremely likely to have intimate contacts with the source case. Of course, each source case is also a potential source of secondary infections, in the general population, via casual contacts. Therefore, the development and study of models of disease dynamics in networks where casual and intimate contacts are common is of importance. In this note, we carry out such a study in the simplest possible setting. Our goals here are to highlight the importance of contact structures based on the quality of contacts. This view is useful in the study of the transmission dynamics of slow communicable diseases like tuberculosis (Aparicio *et al.*, 2000a).

First, we consider a homogeneous population and assume that an infectious individual, the source case, has contacts with susceptible individ-

*Departamento de Investigación, Universidad de Belgrano-CONICET, Zabala 1851, Piso 12, 1426 Buenos Aires, Argentina.

†Department of Biometrics & Mathematical and Theoretical Biology Institute, Cornell University, 431 Warren Hall, Ithaca, NY 14853-7801, USA.

‡Laboratorio de Ecología, Universidad Nacional de Luján-CONICET, Ruta 5 y 7, 6700 Luján, Argentina.

§Department of Theoretical and Applied Mechanics, Cornell University, 317 Kimball Hall, Ithaca, NY 14853-7801, USA.

uals in two settings. The source case either has contacts within the local network, cluster or generalized household which he has just activated (by becoming infectious) or within the "world". The local network consists of his close associates while the world is comprised of the rest of the network.

Contacts (with susceptibles) of an infectious individual are classified by their level of intimacy. The quality of the contact is closely connected to its frequency and its duration. We do not define them precisely but rather by their context. Intimate or *generalized household* contacts tend to occur in families, schools, and at work. *Casual contacts* are those that are not intimate, they occur in the "world" and at random. Hence, as soon as an individual becomes infectious then he/she defines two networks of significantly different sizes: a generalized household, a small local network of individuals who have been put at a higher risk of infection by their personal connection to the source case and, global network, a 'place' where infections are generated by "accident". Risk from the local network persists only through the epidemiological life of the source case. It is likely that the number of casual contacts of an infectious individual is a lot greater than his/her average number of intimate contacts. It is also likely that the probability of disease transmission per contact is significantly lower for casual than for intimate contacts.

Traditionally, contacts between susceptibles and infectious individuals are modeled from the point of view of the susceptible, that is, the rate of infection is modeled by a term of the form $\beta S \frac{I}{N}$. It is assumed that the rate of contact between susceptible and infectious individuals is proportional to the infectious prevalence I/N, or, equivalent, to the susceptible frequency S/N. Since typically all contacts are identical (same duration and intensity) then this distinction is irrelevant. That is, the contact process can be interpreted from the point of view of the infectious or the susceptible individuals. On the other hand, since we focus on diseases with low probability of transmission per casual contact and higher probability of transmission per intimate contacts then contacts must be differentiated by duration and strength or intensity. Furthermore, since intimate contacts occur mostly with individuals with whom one has frequent interactions then a modeling approach based on the networks of the (infectious) source case seems the most appropriate as the process is no longer symmetric.

Hence, the focus is on modeling diseases with two-types of frequency dependent contacts: contacts within an epidemiologically-active generalized household or small local network and, contacts within the "world", a huge network, with a lower probability of transmission per contact.

Shifts in social dynamics driven by cultural changes (urbanization) or population dynamics (demography) have generated a dynamic social landscape that fosters disease evolution. Increases in contact rates due to urbanization and mass-transportation have altered the frequency of contacts and possibly their quality. Models that incorporate contact-quality at multiple levels need to be developed and studied. Here we focus exclusively on the impact of local and global networks (see Aparicio *et al.*, 2000b; and this volume for additional approaches and extensions).

2. Modeling cluster transmission. We consider slow diseases with a long latency period and assume that transmission is *only* possible within a generalized household or an epidemiologically-active cluster. We consider four epidemiological classes: susceptible, latent, infectious and recovered. We assume that the recruitment rate Λ is constant in order to exclude the role of demography. We let μ denote the inverse of life expectancy or the per-capita disease induced mortality rate and r the recovery rate. The total removal rate of infectious individuals, denoted by γ, is therefore given by $\gamma \equiv r + \mu_d + \mu$. We keep track of whether or not an individual is in an epidemiologically-active cluster or not. We let $N_c(t)$, denote the population size of individuals in epidemiologically-active generalized households while $N_{nc}(t)$ denotes the population of those who are not. First we neglect the effects of casual infections, that is, we assume that only susceptible persons belonging to the N_c-population may acquire infection. To simplify the notation, non-infectious populations are identified via subscripts. Subscript 1 is used to identify individuals in generalized-households (epidemiologically-active clusters) while subscript 2 is used to identify those who are not. The period of infectiousness, $1/\gamma$, is assumed to be significantly shorter than life expectancy (as is the case in tuberculosis). This last assumption, justifies our decision to neglect births, deaths, and disease progression within the N_c-population. It is further assumed that cluster size is constant and equal to n; that all infectious individuals, or active cases are equally infectious; and, that all generalized household contacts are equivalent. In other words, a constant risk of infection per capita and per unit of time (β) is assumed for all of susceptible individuals who are members of generalized-households. The per capita disease progression rate is denoted by k and, consequently the fraction of infected people who develop the disease is given by $f = k/(k + \mu)$. To highlight the role of epidemiologically-active clusters on disease transmission, we highlight the mechanics of the infection process.

Whenever an infected individual (belonging to the E_2 class) becomes infectious, that is, when he/she moves into the I-class, his/her generalized-household becomes epidemiologically active. A group of people of size n is instantaneously moved from the N_{nc}-population into the N_c-population. How are they be re-distributed among the N_c-epidemiological classes? They are transferred in proportion to their frequencies in the N_{nc}-population, namely, in proportion to S_2/N_2, E_2/N_2, and R_2/N_2-. From the definition of epidemiologically-active cluster, it becomes clear that kE_2 new (epidemiologically-active) generalized households are "born" per unit of time. Hence, the total recruitment rates into the corresponding N_c-susceptible, latent and recovered or treated epidemiological classes are $\frac{S_2}{N_2}nkE_2$, $\frac{E_2}{N_2}nkE_2$ and $\frac{R_2}{N_2}nkE_2$. The recovery or death of the active case makes the generalized household inactive and this occurs at the rate γI. Whenever an epidemiologically active cluster becomes inactive, individuals are returned to their corresponding epidemiological classes in the N_{nc}-population. Since the "death" rate of the epidemiologically-active generalized-household is γI, and the average generalized-household size is n then, $n\gamma I$ individuals must be moved from N_c- into the N_{nc}-population per unit of time. The relation $N_1 = nI$, which holds by definition, implies that $n\gamma I S_1/N_1 = \gamma S_1$. Hence, γS_1 susceptible individuals must be returned per unit of time to the N_{nc}-population, per unit of time. Rates of return for other epidemiological classes are computed in the same way. If we further assume that those treated will never get the disease again (permanent immunity) then we arrive at the following epidemiological model where the mode of transmission is exclusively via generalized households (intimate contacts):

$$\frac{dS_1}{dt} = -(\beta+\gamma)S_1 + \frac{S_2}{N_2}nkE_2, \tag{1}$$

$$\frac{dE_1}{dt} = \beta S_1 - \gamma E_1 + \frac{E_2}{N_2}nkE_2, \tag{2}$$

$$\frac{dR_1}{dt} = -\gamma R_1 + \frac{R_2}{N_2}nkE_2, \tag{3}$$

$$\frac{dI}{dt} = kE_2 - \gamma I, \tag{4}$$

$$\frac{dS_2}{dt} = \Lambda - bS_2 + \gamma S_1 - \frac{S_2}{N_2}nkE_2, \tag{5}$$

$$\frac{dE_2}{dt} = \gamma E_1 - (\mu+k)E_2 - \frac{E_2}{N_2}nkE_2. \tag{6}$$

$$\frac{dR_2}{dt} = rI + \gamma R_1 - \mu R_2 - \frac{R_2}{N_2}nkE_2. \tag{7}$$

For model (1–7), the *Basic Reproductive Number*, defined as the number of secondary cases generated by a typical infectious individual in a population where every one is susceptible, is given by

$$\mathcal{R}_0 = \frac{\beta n}{(\beta+\gamma)}\frac{k}{(\mu+k)} \equiv Q_0 f, \tag{8}$$

where $Q_0 = \frac{\beta n}{\beta+\gamma}$ is the number of secondary infections caused by one infectious individual in a fully susceptible population; and $f \equiv \frac{k}{\mu+k}$, is the fraction of infected individuals who develop the disease (become infectious). From Expression (8) we see that $\mathcal{R}_0$ is always bounded by cluster size (n) regardless of the level of infectiousness or the length of the infectious period. Hence, mean cluster size plays a fundamental role in determining the severity of an epidemic where the main mode of transmission is via generalized households. The elasticity of $\mathcal{R}_0$ with respect to a parameter

λ is $\mid \frac{1}{\mathcal{R}_0} \frac{\partial \mathcal{R}_0}{\partial \lambda} \mid$. It is straightforward to see that cluster size is the most significant parameter.

2.1. Modeling short latency periods. A ('source') case produces secondary infections and some of them will progress into the infectious class ('secondary' cases). It is likely that some proportion of individuals in an epidemiologically-active generalized household were in fact members of a prior epidemiologically-active generalized household. In other words, generalized household overlap is likely and its likelihood must be linked to duration of the latency period. The shorter the latent period the higher the probability of generalized household overlap.

A simple way of modeling generalized cluster overlap is by assuming that the proportion of susceptible individuals in a newly established epidemiologically-active generalized household is given by a weighted average of the proportion of suceptibles from the N_{nc}- and N_c-populations. This simplistic approach that captures cluster overlap in a phenomenological way can be used to model partial overlap between epidemiologically-active generalized-households just by replacing the term $\frac{S_2}{N_2} nkE_2$ with the weighted average $\left((1-\rho)\frac{S_2}{N_2} + \rho\frac{S_1}{N_1}\right) nkE_2$, with $0 < \rho < 1$. Whenever $\rho = 0$, we recover the case where there is no cluster overlap and that corresponds to diseases with extremely long latency (non-infectious) periods followed by very short infectious periods.

2.2. Modeling casual infections. No disease will be transmitted exclusively in generalized households. In fact, there is growing evidence that even diseases with low probability of transmission per contact, like tuberculosis, can be transmitted often via casual contacts. Tuberculosis transmission in public places like bars and airplanes has been documented (see Rafalli *et al.*, 1996, for a recent review; see also Cobelens *et al.*, 2000). We choose to model the rate of casual infections in the classical way, that is, via a term of the form $\beta^* I \frac{S}{N}$. However, for diseases like TB, with *low prevalence of active cases* further approximations are possible. Since, the prevalence of active cases is $I/N \ll 1$ then $N_1 \ll N_2$. Hence, we choose to approximate S/N by S_2/N_2. Using this approximation our model with intimate and casual contacts becomes:

$$\text{(9)} \qquad \frac{dS_1}{dt} = -(\beta+\gamma)S_1 + \left((1-\rho)\frac{S_2}{N_2} + \rho\frac{S_1}{N_1}\right) nkE_2,$$

$$\text{(10)} \qquad \frac{dE_1}{dt} = \beta S_1 - \gamma E_1 + \left((1-\rho)\frac{E_2}{N_2} + \rho\frac{E_1}{N_1}\right) nkE_2,$$

$$\text{(11)} \qquad \frac{dR_1}{dt} = -\gamma R_1 + \left((1-\rho)\frac{R_2}{N_2} + \rho\frac{R_1}{N_1}\right) nkE_2,$$

$$\text{(12)} \qquad \frac{dI}{dt} = kE_2 - \gamma I,$$

$$\frac{dS_2}{dt} = \Lambda - bS_2 + \gamma S_1 - \left((1-\rho)\frac{S_2}{N_2} + \rho\frac{S_1}{N_1}\right) nkE_2 - \beta^* I \frac{S_2}{N_2}, \tag{13}$$

$$\frac{dE_2}{dt} = \gamma E_1 - (\mu + k)E_2 - \left((1-\rho)\frac{E_2}{N_2} + \rho\frac{E_1}{N_1}\right) nkE_2 + \beta^* I \frac{S_2}{N_2}, \tag{14}$$

$$\frac{dR_2}{dt} = rI + \gamma R_1 - \mu R_2 - \left((1-\rho)\frac{R_2}{N_2} + \rho\frac{R_1}{N_1}\right) nkE_2, \tag{15}$$

where now $N_i \equiv S_i + E_i + R_i$. The resulting Basic Reproductive Number for this model is

$$\mathcal{R}_0 = \left(\frac{\beta n(1-\rho)}{\beta + (1-\rho)\gamma} + \frac{\beta^*}{\gamma}\right)\frac{k}{(k+\mu)}. \tag{16}$$

The infectious period determines the time-scale of the disease dynamics in the N_c-population while life expectancy is the characteristic time-scale for the dynamics (including disease dynamics) in the N_{nc}-population.

Whenever the infectious period is a lot shorter than the life-expectancy (as it would be the case for tuberculosis), we approximate the variables S_1, E_1, R_1 and I by their quasi-equilibrium values which are obtained by setting Equations (9–12) equal to zero. They are:

$$S_1(t) \cong \frac{(1-\rho)}{\beta + (1-\rho)\gamma}\frac{S_2(t)}{N_2(t)} nkE_2(t), \tag{17}$$

$$E_1(t) \cong \frac{1}{\gamma}\left(\frac{\beta}{\beta + (1-\rho)\gamma}\frac{S_2(t)}{N_2(t)} + \frac{E_2(t)}{N_2(t)}\right) nkE_2(t), \tag{18}$$

$$R_1(t) \cong \left(\frac{1}{\gamma} + \frac{R_2(t)}{N_2(t)}\right) nkE_2(t), \tag{19}$$

$$I(t) \cong \frac{k}{\gamma}E_2(t). \tag{20}$$

Whenever this approximation is valid the system reduces (9–15) to a 3-dimensional system for the slow variables associated with the disease dynamics in the N_{nc}-population. The reduced system is

$$\frac{dS_2}{dt} \cong \Lambda - \mu S_2 - (\mu + k)\mathcal{R}_0 \frac{S_2 E_2}{N_2}, \tag{21}$$

$$\frac{dE_2}{dt} \cong -(\mu + k)E_2 + (\mu + k)\mathcal{R}_0 \frac{S_2 E_2}{N_2}. \tag{22}$$

$$\frac{dR_2}{dt} \cong \frac{rk}{\gamma}E_2 - \mu R_2, \tag{23}$$

where $\mathcal{R}_0$ is still given by expression (16). Using approximation (20), the rate of infection term becomes $\frac{\gamma}{k}(\mu + k)\mathcal{R}_0 \frac{S_2 I}{N_2} = \gamma Q_0 \frac{S_2 I}{N_2}$. Hence, Model (1–7) can be approximated by a classical epidemic model with a transmission coefficient given by $\beta_{eff} \equiv \gamma Q_0$. However, the number of secondary infections produced by every infectious individual $Q_0 \frac{S}{N}$ does not depend in a multiplicative way on the infectious period $1/\gamma$. Effectively, we have that

$$Q_0 = \frac{\beta n(1-\rho)}{\beta + (1-\rho)\gamma} + \frac{\beta^*}{\gamma}. \tag{24}$$

The last term in Expression (24) gives the contribution of casual infections to secondary cases and depends linearly on the infectious period while the first term (intimate contacts) is bounded by cluster size. The use of a constant rate (or risk) of infection per susceptible individuals in epidemiologically-active generalized-households (β) gives rise to a nonlinear dependence of $\mathcal{R}_0$ on β. Since it is assumed that risk is exponentially-distributed with parameter β in a cluster then risk becomes an epidemiologically-relevant and measurable parameter. Note that the use of a classical modeling approach for transmission via casual contacts renders the parameter β^* non-measurable-a typical problem of classical models. In fact, despite its epidemiological derivation and justification our lack of approaches to estimate contact rates reduces the value of β^*. In fact, β^* becomes mostly a fitting parameter.

In our case, however, we have that $\beta_{eff} \equiv \gamma Q_0$. It is not necessary to know the value of the infectious period $1/\gamma$ because the rate of infection is approximately $(k + \mu)Q_0 \frac{SE}{N}$. Although Q_0 is still a function of the infectious period (see expression (24)), standard epidemiological surveys provide estimates of Q_0 using a direct classification of contacts for the source case. Therefore our formulation uses parameters closer to the those obtained from epidemiological studies.

2.3. Discussion. Our approach allows for the exploration of various sociological settings including the impact of urbanization, mass transportation, and global travel on contact rates and, consequently, on casual infections. For slow diseases like tuberculosis, cluster overlap, here modeled by ρ, is minimal. However, for diseases like influenza or measles cluster overlap is critical. Models like those described here are not appropriate for the study of the role of clusters on the transmission of "fast" and highly infectious diseases. In fact, the results of Watts and Strogatz (1998) support, albeit indirectly, the use of classical models.

In classical network models for the spread of infectious diseases each person is modeled as a node and the links among them are those with potential infective contacts. For the study of disease transmission in small communities an approach based on a full characterization of the entire network of contacts is possible. For large communities, such a global network analysis is not only impractical but unnecessary. Watts and Strogatz (1998) have shown, in some sense, that the spread of an infectious disease in a 'small-world' network is quite similar to the spread of a disease in a randomly connected network, provided that all the contacts are identical and

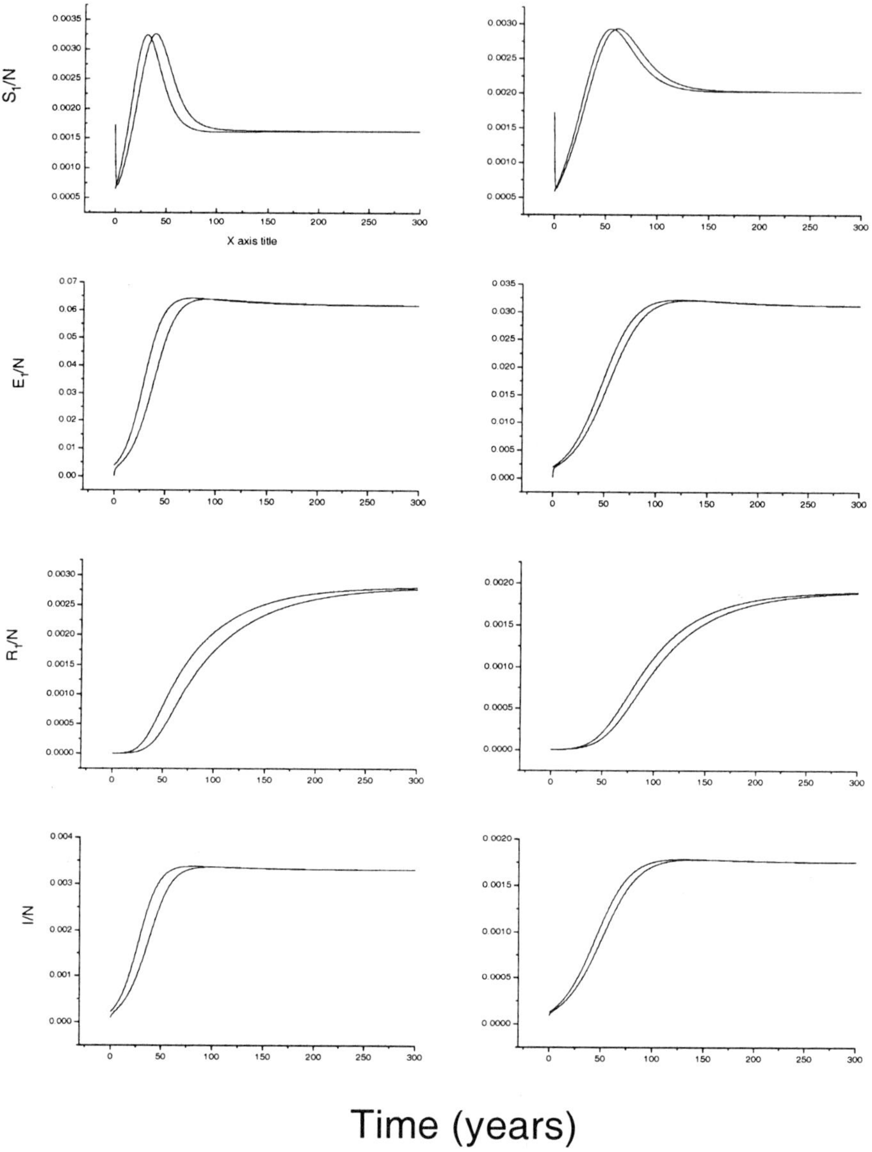

FIG. 1. *Solutions of the full model and those obtained by setting time derivative equal to zero. In figures on the left mean infectious period is as long as 5 years. In the figures on the right infectious period is 2 years. For infectious periods less than one year both solutions are almost identical.*

the number of contacts (cluster size) remains constant (with some minimal cluster overlap). Local network analysis which is based on our knowledge of the links of sampled individuals (see Morris, 1995, for a short review) is close to our work. From the point of view of epidemiological field studies (data) local network approaches appear to be significantly more appropriate than global ones.

In small-world networks, randomly connected networks, and some intermediate networks (considered by Watts & Strogatz) individuals are assumed to have contacts with a fixed number of individuals (nodes). Hence, the network is seen as an inter-connected collection of (almost independent) clusters where transmission is possible only within the cluster. A small-world network can be viewed as a highly clustered network where the probability of contact between two individuals is very high whenever they share a contact (connection to a common node).

Although this network structure is very different from that of a randomly connected network, its structure does not seem to affect significantly the spread of a disease. In other words, randomly connected and small world networks predict qualitatively similar epidemics.

Our work shows that the critical parameter for disease spread is mean cluster size. It seems reasonable to expect that every human community is, at least in some sense, well represented by a small world network. If this is so then our work (when combined with the results of Watts & Strogatz' (1998)) shows that disease spread is highly dependent on the distribution of generalized household (local networks) sizes.

Research on local network analysis has focused mostly on efforts to characterize the mixing of heterogeneous populations (see, for example, Anderson *et al.*, 1990; Blythe *et al.*, 1991; Castillo-Chavez & Blythe, 1989; Jacquez *et al.*, 1989; Hyman & Stanley, 1988; Sattenspiel, 1987; Hethcote & Yorke, 1984). In most of the works just cited, links are identical within homogeneously mixing sub-populations. Our approach considers a homogeneously mixing population but discriminates in the type of links within subpopulations—in the simplest possible way. Sustained contact are different from casual ones. Sustained contacts are more infectious, on the average, than casual contacts. At the population level, casual contacts may still have a significant impact on the spread of a disease. In fact, casual contacts enhance the effect of the "long-distance" rare interactions assumed in small-world networks. Casual contacts reduce the differences between randomly connected and small-world networks. Our work support this view through the incorporation of contact quality (edges between nodes are not identical).

Networks here (fixed in size as in Watts & Strogatz, 1998) allow for dynamic links between nodes. When an individual becomes infectious all the links between the source case and its local network become active (intimate contacts in generalized household) as well as some randomly distributed links outside the local network (casual infections). In other words, individuals are only temporary members of a network.

REFERENCES

[1] Anderson, R.M., Gupta, S., & Ng, W. (1990). The significance of sexual partner contact networks for the transmission dynamics of HIV. *JAIDS* **3**, 417–429.

[2] Aparicio, J.P., Capurro, A.F., & Castillo-Chavez, C. (2000a). Transmission and dynamics of tuberculosis on generalized households. *J. Theor. Biol.* **206**, 327–341. doi:10.1006/jtbi.2000.2129.

[3] Aparicio J.P., Capurro A.F., & Castillo-Chavez C. (2000b). On the fall and rise of tuberculosis. Department of Biometrics, Cornell University, Technical Report Series, BU-1477-M.

[4] Blythe, S., Castillo-Chavez, C., Palmer, J., & Cheng, M. (1991). Towards a unified theory of mixing and pair formation, *Math. Biosc.* **107**, 349–407.

[5] Castillo-Chavez, C. & Blythe, S. (1989). Mixing framework for social/sexual behavior. In: *Mathematical and statistical approaches to AIDS epidemiology* (Castillo-Chavez ed.). Springer, Berlin, 275–288.

[6] Colbelens, F.G.J., van Deutekmon, H., Draayer-Jansen, I.W.E., Scepp-Beelen, A.C.H.M., van Gerven, P.J.H.J., van Kessel, R.P.M., & Mensen, M.E.A. (2000). Risk of infection with *Mycobacterium tuberculosis* in travellers to areas of high tuberculosis endemicity. The Lancet **356**, 461–465.

[7] Hethcote, H.W. & York J.A. (1984). Gonorrhea Transmission and Control. Lectures Notes in Biomathematics 56, Springer, New York.

[8] Jacquez, J.A., Simon, C.P., & Koopman, J. (1989). Structured mixing: heterogeneous mixing by the definition of activity groups. In: *Mathematical and statistical approaches to AIDS epidemiology* (Castillo-Chavez ed.). Springer, Berlin, 275–288.

[9] Hyman, J. & Stanley, E. (1988). Using mathematical models to understand the AIDS epidemics. *Math. Bios.* **90**, 415–473.

[10] Morris, M. (1995). Data driven network models for the spread of disease. In *Epidemic Models: their structure and relation to data*, (Mollison, D. ed.), Cambridge University Press, pp. 302–322.

[11] Raffalli, J., Sepkowitz, K.A., & Armstrong, D. (1996). Community-Based Outbreaks of Tuberculosis. *Arch. Intern. Med.*, **156**, 1053–1060.

[12] Satenspield, L. (1987). Population structure and the spread of disease. *Human Biology*, **59**, 411–438.

[13] Watts, D.J. & Strogatz, S.H. (1998). Collective dynamics of 'small-world' networks, *Nature*, **393**, 440–442.

LONG-TERM DYNAMICS AND RE-EMERGENCE OF TUBERCULOSIS

JUAN P. APARICIO*†, ANGEL F. CAPURRO*‡, AND CARLOS CASTILLO-CHAVEZ*§

Abstract. The issue of disease emergence of re-emergence is central to the study of disease evolution and to the implementation of surveillance and public health policies. In this note, we struggle with the concept of re-emergence and illustrate our thoughts on this issue using partial population growth, mortality, tuberculosis prevalence and incidence data from the United States over the last 150 years. Past and current trends of tuberculosis dynamics are explained via simulations based on US demographic data and under the assumptions of reduced host susceptibility and host-parasite coevolution.

1. Introduction. Despite the fact that tuberculosis (TB) incidence and prevalence have declined during the last century it is still responsible for about 3 million deaths annually (Snider, 1997). This downward trend stopped, in many parts of the world, in the middle 80's. An increase of about 50,000 new cases over the expected number of cases was observed in United States between 1985 and 1992 (Snider, 1997). Denmark, Ireland, Italy, Netherlands, Norway, Spain, and Switzerland experienced an increase in incidence of active-TB in the early 90's (Raviglione *et al.*, 1993). Costly efforts to reduce active-TB incidence in the US began to pay off after 1993. The number of cases of active-TB from 1995 to 1998 were less than those reported in 1985. Patterns of incidence of active-TB in different regions of the world are as follows (WHO, 1999):

- Western Europe and South America had a declining trend until 1989; incidence of active-TB remained stabilized until 1993; a downward trend was re-established in 1994.
- Eastern Europe had a declining trend until 1990 followed by an upward trend.
- Sub-Saharan Africa has had an upward trend since 1981.
- South Asia has experienced no change since 1981.

A glance at these data raises the obvious question: Is the notion of global TB re-emergence supported by data? US's increase in the number of active cases in the 1985–1992 period was attributed to several factors including: immigration from countries with high TB-prevalence; increases in drug abuse and poverty; the HIV-epidemic; and, relapses in TB control programs

*Departamento de Investigación, Universidad de Belgrano-CONICET, Zabala 1851, Piso 12, 1426 Buenos Aires, Argentina.

†Department of Biometrics & Mathematical and Theoretical Biology Institute, Cornell University, 431 Warren Hall, Ithaca, NY 14853-7801, USA.

‡Laboratorio de Ecología, Universidad Nacional de Luján-CONICET, Ruta 5 y 7, 6700 Luján, Argentina.

§Department of Theoretical and Applied Mechanics, Cornell University, 317 Kimball Hall, Ithaca, NY 14853-7801, USA.

(Snider 1997). US recent downward trend has been linked to the successes of programs like the *Directly Observed Treatment Strategy* (McKenna, *et al.*, 1998) and to recent improvements in inner-cities health services.

A study of the long-term dynamics of tuberculosis may increase our understanding of present trends. Changing demographic patterns in the US support the hypothesis that the main causes behind TB reduction must include a considerable reduction on TB-progression rates over the last century. This reduction, regardless of the sources, effectively explains observed trends of incidence of active-TB at least in some parts of the world over the past two centuries.

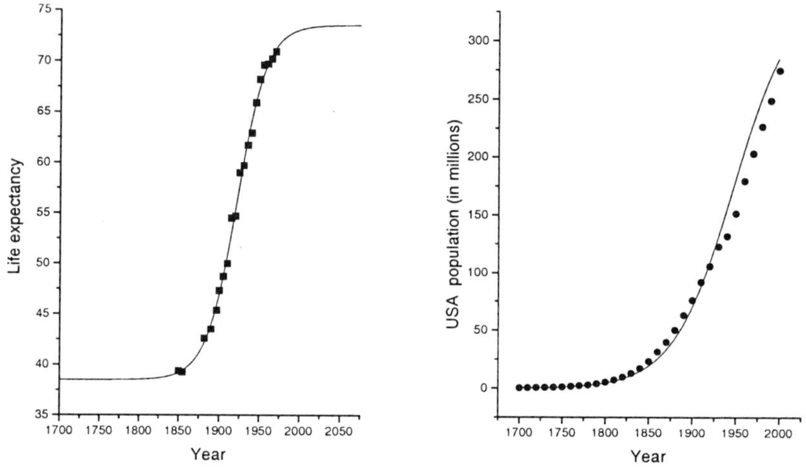

(a) (b)

FIG. 1. *a) Observed (squares) life expectancy at birth (τ) and their best fit to model (5). b) Observed (squares) population growth for the United States and model solution (continuous line). We used a density-dependent birthrate,* $b = a(1 - \frac{N}{K}) + \mu$ *with* $a = 0.0293528yr^{-1}$ *and* $K = 345 \times 10^6$*, the parameter values are obtained from the best fit of data to a logistic model growth. The mortality rate* μ *was estimated as the inverse of life expectancy at birth* τ.

2. What is re-emergence? According to Webster's (1995) dictionary *emerging* means

> "to come forth or rise up from or as if from immersion" or "to become obvious or evident" or "to issue from obscurity" or "to come into existence"

while *disease re-emergence*, according to the World Health Organization (WHO, 1998), is:

> "... due to the reappearance of, and an increase in, the number of infections from a disease which is known, but which had formerly caused so few infections that it had no longer been considered a public health problem."

Active-TB incidence trends (see Fig. 2) show that TB re-emergence – according to WHO's views – is, in part, a function of societies' changing expectations. In the USA, the total number of new cases of active-TB increased from 22,201 in 1985 to a maximum of 26,673 in 1992 before it began to decline as a result of enhanced and costly public health strategies. A 20% increase was observed in a 7 year period! How much can it be attributed to better disease surveillance mechanisms developed in the aftermath of the HIV epidemic? How much can it be attributed to the increase in HIV immuno-suppressed individuals? Increased efforts to fight and detect TB have often been linked to society's efforts to fight HIV co-infections and hence, they are part of the story.

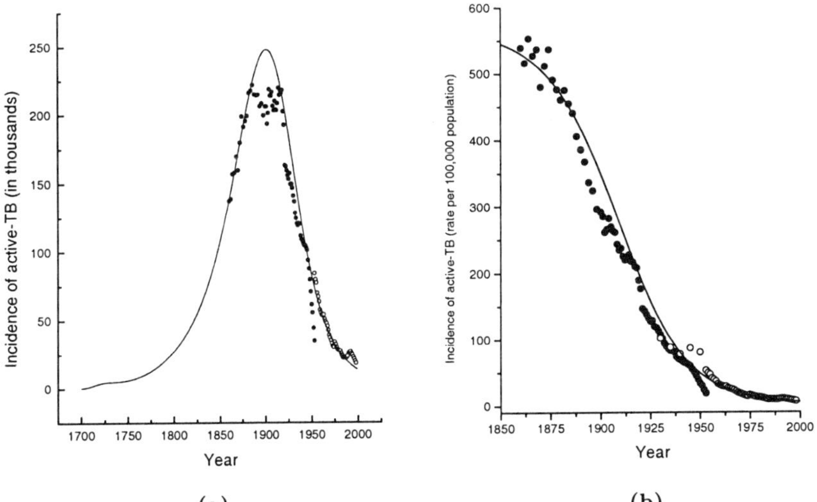

(a) **(b)**

FIG. 2. *Possible incidence of active-TB (number of new cases per year) (a), and the corresponding rate per 100.000 population (b) estimated as 1.5 times mortality the rates between 1860 and 1940 (solid circles). We have overlaid the observed incidence (1930–1998, open circles), and model solutions (continuous line). Between 1850 and 1900, population growth was faster than the increase in the total number of new cases per year and, then the incidence rate (*$\sim kE/N$*) showed a declining trend during this period. Parameter values are* $Q_0 = 10$, $f_i = 0.245$, $f_f = 0.08$.

Wealthy societies may classify a disease as re-emergent as soon as a 'prolonged' downward trend shifts – even minimally – upward. Increases in host contact rates, deterioration of living conditions, or the appearance of drug-resistant strains may all contribute to relatively small changes that either temporarily or 'permanently' change an established trend. The length of the time-scale used to determine whether or not re-emergence has taken place is of importance. In societies like the US, where the implementation of effective public health measures can be extremely fast, the issue of whether or not a disease has re-emerged is difficult to asses. Was the upward trend observed from 1985 to 1992 the result of deep structural changes in social dynamics? Or was this 'minor' upward shift just the result of natural fluctuations from typically small perturbations linked to local or rare events (see Feng *et al.*, 2000)? Or was it the result of better surveillance? A sudden but temporary increase in immigration, from countries with high TB-prevalence, to US cities may provide such a temporary perturbation of the system. Such perturbations typically do not alter the evolutionary (social) landscape and, hence, typically they do not give rise to 'permanent' changes in epidemic patterns. There is not enough data to differentiate between many reasonable hypotheses. How are we to identify critical factors responsible for disease re-emergence using data from nations with quick interventions policies? Global surveillance mechanisms must be part of the equation.

The Twentieth Century saw dramatic increases in contact rates from the birth and growth of cities (urbanization). The growth of public transportation and international travel have resulted in increased levels of interconnectedness between sub-populations. Advances in public health resulted in improved surveillance mechanisms that reduced the infectious life of a large number of individuals. Regardless of the direction of this evidence, during this period of time, *dramatic decreases* of active-TB morbidity and mortality have been observed. Are these changes due to the massive use of antibiotics and/or to better public-health measures and/or to pathogen and host coevolution?

A dynamical systems approach is used to study the long-term dynamics of tuberculosis. A model capable of explaining observed dramatic shifts on the number of cases of active-TB in the US, that began in the nineteenth century, is developed. Population growth and reductions in virulence play a significant role on our reconstruction of observed past and current TB-epidemic patterns.

3. A dynamical system approach to tuberculosis dynamics.

3.1. Basic epidemiology. *Mycobacterium tuberculosis*, the causal agent of tuberculosis, is transmitted mostly through droplets expelled by coughing infectious people. The probability of TB transmission per contact is low when compared to that of airborne transmitted diseases like influenza but the infectious period of TB is longer. The risk of infection is significant only for individuals who have frequent and close contacts with source cases (see Rafalli *et al.*, 1996; Aparicio *et al.*, 2000a). Most individuals' immune system is capable of containing the proliferation of *M. tuberculosis.* Such latently-infected individuals are asymptomatic and non-infectious. Only a fraction of them progress to the infectious stage (active-TB). The risk of progression to active-TB is higher during the first years following infection. Risk of disease progression is also high in situations where an individual's immune system has been compromised (Styblo, 1991). Immune response deterioration may be due to poor nutrition, drug abuse, alcoholism, age, or HIV co-infection, to name some possibilities. Further re-infections with *M. tuberculosis* may also increase the risk of TB-progression (Styblo, 1991; Sutherland, 1975; Feng *et al.*, 2000).

3.2. A simple model for TB dynamics. A simplified picture of TB transmission dynamics is sufficient to highlight the importance of demography and reduced virulence on observed TB patterns over the last two centuries. TB dynamics are modeled via the following $SEIR$ transmission model (Aparicio *et al.*, 2000b):

$$\frac{dS}{dt} = bN - \mu S - \gamma Q_0 \frac{S}{N} I, \tag{1}$$

$$\frac{dE}{dt} = \gamma Q_0 \frac{S}{N} I - (k + \alpha + \mu)E, \tag{2}$$

$$\frac{dI}{dt} = kE - \gamma I, \tag{3}$$

$$\frac{dR}{dt} = rI + \alpha E - \mu R, \tag{4}$$

where S denotes the susceptible class, E the latently-infected class, I the actively-infectious class, and R the recovered class. The birth (b) and death (μ) rates are estimated from available data. Progression from the latent-class E to the active-TB class I occurs at the rate k. Model (1–4) implies that the fraction of latently-infected individuals who develop active-TB is $f = k/(k + \mu + \alpha)$. Re-infection and TB-relapse are disregarded (but see Feng *et al.*, 2000). TB induced mortality is included in the removal rate $\gamma = r + \mu$. Q_0 denotes the mean total number of infections caused by a typical infectious individual during its infectious period in a susceptible population. The value of this parameter varies from population to population and implicitly depends on the average contact rate and the host's susceptibility (probability of becoming infected per contact with an infectious individual). Q_0 is a function of the length of the infectious period $(1/\gamma)$ and the size of the network of close and casual contacts (for additional details see Aparicio *et al.* 2000a, and this volume).

3.2.1. Basic reproduction number. Out of the number of secondary infections Q_0, only the fraction $f = k/(k + \mu + \alpha)$ survives the latency period resulting in new cases of active-TB. The basic reproductive number ($\mathcal{R}_0$), the number of secondary (infectious) cases produced by a 'typical' infectious individual in a population where everyone is susceptible, is given by $\mathcal{R}_0 = Q_0 f$. Typically, if $\mathcal{R}_0 < 1$ the disease goes to extinction while if $\mathcal{R}_0 > 1$ the disease survives. When the population size is constant and $\mathcal{R}_0 > 1$, the infected population typically reaches a stable, steady or endemic state, characterized by the condition $\mathcal{R}_{eff} \equiv \mathcal{R}_0 \frac{S_\infty}{N} = 1$ where $\frac{S_\infty}{N}$ is the susceptible proportion at equilibrium.

When parameters are time-dependent $\mathcal{R}_0^A(t) \equiv Q_0 f(t)$ does not give the basic reproductive number. It is still a useful parameter as its values determine the sign of the incidence rate at each time.

3.3. Understanding TB dynamics.

3.3.1. Can we explain the historical trend? The long-term decline in TB notifications observed during the last two centuries may be mostly explained (using our simple model) through the assumption that drastic reductions on progression and/or transmission rates have taken place. Purely dynamical phenomena generated by classical epidemiological models it is not enough (Blower *et al.*, 1995). Urbanization and population growth over the last century and a half imply an increase in contact rates. However, a reduction in the risk of progression (due to improved living conditions) is quite likely (McKewon and Record, 1962; see also Barnes, 1995).

During the Twentieth Century, a marked increase on the average life expectancy at birth was observed. US data (reference) on life expectancy at birth can be fitted to the model

$$\tau = \tau_f + \frac{(\tau_0 - \tau_f)}{1 + exp[(t - t_{1/2})/wt]} \tag{5}$$

with $\tau_0 = 38.5yr$, $\tau_f = 73.5yr$, $t_{1/2} = 1921.3yr$, and $wt = 18.425yr$. The per-capita risk, per unit of time k, of developing active-TB is associated to the average individual's lifespan since $f = k/(k + \mu + \alpha)$. The functional form (5) is used to model the risk of developing active-TB because we assume that $f(t)$ varies as abruptly as life expectancy at birth τ. Prior shape parameter values, $t_{1/2} = 1921.3yr$ and $wt = 18.425yr$ are therefore used. Hence, $f(t)$ is modeled using only two free parameters, the asymptotic values f_0 and f_f:

$$f(t) = f_f + \frac{(f_0 - f_f)}{1 + exp[(t - t_{1/2})/wt]}. \tag{6}$$

Incidence of active TB was no recorded until recently (1930). Its past values have been inferred conservatively from recorded TB-mortality rates. Fig. 2 shows the simulation results of one 'typical' scenario. Extensive simulation results can be found in Aparicio *et al.* (2000b; 2000c). A reduction on the risk f, attributable to improved living conditions (typically better nutrition), can explain a century and a half of TB dynamics.

$I(t)$ is a fast variable when compared to the others. Hence, it is adiabatically eliminated, that is, its value is set at the quasi-equilibrium ($dI/dt = 0$ at all time t)

$$I(t) \simeq \frac{k}{\gamma} E(t). \tag{7}$$

The approximate dynamics of the remaining variables are studied under (7). Replacing (7) in Equation (2) gives the dynamics of the slow variable E

$$\frac{dE}{dt} \simeq (k + \mu + \alpha)(Q_0 f(t) \frac{S}{N} - 1)E. \tag{8}$$

Solutions of Model (2), with infectious periods ranging from 1 month to 1 year, give almost identical solution curves to those obtained from Equation (8). Hence, the quasi-equilibrium assumption works well in a parameter range that it is appropriate for TB.

The time dependent parameter $\mathcal{R}_0^A(t) \equiv Q_0 f(t)$ is also useful. The expression $\mathcal{R}_{eff}^A(t) \equiv Q_0 f(t) \frac{S}{N}$ dictates the dynamics of the latently-infected population $E(t)$ (see Fig. 3). Whenever $\mathcal{R}_{eff}^A(t) > 1$ in (8), the latently-infected population $E(t)$ grows while, whenever $\mathcal{R}_{eff}^A(t) < 1$, it declines.

3.3.2. Tuberculosis future trends. The incidence of active-TB (per 100,000 population) becomes approximately $100,000k\frac{E}{N}$ per year if variations in k and E over (the short) period of one year are neglected. The incidence rate of active-TB is a useful index of the relative severity of a TB-epidemic. However, it is an inadequate index for disease trends (see Fig. 2). If a constant risk of developing active-TB (k) is assumed then a continuous increase in the number of infected individuals (E), accompanied by declining TB-incidence rates, is possible in growing populations. In fact, it is possible to generate a prevalence of active-TB (proportion of active cases) that goes down while $E(t)$ increases. A spurious re-emergence (if population growth is slower than the growth of the infected population) is also possible. Hence, the time evolution of diseases like TB may be better captured by looking at the number of new cases per unit of time (incidence of active-TB). In our framework the incidence of active-TB is approximately kE. Variations in risk k may play a significant role on the long-term dynamics of TB. Fig. 3 shows the results of the simulations where $\mathcal{R}_0^A(t) > 1$ all the time. The latent population declines for more than a century after 1922, because $\mathcal{R}_{eff}^A(t) = \mathcal{R}_0^A(t)\frac{S}{N}$ is less than one but around 2068 $\mathcal{R}_{eff}^A(t)$ becomes greater than one and, the latent population (and the incidence of active-TB), begins to grow again. This example of re-emergence is interesting because it does not come from the deterioration of epidemiological conditions – epidemiological parameters are nearly constant during this period of time. Hence, re-emergence may be the result of the natural long-term dynamics of an epidemic. A disease may naturally re-emerge many decades after a period where the system experienced dramatic variations in epidemiological conditions (parameters).

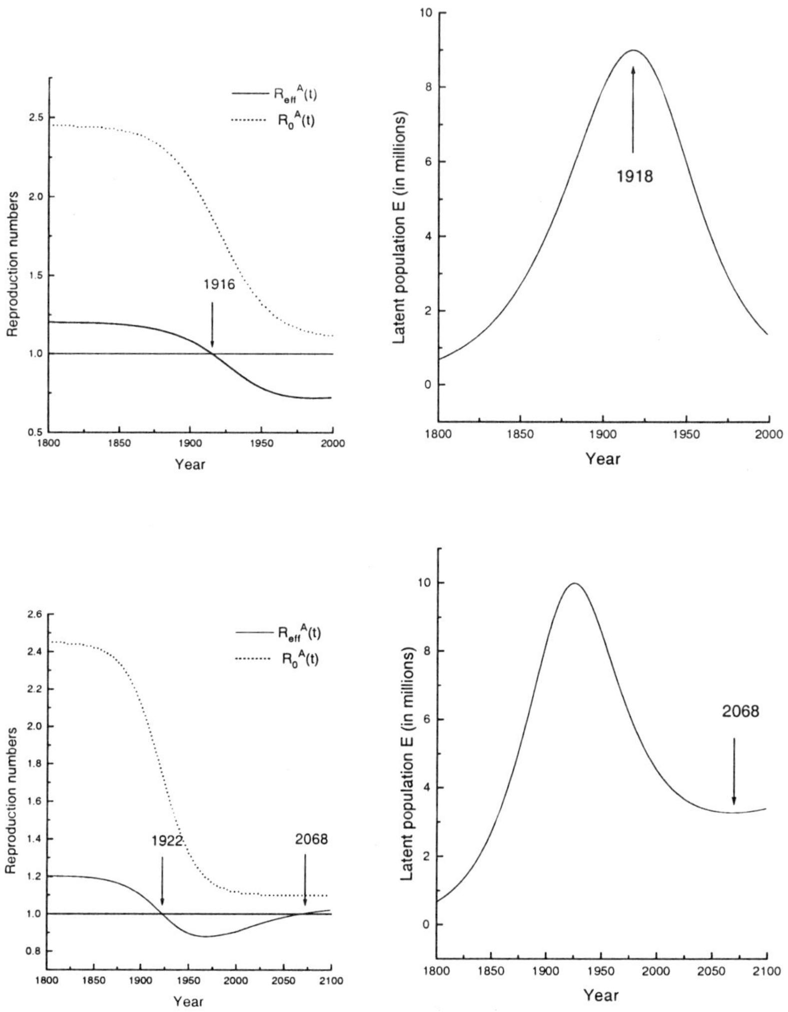

FIG. 3. *Time evolution of* $\mathcal{R}_0^A(t) = Q_0 f(t)$, $\mathcal{R}_{eff}^A(t) = \mathcal{R}_0^A(t)\frac{S}{N}$ *and infected population* $E(t)$. *Here* $Q_0 = 10$ *and* $f(t)$ *is given by (6). Upper figures (case A) correspond to the simulations shown in Fig. 2. Lower figures (case B) correspond to the case where* $\mathcal{R}_0^A(\infty)$ *is greater than one* ($f_f = 0.11$). *Linear population growth for the period 2000–2100 is assumed. Since 1922, and for more than a century,* $\mathcal{R}_{eff}^A(t)$ *is below one, and therefore the latently-infected population shows a declining trend in accord to (8). The small shift in the response of the latent infected population to the changes in* $\mathcal{R}_0^A(t)$ *are of the order of the relaxation time (mean infectious period) of the fast variable* $I(t)$. *After 2068* $\mathcal{R}_{eff}^A(t) > 1$ *and then latent population (E) start a growing phase as expected. Because* f *has been reached the asymptotic value (and then* k *is constant), incidence of active-TB (*kE*) is also growing with time. However incidence rate of active-TB (*$10^5 kE/N$*) is still in a declining phase because the increase in population overcompensate the increase in the number of new cases.*

4. Concluding remarks. Disease re-emergence became a 'hot' topic again after the observed simultaneous rise in the number and prevalence of active tuberculosis at various locations in the world in the middle 80's. The sophistication of current surveillance methods and their associated public health measures and policies (in developed nations like the US) make the characterization of re-emergent patterns difficult. The rise of TB cases around the world is indisputable and the fast response of public health policies in developed countries has been quite impressive. However, we are still left with the question: Why did TB re-emerge? In this article, we have used a simple differential equation model with time-dependent parameters (fitted from data) and realistic demography (variable population size) to show that the main forces behind re-emergence may be just the result of a combination of 'simple' temporal changes in epidemiological and demographic factors. The US population has been growing (this factor has been incorporated in the model) and naturally, contact rates have gone up over the last 150 years (they may be substantially higher today than 50 years ago); yet, the population of latently-infected individuals has gone down considerably (Styblo, 1991). Hence, higher contact rates and a reduced flow of individuals per unit of time into the E-class must be the result of reduced host susceptibility and reduced progression rates. The reduction in progression rates to active-TB must be dramatic. The reduction in host susceptibility (defined as the ability to become infected) is an implicit part of the model because contact rates and susceptibility (probability of becoming infected per contact with an infectious individual) are included (as multiplicative factors) on the definition of Q_0 (Aparicio *et al.*, 2000a; and this volume) – which it is assumed to be constant.

The prevalence of active-TB as well as TB mortality rates (a major source of mortality in the past) have gone down (Sutherland, 1975; see also Barnes, 1995, and Fig. 2). Our model includes TB-mortality, assumes no changes on Q_0 (which includes contacts and host susceptibility). Solution curves (epidemics), using fitted demographic parameters, fit the data only if $k(t)$ experiences dramatic changes during the Twentieth Century. The assumption of reduced progression works very well when data recorded prior to the massive treatment of TB by antibiotics is used. Population growth, a dramatic reduction in progression rates, and an unquantified reduction in host susceptibility can explain the major patterns of TB-dynamics over the last 150 years.

Our results have been corroborated at multiple scales, that is, we have repeated the above analysis using specific cities such as Boston (US) and using specific states (Massachusetts, US). The results are consistent, that is, a reduction decrease in host progression rates, population growth and constant Q_o (that is, a possible reduction in host susceptibility) are enough to reproduce past and current patterns.

Acknowledgments. This work has been partially supported by NSF and NSA grants to the Mathematical and Theoretical Biology Institute at Cornell University, the office of the Provost of Cornell University and CONICET of Argentina.

REFERENCES

[1] Aparicio, J.P., Capurro, A.F., and Castillo-Chavez, C. (2000a). Transmission and dynamics of tuberculosis on generalized households. J. Theor. Biol. **206**, 327–341, doi:10.1006/jtbi.2000.2129.

[2] Aparicio, J.P., Capurro, A.F., and Castillo-Chavez, C. (2000b). Markers of disease evolution: the case of tuberculosis, Department of Biometrics Technical Report Series # BU-1496-M, Biometrics Department, Cornell University.

[3] Aparicio, J.P., Capurro, A.F., and Castillo-Chavez, C. (2000c). The fall and rise of tuberculosis, Department of Biometrics Technical Report Series # BU-1477-M, Biometrics Department, Cornell University.

[4] Barnes D.S. 1995. The making of a social disease: tuberculosis in the nineteenth-century France. University of California Press, pp. 5–13.

[5] Blower, S.M., McLean , A.R., Porco, T.C., Small, P.M., Hopwell, P.C., Sanchez, M.A., and Moss, A.R. (1995). The intrinsic transmission dynamics of tuberculosis epidemics. *Nature Medicine* **1**(8), 815–821.

[6] McKenna, M.T., McCray E., Jones, J.L., Onorato I.M., and Castro K.G. (1998). The fall after the rise: tuberculosis in the United States, 1991 through 1994. Am. J. Public Health, **88**, 1059–1063.

[7] McKewon, T. and Record, R.G. (1962). Reasons for the decline of mortality in England and Wales during the nineteenth century, *Population Studies*, **16**, 94–122 .

[8] Feng, Z., Castillo-Chavez, C., and Capurro, A.F. (2000). A Model for Tuberculosis with exogenous reinfection. Theor. Pop. Biol. **57**, 235–247

[9] Raffalli, J., Sepkowitz, K., and Armstrong, D. (1996). Community-based outbreaks of tuberculosis. Arch Intern Med **156**, 1053–1060.

[10] Raviglione, M.C., Sudre, P, Rieder H.L., Spinaci, S., and Kochi, A. (1993). Secular trends of tuberculosis in western Europe. Bull. WHO **71** 297–306

[11] Snider, G.L. (1997). Tuberculosis then and now: a personal perspective on the last 50 years. Ann Intern Med **126**, 237–243.

[12] Styblo, K. (1991) Epidemiology of tuberculosis, VEB Gustav Fischer Verlag Jena, The Hague

[13] Sutherland, I. (1975). Recent studies in the epidemiology of tuberculosis based on the risk of being infected with tubercle bacilli. Adv. Tuberc. Res. **19**, 1–63.

[14] Webster's II New College Dictionary (1995). Houghton Mifflin Company, Boston, New York.

[15] World Health Organization (1998). Fact Sheet No. **97**, available from http://www.who.ch.

[16] World Health Organization (1999). Global Tuberculosis Control. WHO Report 1999. WHO/CDS/CPT/TB/99.259. Geneva, Switzerland.

EPILOGUE

The evolution of epidemiological phenomena such as cross-immunity, differential susceptibility, differential disease progression and resistance do not take place on the same time scale as disease dynamics or demographic processes. Disease evolution models deal with processes with inherently distinct temporal epidemiological, demographic and evolutionary scales. The situation is more complex once the need to include changes in cultural and social landscapes is recognized. The accelerated birth and growth of urban centers, fast changes in public health policies, unpredictable demographic growth patterns, increases in the rates of antibiotic use and misuse, impact of globalization on populations' movement (growth of mass transportation, international travel and global warming), advances in genomics and the information revolution are but some of the factors that continuously shift the social and cultural landscape in which disease evolves.

These two volumes grew out of the discussions and presentations that began during the Workshop on Emerging and Reemerging Diseases sponsored by the Institute for Mathematics and its Applications (IMA) at the University of Minnesota in May 17–21, 1999. Workshop activities focused on specific diseases and issues connected to disease emergence or reemergence. Researchers' presentations dealt with possible manifestations of such phenomena while group discussions tried to identify the factors that must be considered in their study. Workshop participants did not attempt to precisely define these concepts.

Challenges posed by particular diseases must often be studied at different levels of complexity. The selection of an appropriate epidemiological unit, for example, has to be tailored to specific questions. The dynamics of HIV are studied (at least) at two levels: the level of the individual (immunology) and the population level (epidemiology). The search for answers to HIV questions posed at both levels has brought together teams of immunologists, sociologists, demographers, economists, mathematicians, statisticians, public health officials and evolutionary biologists. The development of preventive and timely vaccines for communicable diseases like influenza, a highly variable and potentially deadly virus, must now include increases in international and regional travel in its development. Renewed threats are being posed by recently observed increases in the number of active cases of tuberculosis (TB) and the number of infected individuals with resistant strains of TB. Factoring the costs associated with the treatment and control of diseases like HIV or TB makes disease control one of the most pressing and challenging issues of our time.

The articles in these two volumes illustrate the role of mathematics in the study of particular diseases and, in the process, highlight important mathematical methods and modeling approaches. It is unfortunate that, for the most part, these volumes have ignored the study of vector-transmitted (malaria, Chagas, etc.) and macroparasitic diseases. There are no articles addressing the study of one of the most scariest diseases, Ebola, the study of animal diseases or the role of humans on the spread of diseases that can devastate local, national and global economies ("foot and mouth disease"). The methods and modeling approaches found in these volumes, particularly those in the tutorial papers, provide a useful starting point for the development of models that may help us gain some understanding on the transmission dynamics and control of these diseases that are ignored in these volumes.

We hope that those interested in the study of communicable diseases will find the methods and tools provided in these volumes useful.

Carlos Castillo-Chavez, Sally Blower, Pauline van den Driessche, Denise Kirschner, and Abdul-Aziz Yakubu.

LIST OF TUTORIAL/WORKSHOP PARTICIPANTS

- Linda Allen, Department of Mathematics, Texas Tech
- Kevin Anderson, Institute for Mathematics and its Applications
- Viggo Andreasen, Department of Matematik, Roskilde University
- Bruce Ayati, Institute for Mathematics and its Applications
- Frank Ball, School of Mathematical Sciences, University of Nottingham
- Joan Bechtold, Midwest Orthopedic Research Foundation
- Robert Berry, Department of Mathematics, University of Houston
- Sally Blower, Department of Biomathematics, UCLA School of Medicine
- Mary E. Bradley, Department of Mathematics, University of Louisville
- Fred Brauer, Department of Mathematics, University of British Columbia
- Angel Capurro, Departamento de Investigacion, Universidad de Belgrano
- Carlos Castillo-Chavez, Departments of Biometrics, Statistics and Theoretical and Applied Mechanics, Cornell University
- Lester F. Caudill, Department Mathematics and Computer Science, University of Richmond
- Kenneth Cooke, Pomona College
- Fred Dulles, Institute for Mathematics and its Applications
- Jonathan Dushoff, Institute of Physics, Academia Sinica
- Lourdes Esteva, Departamento de Matematicas, Fac. de Ciencios, University Nac Autonoma de Mexico
- Zhilan Feng, Department of Mathematics, Purdue University
- Neil Ferguson, Imperial College
- K. Renee Fister, Department of Mathematics and Statistics, Murray State University
- John Gardner, University of Houston,
- Don Gaver, Naval Postgraduate School
- M. Gabriela M. Gomes, Department of Biological Sciences, University of Warwick
- Kimber Gross, Department of Mathematics, University of Houston
- Mats Gyllenberg, Department of Applied Mathematics, University of Turku
- Carlos Hernandez, Department of Biomathematics, Cornell University

- Herb Hethcote, Department of Mathematics, University of Iowa
- Janda Holmes, Department of Mathematics, University of Tennessee
- Sarah Holte, Department of Biostatistics, Fred Hutchinson Cancer Research Center
- Mary Ann Horn, Department of Mathematics, Vanderbilt University
- Shu-Fang Hsu-Schmidt, Institute of Mathematical Statistics, University of Bern
- Wenzhang Huang, Department of Mathematical Sciences, University of Alabama, Huntsville
- Hisashi Inaba, Department of Mathematical Sciences, University of Tokyo
- Yoh Iwasa, Department of Biology, Kyushu University
- John Kemper, University of St. Thomas
- Denise Kirschner, Department of Microbiology and Immunology, University of Michigan Medical School
- Steve Krone, Department of Mathematics, University of Idaho
- Suzanne Lenhart, Department of Mathematics, University of Tennessee
- Jia Li, Department of Mathematical Science, University of Alabama, Huntsville
- Michael Li, Department of Mathematical Sciences, University of Alberta, Edmonton
- Tom Lietman, F.I. Proctor Foundation, University of California-San Francisco
- Frithjof Lutscher, Lehrstuhl fur Biomathematik, Universitat Tubingen
- Maia Martcheva, Department of Mathematics, Polytechnic University
- Gustavo Martinez-Meckler, Centro de Ciencias Fiscas, UNAM
- Douglas Meade, Department of Mathematics, University of South Carolina
- Willard Miller, Institute for Mathematics and its Applications
- Fabio Milner, Department of Mathematics, Purdue University
- Olivier Monzin, MORF
- Johannes Mueller, Biomathematics - C5P13, University of Tubingen
- Ingemar Nasell, Department of Mathematics, Royal Institute of Technology
- Patrick Nelson, Department of Mathematics, University of Michigan
- Douglas Norton, Mathematical Sciences, Villanova University
- Mouzin Olivier, Biomechanics Orthopaedic Laboratory

- Andrea Pugliese, Dipartmimento di Matematica, Universita degli Studi di Trento
- Kathleen Rogers, Mathematics Department, University of Maryland Baltimore County
- Sonja Sandberg, Department of Mathematics, Framingham State College
- Lisa Sattenspiel, Department of Anthropology, University of Missouri
- Matthew Schuette, Applied Mathematics and Computational Sciences, University of Iowa
- Carl P. Simon, Department of Mathematics, University of Michigan
- Zachariah Sinkala, Middle Tennessee State University
- Baojun Song, Department of Biometrics, Cornell University
- Angela Stevens, Max-Planck-Institute for Mathematics in the Sciences
- Moxun Tang, School of Mathematics, University of Minnesota
- Horst Thieme, Department of Mathematics, Arizona State University
- Dean T. Tsukayama, Department of Medicine, Hennepin County Medical Center
- Pauline van den Driessche, Department of Mathematics and Statistics, University of Victoria
- Jorge X. Velasco-Hernandez, Department of Mathematics, UAM-Iztapalapa
- Liancheng Wang, Department of Mathematics and Statistics, Mississippi State University
- James Watmough, Department of Mathematics and Statistics, University of New Brunswick
- Glenn F. Webb, Department of Mathematics, Vanderbilt University
- Kathryn Weld, Department of Mathematics and Computer Science, Manhattan College
- Ralf Wittenberg, Department of Mathematics, University of Michigan
- Lih-Ing Wu, Department of Mathematics, Purdue University
- Abdul-Aziz Yakubu, Department of Mathematics, Howard University
- Zhou Yicang, Department of Applied Mathematics, Xi'an Jiaotong University
- Mary Lou Zeeman, Department of Mathematics and Statistics, University of Texas at San Antonio

IMA VOLUME 126 CONTENTS

MATHEMATICAL APPROACHES FOR EMERGING AND REEMERGING INFECTIOUS DISEASES: MODELS, METHODS AND THEORY

EDITORS: CARLOS CASTILLO-CHAVEZ WITH SALLY BLOWER, PAULINE VAN DEN DRIESSCHE, DENISE KIRSCHNER, AND ABDUL-AZIZ YAKUBU

IMA SUMMER PROGRAMS

1987 Robotics
1988 Signal Processing
1989 Robust Statistics and Diagnostics
1990 Radar and Sonar (June 18–29)
New Directions in Time Series Analysis (July 2–27)
1991 Semiconductors
1992 Environmental Studies: Mathematical, Computational, and Statistical Analysis
1993 Modeling, Mesh Generation, and Adaptive Numerical Methods for Partial Differential Equations
1994 Molecular Biology
1995 Large Scale Optimizations with Applications to Inverse Problems, Optimal Control and Design, and Molecular and Structural Optimization
1996 Emerging Applications of Number Theory (July 15–26)
Theory of Random Sets (August 22–24)
1997 Statistics in the Health Sciences
1998 Coding and Cryptography (July 6–18)
Mathematical Modeling in Industry (July 22–31)
1999 Codes, Systems, and Graphical Models (August 2–13, 1999)
2000 Mathematical Modeling in Industry: A Workshop for Graduate Students (July 19–28)
2001 Geometric Methods in Inverse Problems and PDE Control (July 16–27)
2002 Special Functions in the Digital Age (July 22–August 2)

IMA "HOT TOPICS" WORKSHOPS

- Challenges and Opportunities in Genomics: Production, Storage, Mining and Use, April 24–27, 1999
- Decision Making Under Uncertainty: Energy and Environmental Models, July 20–24, 1999
- Analysis and Modeling of Optical Devices, September 9–10, 1999
- Decision Making under Uncertainty: Assessment of the Reliability of Mathematical Models, September 16–17, 1999
- Scaling Phenomena in Communication Networks, October 22–24, 1999
- Text Mining, April 17–18, 2000
- Mathematical Challenges in Global Positioning Systems (GPS), August 16–18, 2000
- Modeling and Analysis of Noise in Integrated Circuits and Systems, August 29–30, 2000
- Mathematics of the Internet: E-Auction and Markets, December 3–5, 2000
- Analysis and Modeling of Industrial Jetting Processes, January 10–13, 2001

• Wireless Networks, August 6–10 2001

SPRINGER LECTURE NOTES FROM THE IMA:

The Mathematics and Physics of Disordered Media
Editors: Barry Hughes and Barry Ninham
(Lecture Notes in Math., Volume 1035, 1983)

Orienting Polymers
Editor: J.L. Ericksen
(Lecture Notes in Math., Volume 1063, 1984)

New Perspectives in Thermodynamics
Editor: James Serrin
(Springer-Verlag, 1986)

Models of Economic Dynamics
Editor: Hugo Sonnenschein
(Lecture Notes in Econ., Volume 264, 1986)

Current Volumes:

1 **Homogenization and Effective Moduli of Materials and Media** J. Ericksen, D. Kinderlehrer, R. Kohn, and J.-L. Lions (eds.)
2 **Oscillation Theory, Computation, and Methods of Compensated Compactness** C. Dafermos, J. Ericksen, D. Kinderlehrer, and M. Slemrod (eds.)
3 **Metastability and Incompletely Posed Problems** S. Antman, J. Ericksen, D. Kinderlehrer, and I. Muller (eds.)
4 **Dynamical Problems in Continuum Physics** J. Bona, C. Dafermos, J. Ericksen, and D. Kinderlehrer (eds.)
5 **Theory and Applications of Liquid Crystals** J. Ericksen and D. Kinderlehrer (eds.)
6 **Amorphous Polymers and Non-Newtonian Fluids** C. Dafermos, J. Ericksen, and D. Kinderlehrer (eds.)
7 **Random Media** G. Papanicolaou (ed.)
8 **Percolation Theory and Ergodic Theory of Infinite Particle Systems** H. Kesten (ed.)
9 **Hydrodynamic Behavior and Interacting Particle Systems** G. Papanicolaou (ed.)
10 **Stochastic Differential Systems, Stochastic Control Theory, and Applications** W. Fleming and P.-L. Lions (eds.)
11 **Numerical Simulation in Oil Recovery** M.F. Wheeler (ed.)
12 **Computational Fluid Dynamics and Reacting Gas Flows** B. Engquist, M. Luskin, and A. Majda (eds.)
13 **Numerical Algorithms for Parallel Computer Architectures** M.H. Schultz (ed.)
14 **Mathematical Aspects of Scientific Software** J.R. Rice (ed.)
15 **Mathematical Frontiers in Computational Chemical Physics** D. Truhlar (ed.)
16 **Mathematics in Industrial Problems** A. Friedman
17 **Applications of Combinatorics and Graph Theory to the Biological and Social Sciences** F. Roberts (ed.)
18 ***q*-Series and Partitions** D. Stanton (ed.)
19 **Invariant Theory and Tableaux** D. Stanton (ed.)
20 **Coding Theory and Design Theory Part I: Coding Theory** D. Ray-Chaudhuri (ed.)
21 **Coding Theory and Design Theory Part II: Design Theory** D. Ray-Chaudhuri (ed.)
22 **Signal Processing Part I: Signal Processing Theory** L. Auslander, F.A. Grünbaum, J.W. Helton, T. Kailath, P. Khargonekar, and S. Mitter (eds.)

23 **Signal Processing Part II: Control Theory and Applications of Signal Processing** L. Auslander, F.A. Grünbaum, J.W. Helton, T. Kailath, P. Khargonekar, and S. Mitter (eds.)
24 **Mathematics in Industrial Problems, Part 2** A. Friedman
25 **Solitons in Physics, Mathematics, and Nonlinear Optics** P.J. Olver and D.H. Sattinger (eds.)
26 **Two Phase Flows and Waves** D.D. Joseph and D.G. Schaeffer (eds.)
27 **Nonlinear Evolution Equations that Change Type** B.L. Keyfitz and M. Shearer (eds.)
28 **Computer Aided Proofs in Analysis** K. Meyer and D. Schmidt (eds.)
29 **Multidimensional Hyperbolic Problems and Computations** A. Majda and J. Glimm (eds.)
30 **Microlocal Analysis and Nonlinear Waves** M. Beals, R. Melrose, and J. Rauch (eds.)
31 **Mathematics in Industrial Problems, Part 3** A. Friedman
32 **Radar and Sonar, Part I** R. Blahut, W. Miller, Jr., and C. Wilcox
33 **Directions in Robust Statistics and Diagnostics: Part I** W.A. Stahel and S. Weisberg (eds.)
34 **Directions in Robust Statistics and Diagnostics: Part II** W.A. Stahel and S. Weisberg (eds.)
35 **Dynamical Issues in Combustion Theory** P. Fife, A. Liñán, and F.A. Williams (eds.)
36 **Computing and Graphics in Statistics** A. Buja and P. Tukey (eds.)
37 **Patterns and Dynamics in Reactive Media** H. Swinney, G. Aris, and D. Aronson (eds.)
38 **Mathematics in Industrial Problems, Part 4** A. Friedman
39 **Radar and Sonar, Part II** F.A. Grünbaum, M. Bernfeld, and R.E. Blahut (eds.)
40 **Nonlinear Phenomena in Atmospheric and Oceanic Sciences** G.F. Carnevale and R.T. Pierrehumbert (eds.)
41 **Chaotic Processes in the Geological Sciences** D.A. Yuen (ed.)
42 **Partial Differential Equations with Minimal Smoothness and Applications** B. Dahlberg, E. Fabes, R. Fefferman, D. Jerison, C. Kenig, and J. Pipher (eds.)
43 **On the Evolution of Phase Boundaries** M.E. Gurtin and G.B. McFadden
44 **Twist Mappings and Their Applications** R. McGehee and K.R. Meyer (eds.)

45 **New Directions in Time Series Analysis, Part I**
D. Brillinger, P. Caines, J. Geweke, E. Parzen, M. Rosenblatt, and M.S. Taqqu (eds.)

46 **New Directions in Time Series Analysis, Part II**
D. Brillinger, P. Caines, J. Geweke, E. Parzen, M. Rosenblatt, and M.S. Taqqu (eds.)

47 **Degenerate Diffusions**
W.-M. Ni, L.A. Peletier, and J.-L. Vazquez (eds.)

48 **Linear Algebra, Markov Chains, and Queueing Models**
C.D. Meyer and R.J. Plemmons (eds.)

49 **Mathematics in Industrial Problems, Part 5** A. Friedman

50 **Combinatorial and Graph-Theoretic Problems in Linear Algebra**
R.A. Brualdi, S. Friedland, and V. Klee (eds.)

51 **Statistical Thermodynamics and Differential Geometry of Microstructured Materials**
H.T. Davis and J.C.C. Nitsche (eds.)

52 **Shock Induced Transitions and Phase Structures in General Media** J.E. Dunn, R. Fosdick, and M. Slemrod (eds.)

53 **Variational and Free Boundary Problems**
A. Friedman and J. Spruck (eds.)

54 **Microstructure and Phase Transitions**
D. Kinderlehrer, R. James, M. Luskin, and J.L. Ericksen (eds.)

55 **Turbulence in Fluid Flows: A Dynamical Systems Approach**
G.R. Sell, C. Foias, and R. Temam (eds.)

56 **Graph Theory and Sparse Matrix Computation**
A. George, J.R. Gilbert, and J.W.H. Liu (eds.)

57 **Mathematics in Industrial Problems, Part 6** A. Friedman

58 **Semiconductors, Part I**
W.M. Coughran, Jr., J. Cole, P. Lloyd, and J. White (eds.)

59 **Semiconductors, Part II**
W.M. Coughran, Jr., J. Cole, P. Lloyd, and J. White (eds.)

60 **Recent Advances in Iterative Methods**
G. Golub, A. Greenbaum, and M. Luskin (eds.)

61 **Free Boundaries in Viscous Flows**
R.A. Brown and S.H. Davis (eds.)

62 **Linear Algebra for Control Theory**
P. Van Dooren and B. Wyman (eds.)

63 **Hamiltonian Dynamical Systems: History, Theory, and Applications**
H.S. Dumas, K.R. Meyer, and D.S. Schmidt (eds.)

64 **Systems and Control Theory for Power Systems**
J.H. Chow, P.V. Kokotovic, R.J. Thomas (eds.)

65 **Mathematical Finance**
M.H.A. Davis, D. Duffie, W.H. Fleming, and S.E. Shreve (eds.)

66 **Robust Control Theory** B.A. Francis and P.P. Khargonekar (eds.)
67 **Mathematics in Industrial Problems, Part 7** A. Friedman
68 **Flow Control** M.D. Gunzburger (ed.)
69 **Linear Algebra for Signal Processing**
A. Bojanczyk and G. Cybenko (eds.)
70 **Control and Optimal Design of Distributed Parameter Systems**
J.E. Lagnese, D.L. Russell, and L.W. White (eds.)
71 **Stochastic Networks** F.P. Kelly and R.J. Williams (eds.)
72 **Discrete Probability and Algorithms**
D. Aldous, P. Diaconis, J. Spencer, and J.M. Steele (eds.)
73 **Discrete Event Systems, Manufacturing Systems, and Communication Networks**
P.R. Kumar and P.P. Varaiya (eds.)
74 **Adaptive Control, Filtering, and Signal Processing**
K.J. Åström, G.C. Goodwin, and P.R. Kumar (eds.)
75 **Modeling, Mesh Generation, and Adaptive Numerical Methods for Partial Differential Equations** I. Babuska, J.E. Flaherty, W.D. Henshaw, J.E. Hopcroft, J.E. Oliger, and T. Tezduyar (eds.)
76 **Random Discrete Structures** D. Aldous and R. Pemantle (eds.)
77 **Nonlinear Stochastic PDEs: Hydrodynamic Limit and Burgers' Turbulence** T. Funaki and W.A. Woyczynski (eds.)
78 **Nonsmooth Analysis and Geometric Methods in Deterministic Optimal Control** B.S. Mordukhovich and H.J. Sussmann (eds.)
79 **Environmental Studies: Mathematical, Computational, and Statistical Analysis** M.F. Wheeler (ed.)
80 **Image Models (and their Speech Model Cousins)**
S.E. Levinson and L. Shepp (eds.)
81 **Genetic Mapping and DNA Sequencing**
T. Speed and M.S. Waterman (eds.)
82 **Mathematical Approaches to Biomolecular Structure and Dynamics**
J.P. Mesirov, K. Schulten, and D. Sumners (eds.)
83 **Mathematics in Industrial Problems, Part 8** A. Friedman
84 **Classical and Modern Branching Processes**
K.B. Athreya and P. Jagers (eds.)
85 **Stochastic Models in Geosystems**
S.A. Molchanov and W.A. Woyczynski (eds.)
86 **Computational Wave Propagation**
B. Engquist and G.A. Kriegsmann (eds.)
87 **Progress in Population Genetics and Human Evolution**
P. Donnelly and S. Tavaré (eds.)
88 **Mathematics in Industrial Problems, Part 9** A. Friedman
89 **Multiparticle Quantum Scattering With Applications to Nuclear, Atomic and Molecular Physics** D.G. Truhlar and B. Simon (eds.)

90 **Inverse Problems in Wave Propagation** G. Chavent, G. Papanicolau, P. Sacks, and W.W. Symes (eds.)

91 **Singularities and Oscillations** J. Rauch and M. Taylor (eds.)

92 **Large-Scale Optimization with Applications, Part I: Optimization in Inverse Problems and Design** L.T. Biegler, T.F. Coleman, A.R. Conn, and F. Santosa (eds.)

93 **Large-Scale Optimization with Applications, Part II: Optimal Design and Control** L.T. Biegler, T.F. Coleman, A.R. Conn, and F. Santosa (eds.)

94 **Large-Scale Optimization with Applications, Part III: Molecular Structure and Optimization** L.T. Biegler, T.F. Coleman, A.R. Conn, and F. Santosa (eds.)

95 **Quasiclassical Methods** J. Rauch and B. Simon (eds.)

96 **Wave Propagation in Complex Media** G. Papanicolaou (ed.)

97 **Random Sets: Theory and Applications** J. Goutsias, R.P.S. Mahler, and H.T. Nguyen (eds.)

98 **Particulate Flows: Processing and Rheology** D.A. Drew, D.D. Joseph, and S.L. Passman (eds.)

99 **Mathematics of Multiscale Materials** K.M. Golden, G.R. Grimmett, R.D. James, G.W. Milton, and P.N. Sen (eds.)

100 **Mathematics in Industrial Problems, Part 10** A. Friedman

101 **Nonlinear Optical Materials** J.V. Moloney (ed.)

102 **Numerical Methods for Polymeric Systems** S.G. Whittington (ed.)

103 **Topology and Geometry in Polymer Science** S.G. Whittington, D. Sumners, and T. Lodge (eds.)

104 **Essays on Mathematical Robotics** J. Baillieul, S.S. Sastry, and H.J. Sussmann (eds.)

105 **Algorithms For Parallel Processing** M.T. Heath, A. Ranade, and R.S. Schreiber (eds.)

106 **Parallel Processing of Discrete Problems** P.M. Pardalos (ed.)

107 **The Mathematics of Information Coding, Extraction, and Distribution** G. Cybenko, D.P. O'Leary, and J. Rissanen (eds.)

108 **Rational Drug Design** D.G. Truhlar, W. Howe, A.J. Hopfinger, J. Blaney, and R.A. Dammkoehler (eds.)

109 **Emerging Applications of Number Theory** D.A. Hejhal, J. Friedman, M.C. Gutzwiller, and A.M. Odlyzko (eds.)

110 **Computational Radiology and Imaging: Therapy and Diagnostics** C. Börgers and F. Natterer (eds.)

111 **Evolutionary Algorithms** L.D. Davis, K. De Jong, M.D. Vose, and L.D. Whitley (eds.)

112 **Statistics in Genetics** M.E. Halloran and S. Geisser (eds.)

113 **Grid Generation and Adaptive Algorithms** M.W. Bern, J.E. Flaherty, and M. Luskin (eds.)

114 **Diagnosis and Prediction** S. Geisser (ed.)

115 **Pattern Formation in Continuous and Coupled Systems: A Survey Volume** M. Golubitsky, D. Luss, and S.H. Strogatz (eds.)

116 **Statistical Models in Epidemiology, the Environment, and Clinical Trials** M.E. Halloran and D. Berry (eds.)

117 **Structured Adaptive Mesh Refinement (SAMR) Grid Methods** S.B. Baden, N.P. Chrisochoides, D.B. Gannon, and M.L. Norman (eds.)

118 **Dynamics of Algorithms** R. de la Llave, L.R. Petzold, and J. Lorenz (eds.)

119 **Numerical Methods for Bifurcation Problems and Large-Scale Dynamical Systems** E. Doedel and L.S. Tuckerman (eds.)

120 **Parallel Solution of Partial Differential Equations** P. Bjørstad and M. Luskin (eds.)

121 **Mathematical Models for Biological Pattern Formation** P.K. Maini and H.G. Othmer (eds.)

122 **Multiple-Time-Scale Dynamical Systems** C.K.R.T. Jones and A. Khibnik (eds.)

123 **Codes, Systems, and Graphical Models** B. Marcus and J. Rosenthal (eds.)

124 **Computational Modeling in Biological Fluid Dynamics** L.J. Fauci and S. Gueron (eds.)

125 **Mathematical Approaches for Emerging and Reemerging Infectious Diseases: An Introduction** C. Castillo-Chavez with S. Blower, P. van den Driessche, D. Kirschner, and A.A. Yakubu (eds.)

126 **Mathematical Approaches for Emerging and Reemerging Infectious Diseases: Models, Methods, and Theory** C. Castillo-Chavez with S. Blower, P. van den Driessche, D. Kirschner, and A.A. Yakubu (eds.)

127 **Mathematics of the Internet: E-Auction and Markets** B. Dietrich and R.V. Vohra (eds.)

Forthcoming Volumes:

1998–1999: Mathematics in Biology

Membrane Transport and Renal Physiology

Decision Making Under Uncertainty: Energy and Environmental Models

1999–2000: Reactive Flow and Transport Phenomena

Confinement and Remediation of Environmental Hazards and Resource Recovery

Atmospheric Modeling

Dispersive Corrections to Transport Equations, Simulation of Transport in Transition Regimes/Multiscale Models for Surface Evolution and Reacting Flows

2000-2001: Mathematics in Multimedia

Mathematical Foundations of Speech Processing and Recognition/Mathematical Foundations of Natural Language Modeling

Mathematical Methods in Speech and Image Analysis/ Image Processing and Low Level Vision/Image Analysis and High Level Vision

Fractals in Multimedia

2001 Summer Program

Geometric Methods in Inverse Problems and PDE Control